FOOD IS BETTER
MEDICINE
THAN DRUGS

Also by Patrick Holford

The New Optimum Nutrition Bible
The Holford Low-GL Diet
The Holford Low-GL Diet Cookbook
The Optimum Nutrition Cookbook
Optimum Nutrition for the Mind
Optimum Nutrition for Your Child's Mind (with Deborah Colson)
The Alzheimer's Prevention Plan (with Shane Heaton and
Deborah Colson)
Hidden Food Allergies (with Dr James Braly)
Say No to Heart Disease
Balancing Hormones Naturally (with Kate Neil)
Boost Your Immune System (with Jennifer Meek)
Say No to Cancer
Beat Stress and Fatigue
Say No to Arthritis
Improve Your Digestion
Solve Your Skin Problems (with Natalie Savona)
Six Weeks to Superhealth
Natural Highs (with Dr Hyla Cass)
The H Factor (with Dr James Braly)
Optimum Nutrition Before, During and After Pregnancy
(with Susannah Lawson)
500 Top Health & Nutrition Questions Answered
The Holford Diet GL Counter

FOOD IS BETTER MEDICINE THAN DRUGS

Your prescription for drug-free health

PATRICK HOLFORD and JEROME BURNE

PIATKUS

Visit the Piatkus website!

Piatkus publishes a wide range of best-selling fiction and non-fiction, including books on health, mind, body & spirit, sex, self-help, cookery and biography.

If you want to:
- read descriptions of our popular titles
- buy our books over the Internet
- take advantage of our special offers
- enter our monthly competition
- learn more about your favourite Piatkus authors

VISIT OUR WEBSITE AT: www.piatkus.co.uk

First published in Great Britain in 2006 by
Piatkus Books Ltd
5 Windmill Street, London W1T 2JA
email: info@piatkus.co.uk

Reprinted 2006, 2007

The moral right of the author has been asserted

A catalogue record for this book is available from the British Library

ISBN 978 0 7499 2766 0

Text design by Paul Saunders
Edited by Barbara Kiser
Proofread by Anthea Matthison
Illustrations by Rodney Paull

This book has been printed on paper manufactured
with respect for the environment using wood from
managed sustainable resources

Typeset by Phoenix Photosetting, Chatham, Kent
www.phoenixphotosetting.co.uk
Printed and bound in Great Britain by William Clowes Ltd, Beccles, Suffolk

About the authors

Patrick Holford is one of Britain's leading nutrition experts. In 1984 he founded The Institute for Optimum Nutrition (ION) in London, with his mentor, twice Nobel Prize winner Dr Linus Pauling, as patron. ION is an independent educational charity that has been researching and defining exactly what it means to be optimally nourished for the past 20 years. Now the largest and most respected educational establishment for training degree-accredited nutritional therapists in Europe, the ION method for assessing a person's optimal nutrition needs has been tried and tested on over 100,000 people.

In the UK Patrick is frequently involved in government campaigns and debates and is invited to the House of Commons, the Food Standards Agency and Oxford University as an expert in nutrition. In October 2004 he co-authored Britain's largest ever health and diet survey (ONUK), comparing the health and diet of 37,000 people. Patrick's landmark book, *The Optimum Nutrition Bible*, the result of 20 years of intensive research, is a worldwide bestseller, with over one million copies sold.

Jerome Burne is a leading medical and science journalist. For the past 15 years he has been writing regularly for the *Independent*, the *Guardian*, the *Financial Times*, the *Observer*, the *Sunday Telegraph* and, more recently, *The Times*. For three years he edited the award-winning newsletter *Medicine Today*, which provided accurate and vivid accounts of cutting-edge science.

His desire to write this book was inspired by the way the Internet has transformed the reporting of health and medicine. The web means that the medical profession no longer has exclusive access to the latest research. While writing about the latest breakthroughs in science and medicine, he realised that something had gone badly wrong with an exclusively drug-based approach to health. In the past, studies and reports detailing the failures would have remained largely confined within medical journals, a matter for private professional concern. By bringing this research to a wider audience and showing that 'science-based' doesn't just mean drug-based, he hopes to provide an impetus for change.

Contents

Acknowledgements

A book of this size involves calling on the research and expertise of dozens of top scientists, including Dr Stephen Sinatra, Dr David Haslam, Dr Fedon Lindberg, Dr Andrew McCulloch, Richard Brookes, Dr Hyla Cass, Dr James Braly and Dr Shirley Bond, and too many more to thank by name. We are immensely grateful to them all. Particularly, we would like to thank Martin Walker for checking the political information, and for his help researching and contributing to Chapter 9: Balancing Hormones in the Menopause. Deborah Colson for her epic work on research and referencing, Charlotte for her support, and our respective wives, Gill and Gaby, and children, for their valuable input and putting up with us burning the candle at both ends. We would also like to thank the editorial team at Piatkus, especially Gill, Jo and Barbara.

Guide to Abbreviations, Measures and References

Abbreviations and measures

1 gram(g) = 1,000 milligrams (mg) = 1,000,000 micrograms (mcg, also written μg).

All vitamins are measured in milligrams or micrograms. Vitamins A, D and E used to be measured in International Units (ius), a measurement designed to standardise the various forms of these vitamins that have different potencies.

6mcg of beta-carotene, the vegetable precursor of vitamin A is, on average, converted into 1mcg of retinol, the animal form of vitamin A. So, 6mcg of beta-carotene is called 1mcgRE (RE stands for retinol equivalent). Throughout this book beta-carotene is referred to in mcgRE.

1 mcg of retinol (mcgRE) = 3.3ius of vitamin A
1 mcgRE of beta-carotene = 6mcg of beta-carotene
100ius of vitamin D = 2.5mcg
100ius of vitamin E = 67mg
1 pound (1b) = 16 ounces (oz)
2.2lb = 1 kilogram (kg)
1 pint = 0.6 litres
1.76 pints = 1 litre
In this book 'calories' means kilocalories (kcals)

References

Hundreds of references from respected scientific literature have been used in writing this book. Details of specific studies referred to are listed starting on page 409. Other supporting research for the statements made is available from the library at the Institute for Optimum Nutrition (ION) (see pages 403–04) for members of ION. ION also offers information services, including literature search and library search facilities, for readers who want to access scientific literature on specific subjects. On pages 398–400 you will find a list of the best books to read, linked to each chapter, to enable you to dig deeper into the topics covered. You will also find many of the topics touched on in this book covered in detail in feature articles available at www.patrickholford.com. If you want to stay up to date with all that is new and exciting in this field, we recommend you subscribe to the *100% Health* newsletter, details of which are on the website www.foodismedicine.co.uk.

Introduction

THESE DAYS IT'S practically impossible to turn on the TV or open a paper without seeing some kind of evidence that eating poor-quality food can make you ill or at least below par, while eating fresh, wholesome food gives you a much better chance of staying fit and healthy.

Morgan Spurlock's movie *Super Size Me* was a vivid and shocking illustration of just how bad a month's worth of hamburgers, cola and milkshakes can make you feel, while Jamie Oliver's British TV series chronicling his heroic attempts to provide decent food for school-children made it clear not just how hard it is to turn round an institution, but also what a difference proper food can make in our children. Shortly before we finished this book, a report was published in the US showing that a teenager drinking one can of fizzy drink a day could put on 14lbs (6.4kg) a year[1] – thus moving a step closer to developing diabetes or heart disease later in life.

Meanwhile, studies showing more specific benefits from the right sort of nutrition are proliferating, too. Last January, scientists on a very big UK project – 14,000 women followed up over 15 years – reported that the amount of omega-3 essential fats in a pregnant woman's diet helps to determine her child's intelligence and fine motor skills as well as their 'propensity to anti-social behaviour'.[2]

So food is powerful stuff. Even so, it's well known that many of us don't eat that well and that we also have low levels of various essential vitamins and minerals. And this ties in with statistics showing that quite a few of us – like that teenager clutching a daily bottle of cola – are heading for various chronic diseases as we get older.

For example, one in six are set to develop diabetes, and one in six are expected to die prematurely, the most likely cause being heart disease, strokes or cancer. Obesity, linked to type 2 diabetes and a range of other health problems, is becoming more common too: by the age of 50, one in three of us will be officially obese. And it gets worse. A quarter of us will spend the last 30 years of our lives with the pain of arthritis, and a quarter of those who make it through to 80 will have Alzheimer's. Perhaps most depressing of all is the statistic that on any given day in the UK, three in ten people are sick or in pain. Precise figures may vary a bit in other Western countries, but the general picture is much the same.

That's the bad news. The good news is that it doesn't have to be like this. We can prevent these disorders, and we can also change the way we treat them in people who do develop them. This book is all about what needs to be done and why.

Bitter pill

At the moment, what happens to all these people hit by disease? In a word, drugs – perhaps two or three to start with, then a dozen or more towards the end to help deal with the symptoms of these diseases. Many more of us will be put on drugs for less serious conditions such as high blood pressure or raised cholesterol, with the promise that they will reduce our chances of joining the ranks of the chronically ill. But is this really the best way to deal with the rising tide of poor health?

So many of us view doctors as a kind of one-stop pill dispensary that we rarely consider how limited this way of thinking is. To begin with, the drugs almost never do anything about the underlying cause. They're designed to treat symptoms – raised blood pressure, the pain in your joints. And in the end, they don't do the job. Imagine that your health problem was a leaking roof and the symptom was water dripping into the bedroom. Putting buckets under the drips year after year would treat the symptom, but a more sane and satisfactory solution would be to replace the missing tile.

Suppose you've been to your doctor and have been told that your blood-sugar level is getting dangerously high – in fact, that you have type 2 diabetes. You will very likely be given a drug called metformin, which will bring your blood-sugar level down fast. Once it's done its job, however, metformin will obviously not get to the root of why you've got blood-sugar problems in the first place. It's the classic 'bucket' approach.

Getting to grips with your illness – replacing the tile – demands a solution that goes much deeper. A drugless, and painless, way to treat the specific condition while enhancing overall health. In essence, you need to avoid foods that raise blood sugar. But just handing out diet sheets, as many doctors now do, is worse than useless. We need to know how specific foods can fix specific conditions, and how we can put both the basics of good health together with those to make a nutritional blueprint that's best for us.

Food for thought

More and more of us realise that the chronic diseases of the West are caused by poor diet and an unhealthy lifestyle. As the evidence in this book will make crystal-clear, we are digging our own graves with a knife and fork. So for both prevention and cure, the logical route is to change what you put in your mouth. And, as we'll see, exercise more, and learn to handle stress better.

This is the approach that I (Patrick) have been championing for the last 20 years. For me it all began when I heard that a Canadian doctor was using nutritional therapy to treat schizophrenia, with extraordinary success. I went to meet Dr Abram Hoffer, the director of psychiatric research in Saskatchewan. Hoffer had treated over 5,000 schizophrenic patients. I asked him what his success rate was. He said, 'Eighty-five per cent cured.'

As I am also a psychologist specialising in mental illness, I knew that the drugs given for schizophrenia don't cure anything, but act as a kind of chemical straitjacket. This means they help the relatives more than the patient! Hoffer's definition of cure was 'free of symptoms, able to socialise with family and friends and paying income tax'. I was so impressed that I became his student and learned how the right combination of diet and supplements really can cure a wide range of serious health problems.

As you'll see the further you get into this book, most doctors know very little about this sort of detailed nutritional approach to preventing and treating chronic diseases. They rely almost exclusively on drugs. But the problem with instantly reaching for the prescription pad isn't just that pharmaceuticals generally only target symptoms. It's also that many of the most widely used drugs turn out to have dangerous and debilitating side effects. One of the revelations of this book is that not only are adverse drug reactions or ADRs more common than most people believe – but that the drug companies go to remarkable lengths to conceal them from both doctors and their patients for as long as possible.

This is one of the areas that I (Jerome) have been researching. I first realised just how extensive and determined a drug company's cover-up of a dangerous side effect could be about six years ago, when I spent an evening interviewing the psychiatrist David Healy in Wales. For several years he had been campaigning to have a possible link between the anti-depressant SSRI drugs and suicide officially recognised and properly investigated by the drug regulatory agency. During the evening he regularly amazed me with the amount of data he had uncovered – internal company memos, clinical trials that had never been published. All pointed to the fact that in a small proportion of patients these drugs could increase the risk of suicide, and that the companies were going to alarming lengths to conceal it. It took about five years before the regulators acknowledged there was a problem.

As a journalist, I felt this was a shocking story that wasn't being told properly, and at a basic human level it just seemed wrong. The more I researched it, the more it became clear that the way the truth about SSRIs had been concealed was not an aberration but the norm. If people are going to make real choice about how to treat health problems and disease, they should be aware of just how much of the bad news about drugs is kept from them – and how much of the good news owes more to marketing than science.

None of this is to say that drugs don't have a major part to play in medicine. If you had just been in a serious accident or needed a hip replacement or a coronary bypass, there is little doubt that you would get expert and possibly life-saving treatment at your local hospital. But what if, like millions of others, your problem wasn't acute? What if instead you were developing the early signs of one of those chronic diseases that have now been indisputably linked with poor nutrition?

Raised risks

Christine, for example, suffered from arthritis – nasty but not life-threatening – and was given a prescription for the anti-inflammatory drug Vioxx. Her doctor recommended it as a great improvement over aspirin. Shortly after starting on the drug, she suffered a stroke which left her blind and paralysed on one side and epileptic. She believes the drug, later withdrawn because it raised the risk of cardiovascular problems (see Chapter 1), was responsible. Had she been treated nutritionally, her story would have been quite different.

A clinical nutrition centre like the one run by Patrick would have advised her to make sure she included good amounts of fish and fish oils in her diet and to cut back on meat. She might have been given an allergy test to see if there were any foods she should avoid, and she would also be advised to up her intake of both antioxidants and B vitamins, and to take glucosamine. Natural painkillers such as curcumin – an extract from the spice turmeric – and ginger might have been suggested.

Ed Smith, who had suffered from arthritis for years, gave up anti-inflammatory drugs and switched to a similar regime. 'I used to have constant pain in my knees and joints and I couldn't play golf or walk more than ten minutes without resting my legs,' he says. 'Since following your advice my discomfort has decreased 95 to 100 per cent.'

In this book we look at evidence, often hidden away in medical journals, suggesting that bestselling drugs for chronic diseases – such as anti-inflammatories for joint pain, cholesterol-lowering drugs and anti-depressants – may not be as safe and effective as we are led to believe. It's only when you know about this research that you can decide how taking the drugs compares to an approach involving diet, supplements and simple lifestyle changes. In essence, we're giving you the basics for making choices in how you look after your health.

We realise that making changes in the most fundamental aspects of life – eating, exercising, dealing with day-to-day challenges – might seem much more daunting than popping a pill. It's not the usual default path. Many people only make a move to change the way they've been living when they suddenly experience, say, severe pain. So they'll visit their doctor.

And rightly so. Doctors go through lengthy training to learn how to diagnose disease. You need to get yourself properly checked out so that you know what you are dealing with. If you've become ill, you need to understand its origins – why you've lost blood-sugar control or thyroid function, or why your arteries have deteriorated in such a way that you are now more vulnerable to heart attack or stroke.

But once you've got a diagnosis, we hope you'll use this book to make a more informed choice about what course to take. Your doctor may well tell you that this choice is between scientific, properly tested medicine (drugs, in short) and untested 'folk' medicine that depends on exaggerated claims and ignorance, and works – if at all – only through the placebo effect. We view that choice very differently.

Good vs profitable

One of the most striking findings of this book is that much of the supposed scientific basis for the top-selling drugs owes more to skilful marketing than a detached assessment of the evidence. We too believe in scientific medicine – in properly conducted controlled trials and accurate reporting of results. Unfortunately, many drugs never go through this process – as we will show. So the real distinction is actually between good medicine and profitable medicine.

We define good medicine very simply.

- It works – relieves the pain *and* removes the cause of the disease
- It's safe – has minimal side effects or risk of harm
- It's doable – doesn't cost too much and is practical.

Profitable medicine is just as easy to define, but completely different.

- It's hugely expensive
- It's synthetic because it must be to be patentable
- It's designed only to relieve symptoms, so patients have to keep taking it
- It's supported by multi-million dollar marketing campaigns.

We have plenty of evidence that many of today's bestselling medicines are money-making devices rather than effective, safe, affordable and practical remedies. A large number of drugs, as will become clear, are brought on to the market not because they represent a significant improvement over what is there already, but simply so that the company can continue charging high prices for a drug covered by a new patent.

What you need is some way of telling good medicine from profitable medicine, so in Chapter 4 we set out the ten questions you need to ask your doctor to find out which sort you are being offered.

We also believe in the Hippocratic principle – 'First do no harm' – so that if there is a nutritional treatment that works just as well as a drug but is safer, then we recommend it as a priority.

If you are fortunate enough to be fit and healthy, and plan to stay that way, this book will help you to define the diet and lifestyle most likely to keep you disease-free and drug-free.

How this book is organised

In Part 1 you will find out how modern pharmaceutical medicine, and especially drugs aimed at the most common major diseases, has strayed away – for reasons largely to do with profit and power – from the true science of healing and keeping people healthy and free of pain. You will find out how, after the dazzling discoveries of valuable new drugs in the middle of the twentieth century, the relentless search for a new pill for every ill has given us a prescription-based approach to chronic disease that owes more to marketing than science. You'll see how the truth about many of these drugs has been kept from patients and doctors alike, making it impossible to practise a true science of healing. This part of the book is for the many people who would like to handle chronic conditions without the long-term use of drugs, but have up to now lacked the right information to question the value of the drugs they are offered.

In Part 2, we explain why food really is better medicine than drugs, and how to build your own perfect nutrition plan. You will discover a different way of looking at your body and your health. Prescription drugs are often said to be 'scientific' because they contain one purified substance and target a single pathway in the body. This is essentially a nineteenth-century view of the body as machine: pull a lever here, shut off a valve there. But the body doesn't work like that at all.

Cutting-edge science now sees it more as an ecosystem, like a forest or a coral reef, where all parts eventually affect all the others. A food such as an omega-3 fat affects many parts of this system in a healing way: the walls of your cells, your brain tissue, the stickiness of your blood, even the rhythm of your heart. Most drugs actually affect more than one pathway, but the effect on most of the unintended ones can cause harm – in other words, side effects. In this part you'll also find out how to give yourself a health check-up, and what needs to change for you to pass the test.

In Part 3 we look in detail at the top nine chronic disorders, including diabetes, depression, heart disease, joint pain and asthma and eczema. (We have not addressed the many types of cancer because of its complexity, both in prevention and treatment – a subject that warrants a book in its own right.) We describe the main drugs you would normally be prescribed for them, and tell you honestly just how good the evidence is that they are safe and effective. We then go through the evidence for a range of non-drug treatments, concentrating on nutrition and supplements. You will learn, for instance, how and why chromium can be very effective in treating diabetes, why niacin is more effective in normalising your cholesterol than statins, and just how poor the evidence is, in comparison to safer nutritional alternatives, for anti-depressants, sleeping pills and the Ritalin-type drugs often prescribed for ADHD (Attention Deficit Hyperactivity Disorder).

Finally, in Part 4, we look to the future and how we might all benefit from a better system of medicine – one that is primarily committed to improving people's health rather than solely concerned with profits. We suggest some of the changes that need to happen to make this a reality, such as significantly increasing the tiny amount currently spent on researching the alternatives to drug therapies. We expose the shoddy science behind the various vitamin scares – for instance, the ones proclaiming that vitamin E is no good for protecting against heart disease or that vitamin C can be damaging in large doses. We also describe the work of a number of doctors who are already practising a form of medicine that integrates nutrition, exercise and drugs. In these medical practices, serious attention is paid to helping people change rather than just giving them offhand lifestyle advice and then resorting to drugs when that, unsurprisingly, fails.

We all want to keep ourselves and our family and friends free of pain and illness. And very few people want to keep taking drugs on a daily basis. Yet many continue to swallow them, because they believe they're safe and effective and that other treatments can't possibly pack the same scientific punch.

We wrote this book, however, to put the evidence that this isn't the case into your hands. We hope the advice in this book will restore your health if you are unwell, and keep you healthy if you are free from disease. We invite you to show this book to your doctor, your family and anyone you care about who is currently suffering from any of the health problems or taking any of the medications we cover. In this way, you will be playing your part in creating a better future.

Mark Twain once said, 'Everybody complains about the weather but no one does anything about it.' Here's your chance. You don't have to swallow what the drug companies tell you and you don't have to suffer. Food really is better medicine.

Wishing you the best of health,

Patrick Holford and Jerome Burne

Part **1**

The Truth about Drugs

1.

The Prescription Addiction
Why we need to kick the habit

HAVE YOU EVER fantasised about going back in time to an earlier, simpler age? You may have dreamed of life as an Edwardian aristocrat, a citizen of ancient Rome or a scion of the Baghdad caliphate. But whatever the era, there is one modern advance you would find yourself missing desperately – medical care.

Scientific medicine is undoubtedly one of the triumphs of the late twentieth century. It is extraordinary to think that just under 70 years ago, on the eve of the Second World War, doctors were relatively powerless at staving off disease. They could make a careful diagnosis and say what the likely outcome was, but after that nature was pretty much allowed to take her course.[1]

About the only effective remedies in British medicine cabinets at the time were aspirin from willow bark, given for rheumatic fever; digoxin from foxglove, a remedy for heart conditions; immunisation for some infections; and salvarsin for syphilis. Meanwhile, children were dying from diseases like polio, diphtheria and whooping cough, while adults succumbed to various infectious diseases such as tuberculosis or puerperal fever, which killed 1,000 women a year during childbirth.

Over the next 30 years, this bleak scenario was utterly transformed through a series of remarkable discoveries. Among the treatments and medical breakthroughs that emerged were penicillin, kidney dialysis, general anaesthesia with curare, cortisone, a cure for tuberculosis, open-heart surgery, polio vaccination, the contraceptive pill, hip replacements, kidney transplants, heart transplants and the cure for childhood cancer.

The most highly publicised drugs coming out of this medical revolution were antibiotics, which vanquished such major killers as septicaemia, meningitis and pneumonia. But they didn't only save lives. They also created the potent myth that drugs would soon be able to cure most if not all of our illnesses and afflictions. Folklore, luck and personal skill would give way to treatments based on scientific principles that were testable and repeatable. It was a noble vision – the application of science to benefit the health of humanity – and it is one that most people still believe in today.

A darker side

But for all its remarkable successes in medical emergencies such as physical trauma after a car crash, the performance of drug-based medicine has been far less impressive in preventing and treating the chronic conditions that now plague us – arthritis, depression, diabetes, heart disease. Not only do the drugs concentrate on alleviating the symptoms rather than tackling the underlying cause, but they inevitably have unpleasant and sometimes deadly side effects. And these side effects are made even more damaging by drug companies' practice of down-playing and concealing them.

Fred Myers, who is 68 and from Mattishall in Norfolk, used to love golf, but now, following a heart attack, just practising his golf swing leaves him breathless. He is one of 500,000 people in the UK who took the anti-inflammatory drug Vioxx, which was withdrawn from the market in 2004 after research showed that it doubled the risk of heart attacks. 'I've kept fit all my life – and done all the things doctors tell you you should do,' he says. 'I don't smoke, don't drink too heavily, don't eat fatty food. The heart attack has altered my life so much in the things I can do.' Myers started taking the drug for his arthritis because he was told it wouldn't cause the side effects he experienced with traditional painkillers. Nineteen months later, he suffered a heart attack.[2]

There are now an estimated 10,000 court cases outstanding against Merck – the makers of Vioxx – brought by patients in the US who claim to have been damaged by the drug and not properly warned about the risks. One expert estimates that 140,000 Americans were killed or now suffer from vascular problems as a result of the drug, and the cost of legal actions to Merck has been put at between $5 and $50 billion.[3] As of April 2006, just six cases had been heard. In three, the plaintiffs were awarded damages running into millions of dollars. Myers is among 400 people from the UK who are now trying to sue Merck in the American courts. No cases can be brought in the UK because claimants have been refused legal aid and insurers will not fund no-win, no-fee cases.

However, the Vioxx scandal is just one of a series involving widely used drugs whose damaging side effects, it is claimed, were concealed from doctors and public alike for years.

The SSRI (selective serotonin reuptake inhibitor) anti-depressants are a well-known case in point. Research done in the mid-1990s revealed a link between these drugs and suicide in children, but no formal warning was issued until 2003, by which time tens of thousands of young people had been prescribed them. According to one study summarising a number of trials, the total number of children who experienced a 'suicide related event' was 74 of the 2,298 on the drug, versus 34 of the 1,952 on the placebo.[4] Though small, the risk is there. Very recently, the makers of the SSRI Seroxat announced that, despite previous statements, the drug could also cause a raised risk of suicide in young adults.[5]

An earlier disaster involved the heartburn medication Propulsid, which could cause irregular heart rhythms. This was also widely prescribed to very young children, even though there was never any evidence that it was effective and it had been linked with a number of deaths. It was withdrawn from sale in 2000. For more details see page 49.

'The public are being allowed to believe that their drugs are safer and more effective than they really are,' says Dr Marcia Angell, who for two decades was editor-in-chief of the *New England Journal of Medicine* and is now a trenchant critic of the pharmaceutical industry. 'Journalists as well as the public and physicians have bought, hook, line and sinker, the idea that these drugs are getting better.'[6]

Food finds a way

The fact that people are being damaged unnecessarily by drugs that are being prescribed to millions is bad enough. But the myth that these drugs are all firmly science-based has led to another, possibly even more harmful long-term effect on our health. It has meant that any non-drug treatments that do tackle the underlying problem and don't inevitably have side effects are not researched properly, and end up regarded by mainstream doctors as unscientific and ineffective.

After the drug revolution in the 1960s and 1970s, it became clear that food and supplements directly affect many of the same biochemical pathways in the body that drugs target, but with far fewer side effects. But patients are rarely told about this. For instance, omega-3 fats lower production of the same inflammatory chemicals that Vioxx does – without damaging the heart. Yet this information is still only filtering through to public consciousness, and is certainly not widely distributed by doctors. That diet, nutrition and supplements can do much, much more – alleviate arthritis, as well as a range of other chronic conditions like depression, angina, high cholesterol or high blood pressure – is almost certainly never passed on, partly because the vast majority of doctors have no training in nutritional medicine.

If your doctor qualified more than ten years ago, chances are he or she had fewer than 12 hours of training in nutrition per se. Of course every doctor will advise patients to eat healthily and take exercise, but with no specialist knowledge, their advice can be too general to effectively target what's actually, specifically wrong. And it is important to get up to speed with this, as we'll be seeing throughout this book. When combined with other non-drug approaches such as exercise and stress reduction, nutritional medicine has the potential to cure many chronic conditions rather than just calm symptoms. And there is plenty of evidence to back this up.

For instance, as we'll see later, more drugs are dispensed to reduce the risk of heart disease than anything else, yet omega-3 fatty acids are pretty effective at this. To take just one study from dozens, a follow-up study of 84,000 nurses over 16 years – that's a large number over a long period – found that 'higher consumption of fish and omega-3 fatty acids is associated with a lower risk of coronary heart disease (CHD), particu-larly CHD deaths'.[7] Drugs for depression are also prescribed in large quantities but again there are plenty of studies showing that omega-3 can have a beneficial effect on mood as well. Another study compared 264 depressed elderly people in a home with 461 from the general population and found a link between the amount of omega-3 in their blood and how depressed or cheerful they felt. 'There is a direct effect of fatty acid composition on mood', the authors concluded.[8]

STATINS VS THE MEDITERRANEAN DIET

Statins work by reducing the amount of cholesterol in the blood through inhibiting a pathway in the liver that produces an enzyme that helps produce cholesterol. These drugs are supposed to work best in people who have already had a heart attack. But how well do they work when compared with a change in diet?

A study published in 2002 gave patients either regular dietary advice about low-fat eating from their doctor, or advice on eating a Mediterranean diet. (This features fresh vegetables and fruit, fish, beans, seeds and nuts, olive oil and moderate amounts of dairy products such as yogurt.) After four years, those on the Mediterranean diet had a 70 per cent lower incidence of heart disease – three times better than the usual risk reduction in similar patients given statins.[9]

Another study published in 2005[10] looked at 74,000 people to see how closely they were following the Mediterranean diet and what effect that had on how long they lived. The patients were rated using a scale of one to ten – a point for so much fish, one for grains and so on.

It was found that for every two points they got closer to the ideal Mediterranean diet, their chances of dying within a period set by the trial went down by eight per cent. People who followed the full Mediterranean diet cut their chances of dying in the set period by 40 per cent. In many groups of people, even though statins reduce heart attacks, they don't cut mortality rates at all.

The doctors' view

At this point, you might be feeling real concern about what we're saying – that nutrition can prevent heart attacks more effectively than a drug marketed to do the job. How can olive oil, fish, tomatoes and beans possibly quell a killer disease better than these drugs? Many doctors think this way, and your doctor may be one of them. After all, our view goes against many aspects of traditional medical training.

Let's look at the classic objections to a regime of optimal nutrition, supplements, exercise and stress reduction as an alternative to pharmaceutical drugs.

Argument 1 – Isn't the nutritional approach simply unworkable?

There's nothing new about eating healthily! After all, Hippocrates himself came up with the phrase 'Let food be your medicine.' Everyone knows that you should eat well and exercise to avoid heart disease or diabetes. The problem is that people don't do it, and only a few would put up with all that nannying and checking up that would be needed to make it work on a large scale. Anyway, even if it did work, it would be hugely expensive and completely impractical.

All you need to stay healthy is a proper balanced diet. We don't know what the long-term effects of taking lots of supplements are, although we do know that some of them, like vitamin E to prevent heart attacks, don't work. And while there may be some impressive case histories about people who cured themselves by having lots of fruit juice or cutting out potatoes, you can't base a whole system of medicine on that.

Argument 2 – The medical approach is tried and tested

Modern medicine has made enormous strides and saved millions of lives over the past 60 years. The whole point of modern medicine is that it's based on rigorous testing of drugs which are trialled first on animals and then in large-scale, double-blind trials on humans to make sure that they are both safe and effective. Only then are they given a licence. The trouble with trying to treat illnesses with special diets and supplements is that the evidence that they work just isn't there. Many of the claims just haven't been tested properly.

Then there's a whole range of new drugs, based on the latest genetic research, just around the corner, which will make a drug regime even more effective. If all this diet and supplement stuff really works, then the people involved should test it properly – and if it passes the tests it will become part of regular medical practice.

What needs to change and why

As you may well have heard your doctor saying some of the above, it might sound very familiar and reasonable. However, we believe that it is wrong – and moreover, that it's actually damaging.

We will be showing how nutrition-based, non-drug approaches to illness are far safer and often demonstrably more effective than prescription drugs for chronic diseases – and how, if this approach were taken up in a big way, it would mean a dramatic reduction in the national drugs bill and in the numbers of people damaged by drugs. If this happened, many more people could live healthy, active lives rather than joining the ranks of the walking wounded.

But first, we will all need to look clearly at the available evidence for the relative efficacy of drug regimes and the nutritional approach. We go into this below, and investigate it in detail in Part 3. But beyond this, there will have to be a number of changes in the way medicine is practised.

Optimum nutrition – getting the real message out

Doctors need to understand 'healthy eating' beyond the level of basic food pyramids and often outdated nutritional advice. Many talk confidently about the lack of evidence for the nutritional approach but, as we indicated above, they receive next to no training in nutrition. If pushed they will talk about a 'balanced diet', but give very few details about what that actually is, and how best to help the many people who are living on unhealthy diets – fast foods, sugary or starchy snacks and stimulants such as coffee and cola.

We propose that doctors could benefit from working much more closely with nutritionists. Once a critical mass of such clued-up doctors is reached, the idea of entire populations living healthier, more energetic, drug-free lives becomes a distinct possibility.

Drug-based regimes – getting at the truth

Doctors need to stay abreast of findings about drugs, and take a more disinterested approach to them. Many tend to be rather casual about side effects – some studies show that they are not as concerned about them as patients. Yet side effects are a far more serious issue than is generally accepted, as we will reveal. We are calling for a proper monitoring and tracking of side effects and a full investigation when a drug has been found to cause serious problems.

The claim that drug-based medicine is based firmly on science is clearly often not the case, as we'll see shortly. We are in favour of scientific, evidence-based medicine and believe that drug companies' marketing regularly conceals or distorts inconvenient scientific findings. This needs to be controlled in patients' interests.

Another problematic issue is that a large proportion of doctors' ongoing education about the effectiveness and safety of drugs is paid for by drug companies. As you will see, much of this information is heavily spun and biased, and this needs to change.

Drug companies also claim that much of their income goes on developing new and valuable drugs. In fact, the number of genuinely innovative drugs they produce is small and declining. Much of their resources go on producing copycat versions of bestselling existing drugs so they can keep selling a patented product at much higher prices. This provides very little benefit to patients and also needs to be changed.

Becoming an informed medical consumer

If you're shocked or confounded by what we've said, it's not surprising. These are the kinds of things we don't really want to hear. When you are ill or worried about being ill, you want to be able to trust your doctor and believe that the treatment they recommend is designed only to make you better. But in the real world, marketing can oversell any product – people are given bad financial advice, products don't do what they claim to – and as grown-up consumers, you have to seek out unbiased information before you buy. The same is now true of medicine, and we hope this book will give you the knowledge to make informed choices.

One thing we must stress again is that drugs per se are not 'bad'. They have a vital part to play in medical treatment and are indispensable in acute situations: no one would wish to be without antibiotics when faced with meningitis, for instance. Drugs have made a big difference in the treatment of AIDS, multiple sclerosis and the kidney damage that can come with diabetes. But the old adage about a man with a hammer seeing everything as a nail applies especially to drugs.

They can work brilliantly, but they're not the only way to provide medicine, and especially not as the starting point to treat or prevent the chronic diseases that increasingly affect us. There are good reasons why drugs have come to dominate medicine and we'll look at some of them later, but first let's look at scientific medicine's scorecard. It claims to be safe, effective and based in well-conducted research. Is it?

Vioxx: a cautionary tale

The story of what happened to the painkiller Vioxx provides a valuable lens through which to look at just how the drug industry, governmental agencies and the medical profession actually behave in the real world. In 2004, Vioxx was withdrawn because of links with heart problems. The events that led up to that are a disturbing eye-opener for anyone who believes our safety always wins out in the face of commercial interests.

The big selling point of Vioxx, as with many other drugs as we will see, was that it didn't cause a side effect that had plagued the previous generation of painkillers, NSAIDs (nonsteroidal anti-inflammatory drugs), which include aspirin. This side effect is gastrointestinal damage bad enough to put 12,000 people in hospital and cause 2,600 deaths in the UK annually.[11] NSAIDS work by inhibiting an enzyme – cyclo-oxygenase-2 or COX-2 for short – that causes inflammation and pain. The trouble is, they also block another version of the enzyme, COX-1, which is needed to produce protective mucus in the gut. Hence the gastrointestinal damage. COX-2 inhibitors like Vioxx promised reduced inflammation without gut damage because they only block COX-2.

However, as also regularly happens with new drugs, this caused a different adverse drug reaction, or ADR. Blocking only COX-2 had a side effect: it boosted the ability of the body to produce blood clots. Throwing a spanner in the works of a system as complex and interdependent as our bodies invariably has unexpected effects somewhere else. (We'll find out more about this – and why non-drug treatments rarely suffer from it – in Chapter 5.)

To the general public and many doctors, the withdrawal of Vioxx came as a shock. After five years on the market it was a billion-dollar blockbuster, prescribed to 80 million people worldwide, including 20 million Americans and 400,000 in the UK. It had been dubbed 'super aspirin', a drug that gave you better pain relief and no gut problems.

Ignoring the link

Given Vioxx's high profile, you might have reasonably assumed that its safety was backed up by plenty of evidence. Not so. It rapidly emerged that quite the opposite was the case. In fact, behind the scenes and in the medical literature, alarm bells had been ringing for years about the link with heart attacks. It's just that they had been deliberately ignored. Here are just a few of them:

- In 1998 a researcher at the University of Pennsylvania sent the results of a trial to Merck showing the possibility of a link with heart disease. They ignored it.[12]

- In 2000, a big trial involving 8,000 people found that compared with an old NSAID, Vioxx caused between four and five times as many heart attacks.[13]

- In 2001, a big analysis of trials involving 18,000 patients getting Vioxx or another major selling COX-2 drug called Celebrex found increased risk of heart problems.[14]

- In February 2001 the US Food and Drug Administration (FDA) Arthritis Advisory Committee met to discuss concerns about the potential cardiovascular risks associated with Vioxx.[15]

- In May Merck sent out an announcement – 'Merck reconfirms cardiovascular safety of Vioxx' – and ran numerous seminars and 'medical education' symposia to 'debunk' concerns about cardiovascular effects.[16]

- As a result, the US Food and Drug Administration (FDA) ordered Merck to send out a letter to doctors warning them of the dangers. It also said that the company had 'misrepresented the safety profile of Vioxx' in their promotional campaign.[17–18]

- Between 1998 and 2001, two placebo-controlled trials involving over 2,000 Alzheimer's patients and Vioxx found a higher death rate among those on the drug. The result was passed to the FDA but not published until 2004. The FDA did not require the company to warn doctors, nor did the company say anything.[19]

A system in trouble

The precise details of the case are being chewed over in the courts and look like they will be for years but, whatever the legal niceties, it is clear that the system went badly wrong. The drug was clearly not safe nor, as research covered in the next chapter suggests, was it any more effective than the drugs it was supposed to replace. 'Something is very wrong,' writes Dr John Abramson of Harvard University in his brilliant and disturbing book *Overdosed America*,[20] 'with a system that leads patients to demand and doctors to prescribe a drug that provides no better relief and causes significantly more side effects.'

But what should be even more worrying for anyone who believes that we have a scientific system with proper protection and checks and balances is that this disaster has not prompted any very strenuous efforts to make sure it never happens again.

Of course, it could just be that this was an unfortunate accident, the sort that happens in the best-run industries. Planes crash, buildings go up in smoke, but in general we are confident that systems are in place to keep such preventable disasters to an absolute minimum. One of the reasons for our confidence in these cases is that in the wake of such disasters, there is an enquiry to find out what went wrong and what can be done to prevent it in the future.

Unfortunately, however, this kind of enquiry never happens in the wake of drug disasters. To understand why, we need to look at a deal that was struck with the drug companies back in the middle of the last century.

A lack of enquiries

In essence, the companies said we will develop powerful new chemicals that can change the working of the body for good, but may also harm some in the process – because bodies are very varied and unpredictable. Doctors and patients had expected that in return they would be warned about possible problems so they could either find ways round or stop taking the drugs. In fact, drug companies have proved to be extremely 'economical with the truth' while the regulators have all too often looked the other way.

This appears to be precisely what happened with Vioxx. In the UK it was licensed by the MHRA (Medicines and Healthcare products Regulatory Agency, part of the Department of Health) in June 1999. As we have seen, over the next four years, various reports had appeared in scientific literature suggesting there could be a problem. Yet no apparent action was taken.

Quite by chance, immediately after Vioxx was withdrawn, the UK's parliamentary committee for health had just begun hearings on the relationship between the pharmaceutical companies and the NHS and the way it was regulated by the MHRA. It was a wide-ranging investigation with over 50 medical and health experts – including academics, journalists, doctors, NHS officials and government ministers – giving evidence.

The committee's report, *The Influence of the Pharmaceutical Industry*, published in April 2005, received remarkably little coverage and prompted almost no discussion. But it provided for the first time a fascinating and far from reassuring insight into the way the MHRA works. Previously, anyone concerned about drug regulation in the UK could only point to the apparent shortcomings of its far more transparent American equivalent, the Food and Drug Administration (FDA). In the wake of the Vioxx scandal, the FDA had been heavily criticised for not responding fast enough to problems with drugs, for being too close to the drug companies and for not devoting enough attention and resources to safety once a drug had been licensed.

Some in the UK had suggested that the MHRA was no better, but since little information about its workings were ever made public, it was hard to tell. However, the committee's report indicated that the critics were largely right. It concluded that the way drugs are monitored after they are launched was 'inadequate', that medical institutions were 'indifferent' to what happened to patients, and that the MHRA knew very little about 'the overall impact of drug-related illnesses in the community'. Doctors, it said, should take some responsibility for the problems with Vioxx because they were too ready to believe drug company PR.

Almost exactly a year later, in May 2006, a report into the FDA by the US government's General Accounting Office made similar damning criticisms of the American agency. It found that the FDA 'did not have clear policies for addressing drug safety issues and that it sometimes excluded its best safety experts from important meetings'. Not only was it slow to respond but 'the agency's entire system for reviewing the safety of drugs already on the market was too limited and broadly flawed'.[21]

The UK committee's report called for a whole range of changes, among them that the MHRA should actively be on the lookout for problems with ADRs, that there should be a public enquiry whenever a drug is withdrawn, that there should be 'research into adverse health effects of medicalisation' and that non-drug treatments should be investigated properly. The government has chosen not to take action on any of these.

Whether the American government will take any steps to reform the FDA remains to be seen. It seems unlikely that other developed countries have regulatory agencies that are any more robust and proactive, not least because the drug company reactions to such concerns have been steadfastly hard-nosed.

Safety vs 'innovation'

At the beginning of 2005, the Pharmaceutical Research and Manufacturers of America commented: 'It's not clear to us that there needs to be change. Less than 3 per cent of medicines have been withdrawn in the last 20 years.'[22] A spokesman from the Association of the British Pharmaceutical Industry explicitly referred to the existing state of affairs between all the parties concerned – except for patients – and implied that as far as they were concerned, it was working fine. 'The challenge is to acknowledge there is a contract between industry, regulators and health service which recognises that there is a trade-off between risks and benefits.'[23]

In the same article Sir Tom McKillop, recently retired from the drug firm AstraZeneca, was even more blunt, expressing 'frustration that the increased priority over drug safety has eclipsed the importance of innovation and discovering new treatments'.

So we now have a rather clearer idea about what is meant by the trade-off between risks and benefits that lies at the heart of modern medicine. If 140,000 people whose initial problem was aching joints are either killed or made seriously ill, this is actually seen as acceptable and not an indicator of a need for any serious change. Not least because it might put the brakes on innovation.

And how much innovation are we getting in return for putting up with that much death and disability? According to Dr Marcia Angell's *The Truth About Drug Companies*, published in 2004,

> Out of seventy-eight drugs approved by the FDA in 2002, only seventeen contained new active ingredients, and only seven of these were classified by the FDA as improvements over older drugs. The other seventy-one drugs were variations of old drugs or deemed no better than drugs already on the market.[24]

This is an industry that drives a hard bargain, one that you might not want to be part of unless absolutely necessary.

A very modern death rate

So both the regulators and the drug companies regard a certain amount of casualties from drug's 'friendly fire', as it were, to be both inevitable and acceptable. But just how many do they see as OK? The figure might come as a surprise.

In the UK, 10,000 people are killed every year by adverse drug reactions or ADRs – which happen when the prescription drug that is supposed to be curing you kills or harms you instead.[25] That is more than the number of people who die from the following causes combined: cervical cancer (927), taking illegal drugs (1,620), mouth cancer (1,700) and passive smoking by people aged between 20 and 64 (2,700). It is also greater than the number of men who die from prostate cancer (9,937). Yet while all these conditions are the focus of campaigns to cut the numbers, nothing comparable is happening to cut deaths from ADRs, nor are there patient groups to help survivors from drug disasters.

Let's look at the figure in another way. Which is more likely – that you will die in a traffic accident or as the result of a visit to your doctor? Surprisingly to say the least, the answer is visiting your doctor. In 2004, traffic accidents were responsible for a relatively modest 3,221 deaths. ADRs, remember, account for 10,000 deaths in the UK alone, and a further 40,000 people are made sick enough by them to be forced to go to hospital at a cost of £466 million.[26] Then there are all the people who just feel bad after taking a drug, but whose new symptoms are never spotted or recorded.

In the US, the problem of ADRs is even bigger. An estimated 106,000 people die from them every year, and over two million are seriously affected.[27–28]

The extent of the problem is shown in how widespread the lack of concern about ADRs is. The dangers of passive smoking or illegal drugs are frequently aired in health campaigns and outraged newspaper editorials, but ADRs – which exact a far greater toll of misery – very rarely trigger the same level of indignation. And quite apart from the human cost, they are a huge and unnecessary financial drain. In the UK, for instance, the hospital beds the victims of ADRs take up are 4 per cent of the total, and cost the National Health Service nearly half a billion pounds a year.[29]

Yet if you were to ask most doctors about ADRs, you would very probably be told two things. First, that the risks of any one person having a problem is pretty small; and secondly, that if a medicine doesn't have any side effects, it's almost certainly not effective. They might admit that things go wrong occasionally, but say that, thanks to a system of proper scientific trials and regulation, modern medicine by and large success-fully balances the risks of drugs against the undoubted benefits they offer.

Doctors have been trained using the pharmaceutical model, and the vast majority believe in it. In fact, much of their skill comes from juggling a range of drugs for a particular problem so the patients suffer the fewest side effects, or knowing which drugs best alleviate the ADRs caused by the first drug. But is this really a sane or effective approach?

A tale of two drugs

To show you just how unscientific and unhelpful this system can be, let's look at two very different classes of drugs: the hypnotics and the antibiotics.

Bad dream – insomnia 'cures'

The drugs prescribed for people complaining of sleep problems are also known as hypnotics. They have a long charge sheet of side effects,[30] but still regularly feature in the top 20 most prescribed drugs in both the UK and US. Astonishingly, they're not very useful, either, according to a report in the *British Medical Journal*,[31] which concludes that there is plenty of evidence that they cause 'major harm' and that there was 'little evidence of clinically meaningful benefit'.

Despite the rhetoric and these findings, 'evidence-based medicine' is cheerfully jettisoned when there is a billion-dollar market at stake.

So are hypnotics being prescribed because there is nothing else? On the contrary: there is a form of treatment for insomnia that has been shown to be both safe and effective, according an extensive review in *The Lancet*.[32] In this article, various forms of counselling and psychological help were found not only to be much more effective than pills, but also virtually free of side effects.

In any scientific system of medicine that is what patients would be getting. But in fact, counselling for people suffering from insomnia is rarely available outside specialist sleep labs. 'Doctors receive little education about the diagnosis and non-pharmacological treatment of insomnia,' noted the paper in *The Lancet*. And who pays for much of your doctor's further education? The drug companies, as we shall see in Chapter 3.

Many doctors have woken up to the fact that hypnotics pose real problems. But instead of exploring less well-trodden avenues, they have turned to another drug to treat insomnia: sedating anti-depressants. Between 1987 and 1996, the overall use of these drugs went up by 146 per cent. Yet there is no evidence that they work for insomnia – in fact, almost no research has been done on the issue.[33] Prescriptions are written on the basis of the doctor's clinical judgement that they *might* work, a practice known as 'off-label' prescribing. (As we will see in Chapter 2, doctors prescribed SSRIs to children on an off-label basis for years before trials showed they doubled the risk of suicide in that age group.)

So despite an almost total lack of evidence that treating insomnia with drugs is either safe or effective – except as a very temporary measure – the amount spent by the US on advertising hypnotics in 2004 was estimated at $145 million, and sales for these drugs in that country alone is soon expected to hit $5.5 billion.[34] Brilliant marketing – but not 'scientific medicine'.

If you happen to be discussing insomnia treatments with your doctor and you mention nutritional approaches, such as lowering blood-sugar levels or taking a nutritional supplement that increases the amount of the sleep hormone in the brain, the response you are likely to get is that there is really not enough evidence to show that it is effective. That is probably a good time to point out the major holes in that argument – by showing the comparable lack of evidence for hypnotics and sedating anti-depressants doing anything to alleviate insomnia.

The case of the vanishing antibiotics

So far, we've just looked at how doctors prescribe pills that cause ADRs or are ineffective. But this isn't the only absurdity in this scenario. The same commercial imperative that turns sleeping pills into a billion-dollar product also ensures that certain drugs that could save your life simply aren't available. The most striking example of this is the search for new antibiotics needed to counter the growing threat of drug-resistant bacteria such as MRSA. Or rather, the lack of one: as the research has virtually ground to a halt. Why? Because they just don't make enough money.

Antibiotics are the drugs that gave rise to the myth of modern medicine's ability to develop so-called 'magic bullets'. They are the foundation of the drug industry, and yet between 2000 and 2004 many of the large drug companies actually abandoned antibiotic development and closed their microbiology departments.[35] As a result, out of 506 new drugs from major firms in the final stages of testing, only six were antibiotics and none of them was aimed at the new targets (that is, proteins or enzymes) thrown up by genetic research.

There is no pretence about the reason behind this trend – the drugs' inherent unprofitability. As top science journal *Nature* put it: 'Antibiotics are the worst sort of pharmaceutical because they cure the disease.'[36] After all, people generally take a course of antibiotics for a week, then stop. Blockbuster drugs that sell billions, the article says, come from developing treatments that people take for a lifetime, say for chronic disorders like high cholesterol or hypertension.

In a genuinely scientific system of medicine, doctors would prescribe non-drug treatments if they were shown to be more effective than drugs, and research wouldn't be limited to the big sellers. In Part 4, we look at proposals for a public–private partnership to run trials on treatments that could improve your health but that might not have huge commercial potential. At the moment, however, marketing trumps science every time in drug development.

THE POWER OF MARKETING

Some time soon – in 2007 or earlier – it's very likely that a testosterone patch made by Proctor and Gamble will be licensed to treat 'female sexual dysfunction' – that is, a lack of interest in sex which women who suffer from this condition find distressing. It is expected to rack up large sales. Here's how it's done, with the facts taken from an analysis in the *British Medical Journal.*

- Sponsor key scientific meetings in sexual medicine and hire leading researchers, as well as three public relations firms and a major advertising agency.

- Set aside an advertising budget of $100 million.

- Be ready for concerns about ADRs. For the patch, the major ones highlighted by the FDA include heart disease and breast cancer, while minor ones are a small increase in acne, hair growth and weight gain.

- Then simply ignore them at international conferences and describe the patch as 'well tolerated'.

- Don't worry about publishing in peer-reviewed journals – just present papers at conferences instead.

- Put out a press release claiming the patch produces 'a 74 per cent increase in frequency of satisfying sexual activity'.

- Ignore the fact that the absolute numbers were less impressive – an extra two episodes of sex a month on top of a baseline of three episodes. Play down the fact that those getting the placebo had one extra episode a month.

- Emphasise that what is important is the decrease in distress in patients on the patch.

- Ignore the fact that this decrease was only six or seven points on a 100-point scale. Ignore also that the increase in desire with the patch was only five to six points.

- Give yourself a pat on the back when the FDA declares these results are 'clinically meaningful.'

- Feel confident that you will be able to meet the FDA requirement to produce evidence of long-term safety.[37]

Once again, brilliant marketing – but can anyone seriously claim that this is scientific medicine?

What you can do to protect yourself

By now it should be pretty obvious that we have a medical system prepared to accept pretty high casualty rates, and that if you or your family or friends are damaged by their drugs that is – so the argument runs – just the cost we all have to bear for having an innovating and highly profitable pharmaceutical industry. What's more, this is not an attitude that is about to change any time soon. That might be all right, if the drugs were highly effective. But as we've seen, many of the treatments for non-life-threatening disorders are of pretty marginal benefit.

But you aren't locked into this system. If you develop a chronic disorder, you will probably like to handle it with treatments that aren't going to harm you and that, if possible, will tackle the underlying problem. And in many cases, that is precisely what good nutritional medicine can do. This approach will target the same biochemical pathways that drugs do – it's not voodoo. Nutritional therapists are just as keen on good scientific procedure as regular doctors – only you can be sure that what they are offering you hasn't been heavily influenced by a billion-dollar advertising campaign.

2.

The Dark Side of the Blockbusters
What else aren't they telling us?

ALASTAIR HAY REMEMBERS the moment very clearly.

I walked down to the garage, which is about 100 yards from the house. Rather surprisingly, the door was locked but when I tried to unlock it, the key wouldn't go in. I peered into the keyhole and saw it had been locked from the inside. I had a very bad feeling and went round to the side window. Through it I saw a pashmina scarf tied to a ladder. 'Oh my God,' I cried. I just knew. I remember screaming . . .

A professor of environmental toxicology at Leeds University in the UK, Hay was describing for the coroner's court in June 2003 how his wife Wendy had committed suicide a couple of weeks after being prescribed the SSRI anti-depressant drug Prozac for depression. The court heard evidence that depressed people on SSRIs were twice as likely to kill themselves as those not on a drug. Earlier that year a Welsh coroner, Geraint Williams, had asked for an investigation into the safety of another SSRI, Seroxat, after hearing of a suicide case involving it.[38] And two years before that the plaintiffs in a case against GlaxoSmithKline who claimed their father had been driven to kill by the drug Seroxat were awarded $6.4 million.[39]

Hiding the truth

These are just a few of the tens of thousands of people who have had reason to believe they have been damaged by an SSRI – a class of top-selling drugs. And three years after Alastair Hay's ordeal, there is plenty of evidence that not only do SSRIs do harm and are not particularly effective, but that the drug companies were aware of the dangers for some time, and did their best to keep them concealed from doctors and patients.

Dreadful as the SSRI saga has been for those involved, it points to a wider problem with blockbuster drugs (defined as those which sell over $1 billion per year) – the enormous financial pressure to keep them on the market. A year before the anti-inflammatory blockbuster Vioxx was withdrawn (see page 20) and while the company was discussing warnings about heart problems with the US Food and Drug Administration, the advertising budget for the drug was $150 million – more than Pepsi-Cola's.[40] A few years before these two scandals broke, a very similar scenario played out featuring the heartburn drug Propulsid (see page 48). This involved several hundred deaths of both adults and infants, and there was also strong evidence of a cover-up.

To the outside observer, what seems astounding is that none of these failures prompted any kind of independent enquiry to discover what went wrong and how regulation could be improved; a fact that might well make you think twice before taking a blockbuster in the future. In any other industry, when the actions of a private company damage members of the public, there is an attempt to identify the failures and learn from them. The 1999 Paddington rail crash in the UK a few years ago, in which 31 people died, prompted a long enquiry. So did the 1987 capsizing of the UK ferry *Herald of Free Enterprise*, in which some 190 people died. Yet after an estimated 140,000 Americans were damaged by Vioxx,[41] it was business as usual.

As we saw in Chapter 1, the industry sees no need for any change, which means that you as consumers of their products have to ask: 'So what else aren't we being told?' What other inconvenient data – which may pertain to other blockbuster drugs you're taking right now – is being kept from public view?

One of the reasons nothing is being done is that until less than a decade ago, almost no one would dream of even asking such a question. Medical knowledge was carefully guarded by the profession, and patients were expected to take their medicine and follow their doctor's recommendation.

Getting informed

This book is a sign of a major change in that kind of thinking – a change that has been prompted in part by the Internet, which has made all medical research available at the click of a mouse. The safety and effectiveness of medical treatments can now be researched by active consumers in the same way we can find 'best buys' in white goods. Consumers' research is hampered, however, partly by the drug companies' decisions over what gets published and what doesn't, and by the medical profession's solid backing of drug-based treatments. We'll see more on these two points in Chapter 3.

However there are a few independent critics who have studied specific blockbuster drugs and made a serious and carefully argued case against them. We have already encountered David Healy, the Welsh psychiatrist who, after years of warning of the dangers of suicide from taking SSRIs, was finally shown to be correct. The work of such people is invaluable when you are seeking to inform yourself as fully as possible about pharmaceuticals. So this chapter brings together for the first time criticisms of several of the top-selling types of drugs. Such information can be hard to find elsewhere because 'good news' reports on drugs get much greater prominence than the bad.

If you are already taking a drug, you may be doing fine. It may agree with you, keep symptoms at bay and have no troubling side effects. But if you are worried about long-term effects or thinking about taking one of the blockbusters, you might consider these three points:

- Even if the clinical trials show no problems, that tells you nothing about the possibility of a problem emerging when millions of people start taking it.

- If evidence of a problem does show up and the regulatory authority asks the drug company to run a trial to test for it, that is unlikely to be done. A recent report in the US revealed that 66 per cent of such studies requested by the FDA had not even been begun.[42]

- So, if serious problems do emerge for some people, it could be a few years or more before you get to hear about them.

ANATOMY OF A BLOCKBUSTER

What is needed to create a blockbuster drug? As it happens, quite a range of factors play a part.

- It has to be patentable. Once you have found a target that has a health benefit – more serotonin, less cholesterol – the chemical you develop has to be new or it won't make billions. It can't be a drug that is already out there, or some natural product such as fish oil or a vitamin.

- It doesn't have to be better than anything already being used to get a licence. It just needs to be more effective than nothing (that is, a placebo).

- It has to treat something that lots of people have. That's why there are many drugs for depression and heart disease but few for, say, the much rarer Raynaud's disease.

- It should only treat symptoms, so people will need to keep taking it. When you stop, the symptoms return – as is the case with sleeping pills.

- So, by the same token, it mustn't cure anything, which will ensure people have to take it for a long time. A perfect example is metformin or sulfonylurea drugs for type 2 diabetes. Companies are aiming for something similar with statins. The official guidelines say any male over 55 should take a statin a day to prevent heart disease – presumably for life.

- Ideally it should be possible to keep increasing the number of patients it can be prescribed for. One way is by lowering the guidelines – as with statins. Another is by prescribing off-label – that is, without needing trials to show effectiveness.

The upshot of all this is that one of the first things you need to do to protect yourself is to become aware of the problems that have emerged with existing blockbuster drugs. That's not nearly as difficult as it sounds: 24 of the top-selling drugs are targeted at treating or preventing just six disorders, each one the kind of chronic condition that responds to non-drug and nutritional therapies. In 2004, these 24 drugs racked up an astonishing $67 billion in global sales between them.[43] Here are the disorders they are designed to treat:

- High cholesterol (four brands, total worth $20 billion)

- High blood pressure (five brands, total worth $12.5 billion)

- Heartburn and ulcers (six brands, total worth $12 billion)

- Depression (four brands, total worth $10 billion)

- Psychosis (three brands, total worth $9.4 billion)

- Joint pain (two brands, total worth $4.7 billion).

We will be examining some of these in more detail. First let's look at the SSRIs – the iconic drugs of the 1990s.

SSRIs – a tangled web

In the 1990s, when SSRIs first came on to the scene, there were even debates about whether people at work would be at a disadvantage if they didn't take them, because the drugs were thought to be so safe and effective. By the middle of that decade there were clear signs that there was a problem, yet the risks were never made public. In fact, as late as 2002 newspaper articles were still appearing with headlines such as this one: 'Happiness ... Is a Pill that Makes You Lose Weight, Sorts Out PMT, and Really Cheers You Up. Its name? Prozac.'[44] The copy told how SSRI drugs were dubbed 'vitamin P', and had become a 'lifestyle choice' that people turn to at the 'slightest trough in their fortunes'.

You might be one of the millions who received a prescription for an SSRI. However, your doctor might have been less blithe about prescribing them, and you about popping them, had you known some of the facts about SSRIs that at the time were deliberately kept buried in the specialist literature. Here a just a few of many:

- The first study to show a link between an SSRI and suicide was published in 1990.[45]

- When Sweden's drug regulatory body insisted in seeing all the data on SSRI effectiveness in the mid-1990s, they found the companies had been highly selective in publishing the studies, and had not made all of them public.[46]

- Between 1995 and 2002, a psychiatrist worried about the link between SSRIs and suicide sent hundreds of pages of evidence about it to the UK Medicines and Healthcare products Regulatory Agency. The MHRA continued to insist there was no problem.[47]

- In 2000, a patent for a new sort of Prozac was found to have been filed by the manufacturers of the original version. It claimed that the new version did not cause the suicidal thoughts the old version had.[48]

- Also in 2000, a big study based on all the best evidence submitted to the US Food and Drug Administration over ten years for SSRI licence applications concluded that these drugs were no better than the older anti-depressants they had replaced.[49]

For all that time, doctors were writing an ever-larger number of prescriptions for these drugs. In the UK, more adolescents were getting them than anywhere else in Europe,[50] even though the drugs had no licence for treating adolescents (see 'Making kids suicidal', overleaf). Both the manufacturers and the regulators were claiming that side effects were minimal and that there was no cause for alarm. In 2004, 3.5 million people received 20 million prescriptions for SSRIs,[51] and global sales of SSRIs were estimated at about $17 billion.[52]

MAKING KIDS SUICIDAL

In December 2003, the MHRA issued a warning to doctors not to prescribe SSRIs to children because it increased their risk of suicide. This might look like a case of the watchdog doing its job. In fact, it showed just how at risk we all are. For instance:

- The research data showing a suicide risk for children dated back to 1996, but over the next seven years the drugs was prescribed to tens of thousands of children by doctors who were not informed about it.[53]

- That data involved three trials using Seroxat to treat major depression in children, but only one was published. The summary claimed that Seroxat was 'well tolerated and effective'.[54]

- However an analysis of this trial, published in the top journal *Science*, revealed that 6.5 per cent of children on the drug showed 'emotional liability' (which includes suicidal thinking) compared with 1.4 per cent of those on the placebo.[55] The other two unpublished trials showed more actual suicides in the group getting the drug than in those getting a placebo.[56]

- It was this distortion of the data that lead the New York state attorney to sue manufacturers GlaxoSmithKline (GSK), alleging 'persistent fraud'.

- GSK paid $2.5 million to settle the case but claimed the charges were 'unfounded'.[57]

Today, at least some of these facts have become more widely known and the press are no longer so upbeat about SSRIs. Doctors are now advised not to prescribe them for children because they double the risk of suicide (apart from Prozac, which is the one SSRI licensed for use in children). Psychological counselling is recommended instead.[58] According to a major study, SSRIs are no better than a placebo,[59] and the manufacturers of Seroxat have admitted that a least a quarter of patients may have withdrawal problems.

If you took an SSRI you might have found it helped, or it might have made you feel a bit fuzzy. You might have been one of the 40 per cent who have reported sexual problems on it, or you might have suffered something even more serious. But even today, with a greatly raised level of scepticism about these drugs, it is still pretty unlikely that your doctor will spend much or any time discussing the other options for dealing with depression. Fortunately, we can help you there. There is a range of effective routes you can take if you're suffering from depression.

Alternatives to SSRIs – the nutrition path

Take the case of the 48-year-old man who had suffered from depression, with occasional manic spells, all his life. He'd tried both Prozac and Seroxat but they'd made him feel worse and occasionally suicidal. Counselling and homeopathy hadn't helped either. Then he visited the Brain Bio Centre in London, run by Patrick.

At the centre, he scored 22 on the Hamilton Rating Scale (the standard test for depression), indicating major depression. Blood tests, among others, showed he had low serotonin and suboptimum levels of many minerals, plus various food allergies. He was given supplements including essential fatty acids, 5-HTP (a naturally occurring chemical the brain uses to make serotonin) and a vitamin B complex, and he was encouraged to exercise. Eight months later he reported feeling 'happy, healthy and fit' and his score on the Hamilton Rating Scale had dropped by 19 points. An SSRI drug can be licensed if it lowers that score by just 3 points.

It's also worth being aware of the dark history of SSRIs because the problems that have now finally emerged haven't in any way deterred the pharmaceutical companies from developing new ones. In fact, there are currently no fewer than 28 in the pipeline. One already on the market is Cymbalta, which works by targeting not just serotonin but its fellow brain chemical, dopamine. During trials, before it was licensed in 2004, there was at least one 'unexplained' suicide by a 19-year-old girl. In 2005 the FDA warned that a 'higher than expected rate of suicide attempts was observed' among patients taking it.[60] Sales of Cymbalta are expected to be worth £2.6 billion.

Statins – a life sentence?

Cholesterol-lowering statins are among the bestselling drugs of all time. Governments and the medical profession stand firmly behind them. In the UK, the National Institute for Health and Clinical Excellence (NICE) has just recommended that 3.3 million more people should be eligible for them on the NHS.[61] If your cholesterol level is above the recommended level of 5,[62] or even if you are just male and over 55, you could be advised to take statins for the rest of your life.[63]

However, a few criticisms have disturbed this apparently solid consensus. To begin with, there is the question of side effects, although they don't seem to be in the same league as the ones associated with Vioxx or SSRIs. With statins, the best-known ADR is a form of muscle weakness. One brand, Baycol, was withdrawn following a number of deaths linked to it, and there have been calls in the US for the withdrawal of Crestor because of side effects, which can range from nausea to fatal rhabdomyolysis, where muscle tissue is destroyed and the kidneys can eventually fail. Less well known but possibly more serious in the long run is the effect statins have on the natural antioxidant co-enzyme Q10 (see 'Why statins can be bad for your heart', on page 284).

STATINS AND THE HEART – THE Q10 CONNECTION

Statins block a biochemical pathway in the liver that makes cholesterol and also co-enzyme Q10. This worries some, such as Dr Peter Langsjoen of Tyler, Texas, because CoQ10 is involved in producing energy in all the major muscles, including the heart. Langsjoen uses it to treat cardiovascular diseases. 'The heart uses a huge amount of CoQ10,' he says, 'and it's been pretty well documented from biopsies that the severity of heart failure correlates with people who have the lowest levels.'

A small study of Langsjoen's found that 10 out of 14 patients with no history of heart problems developed heart rhythm abnormalities when given statins, while giving CoQ10 reversed the abnormality in eight out of nine of the participants.[64]

Langsjoen has unsuccessfully petitioned the FDA to put a warning on statins packets of the sort now mandatory in Canada, saying that CoQ10 reduction 'could lead to impaired cardiac function in patients with borderline congestive heart failure'.

Dr D. Mantle of Newcastle University in the UK believes that because CoQ10 is involved in energy production, reducing it may be the cause of muscle weakness. CoQ10's other functions – such as the stabilisation of cell membranes – may be linked with other statin-induced ADRs, including gastrointestinal upset, liver problems, cataracts, loss of memory and peripheral nerve damage.

Drug companies are well aware of statins' effect on CoQ10. In fact, Merck has a patent on a statin/CoQ10 combo that has yet to be marketed. If you are on statins, discuss supplementing between 100 and 300mg a day of CoQ10 with an expert (see Resources, page 403, and for the benefits of CoQ10 see page 298).

One of the leading critics of statins is John Abramson,[65] an author and member of the Harvard Medical School clinical faculty who has analysed the evidence usually used to support their ever wider use. Abramson is very sceptical of their benefits. He has looked particularly closely at how effective they are in staving off heart attacks and prolonging life in people who don't have heart disease – so called primary prevention. (It is generally agreed that once you've had an attack, taking statins – in this context called 'secondary prevention' – will reduce your chances of another. See 'Just how many statins do you need?', page 43, for some of Abramson's criticisms about the effectiveness of these drugs.)

Other critics of statins also complain that studies that find evidence in favour of the benefits of lowering cholesterol are six times more likely to be mentioned in the literature than ones that don't.[66]

The debate over statins can get a bit complex, as it is all too easy to become mired in interpretations of trial results and biomedical statistics. There are, however, three vital points about why we should handle them with care.

First off, if you just have raised risk factors for heart disease – for instance, you're overweight, you smoke or you have raised cholesterol –

rather than actual heart disease, the evidence that taking statins will stave off a heart attack is much weaker than is generally presented. Secondly, in very large populations of primary-prevention patients given statins, only a vanishingly small number of heart attacks have been prevented, as we'll see below. And finally, for two groups of people – the elderly and women – there are no proper clinical trials to show that, in primary prevention, statins reduce your chance of having a heart attack. In fact, there is some evidence to show that people over 65 with raised cholesterol actually live longer.[67]

Let's take a look at some of the evidence for these conclusions:

- Statins are taken to reduce high cholesterol, yet 50 per cent of heart-attack patients have normal cholesterol.[68]

- Another marker for heart-attack risk that is as accurate as cholesterol is your blood level of the amino acid homocysteine. The way to reduce it is with B vitamins (see Part 3, page 301, for details on this).

- One recent report says that 19,600 people categorised as having as mild to moderate risk of having a heart attack would need to take a statin every day for five years to prevent one death from heart disease.[69]

- Current guidelines recommend that women and old people take statins. However, according to an open letter signed by 36 senior academics, not only is there no proper evidence that this is beneficial – but a number of studies suggest it could be harmful.[70]

- The UK is the only country where you can go and buy a statin drug over the counter; a move which as been denounced as a nation-wide experiment.[71]

- Treating 250 diabetic patients (who have a raised risk of developing heart disease) with statins would prevent one death. Getting 250 diabetic patients to take exercise saves four times as many lives.[72]

JUST HOW MANY STATINS DO YOU NEED?

Statin supporters claim that they reduce the risk of a heart attack by between 20 and 30 per cent. The West of Scotland Coronary Prevention Study,[73] a classic of its kind, reported a 31 per cent reduction in heart attacks among men at high risk. This may sound good, but as John Abramson of the Harvard Medical School points out, there is another way of looking at these figures.

What hasn't been factored into this scenario is that heart attacks, even among people at risk, are pretty rare. In the West of Scotland study, for every 100 men on statins there was an average of 1.1 heart attacks per year, while those on the placebo had 1.6. That is indeed a 31 per cent reduction, but it's not the sort of benefit that most patients think they are getting when they see the bald statistic.

Abramson analysed another key study, known as AFCAPS/TexCAPS,[74] and found the results equally unimpressive. In this study, 6,600 healthy middle-aged people with slightly raised cholesterol took statins or a placebo for five years. The risk of having heart disease among those who got the drug fell by 37 per cent. That looks impressive – until you take into account that the risk of developing any serious disease (that is, one that requires hospitalisation and/or results in death) was identical for both groups. So a lower risk for heart disease effectively meant the risk of another, equally onerous condition stepped into its place. 'Treating with statins,' commented Abramson, 'simply traded coronary artery disease for some other serious disease.'

You could describe the issue here as a numbers game. From the point of view of the government, giving millions of people statins might be worth it on the ground that they save several thousand lives. But from your position as one person wanting to stay healthy, the odds of one in 90 or perhaps one in several hundred (the figures vary) that they will make a difference to you directly might not seem a worthwhile gamble, especially when non-drug and dietary changes are far more likely to be of direct benefit.

There's another issue here. One of the features of our drug-based medical system is that the number of people who need to take drugs is constantly increasing. Between 2001 and 2004, the number of people officially in need of statins tripled. This boom could be because people are so unhealthy that the drugs are all that stands between them and a heart attack. But there is another way of looking at it. Could it be that the net to catch people at risk of heart disease has been cast so wide that it falls on huge swathes of the population? And if that's the case, do you really need the drug?

Evidence that something like this is going on comes from a recent Norwegian study. The scientists found that when they applied the latest 2003 European guidelines on who was at risk of a heart attack (and so ought to be treated with drugs), 85.9 per cent of the men studied were not just at risk, but at high risk by the age of 40. What's more, three out of four Norwegians aged 20 or older were classed as in need of counselling because of high cholesterol or blood-pressure levels.[75]

Are Norwegians just astoundingly unhealthy? This wasn't what the researchers thought. As they commented in the *British Medical Journal*: 'When guidelines class most adults in one of the world's longest living and healthiest populations as at high risk and therefore in need of maximal clinical attention and follow up, it raises several scientific and ethical questions.'

The drive to bring national cholesterol levels ever lower by prescribing higher doses of statins to more and more people was strongly challenged in the *British Medical Journal* last June.[76] The side effects of these drugs, the authors claim, have been consistently underplayed. In one recent major trial comparing two leading brands, they note the alarming fact that 'almost 60% of the participants in both groups experienced side-effects', nearly half of them serious. What's more, the study failed to comment on this, merely saying side effects were the same in both groups. Among the ADRs discussed are heart failure, muscle weakness, cognitive problems and cancer.

Statins and 'diagnostic creep'

It's not just statins that are effectually blanket-bombing entire populations. Something extraordinary is happening in the US. Dubbed 'diagnostic creep', it is the practice of classifying more and more people as in need of medication because they exceed some guideline – which is, at the same time, constantly being lowered. It is estimated that over 40 per cent of Americans are now taking drugs to prevent one or more disease and that 75 per cent of them are at risk for some lifestyle disorder according to those official guidelines.[77] In the UK, 70 per cent of the population is taking medication to treat or prevent ill health or to enhance well-being.[78]

You don't have to be particularly cynical to see that diagnostic creep is a brilliant marketing tool. The two conditions which have been most affected by it are high cholesterol and high blood pressure – currently Nos 1 and 2 in the bestselling drugs chart. The current spend on drugs for hypertension in the US, for instance, is an astonishing $16 billion dollars a year. The bestselling statin, Lipitor, pulls in $11 billion on its own.

CHOLESTEROL – HOW LOW CAN YOU GO?

At the beginning of 2001, if your cholesterol level was below 5 mmol/l (200mg/dl in the US)[79] you were considered pretty much all right, depending on your other risk factors. Around 13 million Americans had higher cholesterol levels, however, and were said to be at risk from heart disease because of raised cholesterol. They were advised to take statins.

Then a report by the US National Cholesterol Education Program slashed the safe level to 130mg/dl, tripling the number of Americans with an officially raised risk for heart disease. Suddenly, 39 million of them were eligible for treatment with statins.[80] The guidelines were lowered yet again[81] in 2004, recommending them for people with cholesterol levels as low as 100mg/dl.

One of the analyses carried out by John Abramson of the Harvard Medical School on a large statin trial found that tripling the number of people needing to take statins made no difference to the number of heart attacks.[82]

So it has to be relevant that the majority of members of the committees that set the guidelines making these levels of profit possible have financial links with the companies making the drugs. Eight out of nine authors of the most recent set of guidelines setting lower cholesterol targets had financial links with statin manufacturers, as did nine of the eleven members of the committee that set lower levels for hypertension in 2001.[83]

Bringing down blood pressure

The debate around hypertension drugs is nearly as complex as that over statins. Much of it centres round the largest hypertension study ever, known as ALLHAT (the Antihypertensive and Lipid-Lowering Treatment to Prevent Heart Attack Trial). This is funded solely by the US federal government – rather than by a drug company — and has produced several major papers showing that the newer and more expensive drugs are no more effective, and in fact are more likely to cause problems, when compared with the older and far cheaper ones.[84–85]

It's a complicated issue, and if you are interested in finding out more from sources that are sceptical about the value of the drug approach in this case, and which explain why these very respectable findings didn't drive the newer drugs off the market, see an article in the *Seattle Times*, available on the web,[86] and also in John Abramson's book.[87] Abramson comments: 'If medical practice were truly "evidence based" these results would have been a major problem for the manufacturers of the . . . brand-name drugs.'

However, the picture gets even more complex with a recent trial in *The Lancet* that concluded the newer drugs were more effective after all.[88] A press release, dated 5 Sept 2005, from the Blood Pressure Association puts it in layman's language (see www.bpassoc.org.uk/media_centre/ media_centre.htm). It is at this point that you really need an informed and sympathetic doctor. But that certainly isn't the final word. A paper earlier this year made the case for using more psychological treatments, such as cognitive behavioural therapy, which can lower blood pressure 'sometimes more effectively than prescribed drugs'.[89] There is also evidence that hypertension drugs may be doing more harm than good. Research from Sweden involving 1,860 men followed for 17 years found that those who had been treated with beta blockers and diuretics to lower blood pressure actually came out worse than those with no treatment. Not only had their blood-glucose levels gone up, putting them at risk for diabetes, but they had a 'significantly higher' number of heart attacks.[90]

Finally, when looked at from a wider perspective, hypertension drugs may be having no effect at all. A big study called MONICA run by the World Health Organisation involving 21 countries found that between the mid-1980s and mid-1990s blood pressure overall dropped, but it concluded that 'no effect from improving treatment of hypertension was detected'.

But the key point, as with statins, is that an awful lot of people have to take hypertension drugs for just one person to benefit. One study found that 95 per cent of patients who dutifully take their tablets for five years will be no better off.[91]

Is it really a rational system for so many people to be defined as sick, and taking vastly expensive medication for so little return? The notion that the safest and most effective way to treat lifestyle disorders is with lifestyle changes seems so obvious as to hardly be worth saying. Yet unimaginably large sums are spent on trying to do it with drugs of doubtful efficacy and possible dangers.

Take heart: the alternatives to statins

Passing up drugs as a way of lowering cholesterol and blood pressure for a nutritional and non-drug approach not only offers a much wider range of options, but is also likely to have a beneficial effect on any other chronic problems. The B vitamins and exercise that help with the heart, for instance – such as walking, swimming or running – will also reduce your chance of developing Alzheimer's. You'll also get a different treatment depending on what various tests show that you need. You might start to lower your blood pressure by boosting your vitamin C intake, which will make your arteries more flexible, as well as taking more magnesium and calcium.

Omega-3 fish oils thin your blood without the gut-damaging side effects of aspirin – and help balance your moods and alleviate joint pains into the bargain. You would also learn about what cholesterol actually does in the body, and why ever more aggressive attempts to lower it may not be such a good idea, as well the possibility of using niacin to raise your levels of the beneficial HDL cholesterol. Finally, you'd be looking at two other markers for heart disease – homocysteine and lipoprotein (a) –

which rarely get discussed in a doctor's surgery. Yet they can be substantially reduced simply by B vitamins and vitamin C, respectively. (See Chapter 15 for more on working towards heart health without drugs.)

Dying to treat heartburn

Heartburn has become another arena for the blockbuster brigade. This painful condition occurs when acid creeps out of the stomach and up into the oesophagus, the tube leading to the mouth, and an estimated 40 per cent of Americans suffer from it at any one time. Pills that reduce the acid are an easy and effective solution – the most recent and powerful a class called proton pump inhibitors (PPI). PPIs are also given for gastro-intestinal damage in people who regularly take aspirin-like NSAIDs (non-steroidal anti-inflammatory drugs). Given the number of people suffering from these conditions, it adds up to a good recipe for a blockbuster.

However, even if you are familiar with drug company practices, what happened with two of the PPIs still comes as a shock. One of them, Propulsid – also known as cisapride – was sold for years despite evidence about its dangers, while the other, Nexium, was launched as a new drug costing ten times as much as the one it replaced, even though it was virtually chemically identical.

What happened with Propulsid is described in shocking detail in a major investigation by the *New York Times*, published on 10 June 2005. The drug was granted a licence for night-time heartburn in 1993. By 1995, the FDA had received reports that it was linked with 18 cases of severe disruption to heart rhythm and the death of an infant. By the following year the number of adult cases was up to 57 and there were seven more involving children. None of this was made public.

By 1998, the Propulsid-linked death toll was numbered in the dozens, and some hundred people were reckoned to have suffered serious heart problems. That year, the FDA was sufficiently concerned to propose changes to the drug's label so it would say: 'Despite more than 20 clinical trials in pediatric patients, safety and effectiveness has not been demonstrated in pediatric patients for any indication'.

However, this did not stop the company – Johnson & Johnson – from organising 'educational' seminars for paediatricians to tell them of the benefits of Propulsid. By 1998 over 500,000 prescriptions for children were being written a year and 20 per cent of infants in neonatal care were on the drug. When it was finally withdrawn in 2000, following the threat of the first public hearing of these safety concerns, the FDA had reports of 80 deaths and 341 serious heart problems among patients taking Propulsid.[92]

The company later asserted that its 'marketing was appropriate' and that it had withdrawn the drug 'because physicians had continued to promote it inappropriately'.

In 2004 Johnson & Johnson agreed to settle outstanding claims – by then risen to 300 deaths and 16,000 injured – with a total of $90 million. Many of the details contained in the *New York Times* piece about official concern about the safety of the drug only came to light when reporters got to see documents the company had been required to release by the courts. It is hard to see how any of this counts as properly controlled, scientific medicine. No other PPI is currently said to pose this sort of risk – but if it did, how would we know?

A particularly tragic footnote to the Propulsid saga involved women in the UK who were charged with damaging their babies because they, the mothers, suffered from the condition Munchausen's syndrome by proxy (MSBP). In 2004 it emerged that many of the children allegedly harmed by these mothers had been on Propulsid. Children who die from taking the drug often show symptoms that look like suffocation. Since the withdrawal of Propulsid, the number of MSBP cases has dropped dramatically.[93]

It is also hard to see where science or benefit to patients came into the launch of Nexium in 2003. Nexium replaced another PPI, Prilosec, as its patent was just about to run out. (Patents, as we briefly saw on page 19, are at the heart of the drug companies' business model. During the years that a drug is covered by a patent it can be sold at a very high price. Once the patent expires, other companies can copy the drug and sell it far more cheaply. So much of drug-company research and development is devoted to producing new drugs to replace those about to lose their patent protection. (For more details on all this, see Chapter 3.)

However, Nexium was chemically very similar to Prilosec, so it was hard to show that it was worth paying ten times the price. Three studies compared the two, but two found no difference and one found that 90 per cent of the ulcers in patients on Nexium had healed after eight weeks, compared with 87 per cent for those on Prilosec. This was despite the fact that in these studies, the participants were getting double the dose of Nexium. The two negative trials were never released.[94] The day was saved by marketing. A $257 million advertising campaign ensured that Nexium was widely prescribed, and sales are now running at $3.8 billion. In 2004 a case was filed by the American Federation of Labor–Congress of Industrial Organisations (AFL–CIO) alleging that consumers had been misled over the superiority of Nexium by a massive advertising campaign.[95]

How else to heal the gut?

There are many ways to reduce inflammation in a gut damaged by NSAIDs or as a result of indigestion or heartburn with nutrition. These include avoiding what's irritating your gut in the first place – usually coffee, alcohol or an unidentified food allergy. You can also take an inexpensive digestive enzyme to digest your food properly, and various gut-healing nutrients such as a spoonful (5g) of glutamine powder in water the last thing at night. In most cases, simple and safe changes like these can render the need for drugs obsolete.

Building choices

All of the information in this chapter has been reported in proper scientific journals and should form part of any informed discussion about the best way to treat any condition you have. Many doctors are aware of these problems but with drugs as their only form of treatment, there is little they can do to change the situation. You, as an informed patient however, have other options.

The next chapter shows how the drug companies ensure that a positive and optimistic picture of the safety and efficacy of drugs is promoted to doctors. Once you know how it is done, you will be in a much better position to help in making decisions about your own health.

3.

Full Spectrum Dominance
How the drug companies keep control

'FULL SPECTRUM DOMINANCE' is the stated aim of the American military. It involves being ready 'to defeat any adversary and control any situation across the range of military operations'. Not a bad description of what the pharmaceutical industry has achieved across the whole field of prescription drugs, from creating to selling. Besides dominating the clinical trials production line, the drug companies have also found ways of exerting control over such vital theatres of their commercial operations as the researchers, the medical journals and the doctors.

The industry's strategy for maintaining their full spectrum dominance all the way down the drug chain is very simple – they pay for it. Drug companies in America spend around $15 billion a year on marketing, about half the amount they spend on research and development.[96] And just in case you think these companies behave differently elsewhere, in the UK for instance, this is what the 2005 Parliamentary health committee investigation, *The Influence of the Pharmaceutical Industry*, found: '[it] buys influence over doctors, charities, patient groups, journalists and politicians, whose regulation is sometimes weak or ambiguous.'[97]

The sums involved are not small either. The global industry is worth over $600 billion, while the UK industry alone is worth £10 billion and employs 8,000 salespeople. In 2003, the UK drug bill was £7.2 billion, which is about 13 per cent of total National Health Service spending. Some companies spend up to £10,000 per doctor on promotion.[98]

And all of this affects you, because the ultimate aim of these companies is to ensure that when you arrive in the doctor's surgery feeling anxious or with aching joints, you and the doctor believe that there is a safe, effective pill to make it better. However, as we've seen in the last two chapters, there is often a gap between that image and the reality. It's a gap that, quite apart from putting patients' lives at risk, makes it impossible to make an informed choice about the treatment you do want.

Full spectrum dominance is about making that gap invisible. It's an ingenious, if wildly expensive, trick but once you understand how it works, there is a good chance that you won't get fooled again. We hear a lot about how much pharmaceutical companies spend on research. This is the story, and one that is far less well known, about what they spend on getting the results they want.

Where the money goes

So who are the drug companies funnelling money to?

- They pay for the trials that test the safety and effectiveness of their drugs. Commercial drug-testing centres are four times more likely to come up with favourable results than independent ones.[99]

- They pay the medical journals. Besides advertising, they pay for reprints of favourable articles, and the sums involved can be as high as a million dollars.

- They pay the academics. Clinical practice guidelines advise doctors on the drugs to use for various conditions. However, 80 per cent of the academics who write them have financial links with the companies whose products they are recommending.[100–101]

- They pay for doctors' further education. Doctors go regularly to seminars, lectures and courses to keep up to date, and fully 60 per cent or more of that education is paid for by drug companies.

- They pay the regulator. Both the American FDA and the UK's MHRA rely for their income on fees for licensing drugs. Until 2004 there was nothing to stop MHRA members from having financial links with drug companies.

- They schmooze the legislators. Drug companies spend more money than any other industry lobbying Congress in the US – $177 million.[102–103] They also actively lobby the UK Parliament.[104]

Stated as baldly as that, these claims may sound wildly exaggerated to you. If that's the case, think about this. When you buy something like a new computer or a washing machine, you assume it's not going to blow up or electrocute you because it will have passed various independent safety checks. Similarly, if you go out to a restaurant, you know your chances of getting food poisoning are pretty low because there are local food safety inspectors checking up on hygiene.

But suppose you then found out that the companies that made the household goods picked up the tab for the safety checks and that restaurants paid hygiene inspectors. How confident would you feel then? And imagine it then emerged that the regulatory bodies, whose job it was to ensure the safety testers and the hygiene inspectors were following the rules, were also being paid by the business involved. Wouldn't you feel your safety might not be in such good hands after all?

Amazingly, that is precisely the situation when it comes to policing the drug trials that form the basis of scientific medicine. Who checks up they are being done properly? Most people, including most doctors, don't have a very clear idea. If they did, they might not trust these trials to the extent they do.

The semi-secret drug-testing machine

Running clinical trials is a vast and almost invisible $14 billion industry in the US, where there are an estimated 15,000 private drug-testing centres that ran nearly 40,000 trials for the pharmaceutical industry between 2001 and 2004 – amounting to around 75 per cent of the total. But the drug companies don't just pay the testing centres. They also, remarkably, fund up to 5,000 'institutional review boards' in the US, responsible for ensuring the testing centres follow medical and ethical guidelines. Many countries have some form of drug-testing centres, and it is very unlikely that they are more closely regulated.

A lengthy account of this system, published recently on the website bloomberg.com – a leading financial information provider – painted an alarming picture of a setup that is 'poorly regulated and riddled with conflicts of interest'. The few existing independent investigations of this hidden world have found 'poorly trained and unlicensed physicians' running the centres where there are 'significant objectionable conditions'.

What might those be? In one case, the head of the review board was the wife of the man running one of the clinics it was entrusted with overseeing. In another, the same man headed both a trial centre and its review board. Members of the review boards do not have to be trained or certified and many keep the names of their members secret. There has never been an audit of the effectiveness of the review boards, nor are there any records of the number of test subjects injured or killed each year.[105]

This is a system that has a direct impact on your health – and beyond. The results of trials run in the American system can be used to license drugs around the world. Many other countries also have their own commercial testing centres, but the American one is by far the largest. However, the products that come out of it have not been made with your health in mind. The driving force behind this production line is a simple financial imperative – to find replacements for drugs that are about to lose their patent.

As we saw in Chapter 2, when a drug company finds a promising new chemical, it is patented. Once the drug gets a licence, the company can charge high prices for the seven or so years the patent has to run to recoup their costs. Then, when the patent expires, the price per pill plummets from maybe $5 to 50 cents because anyone can make copies. Between 2003 and 2008, a total of 28 of the top-selling drugs are coming off patent, losing the drug companies around $50 billion. But there's that safety net: the system is designed to produce results that will allow patented replacements to be brought to market.

As we saw with Nexium (page 49), it is sometimes a tricky business to show that the new drug is actually any better. The official reason for this

system – to generate new life-saving drugs – is a secondary considera-
tion, as will soon become clear.

How clinical trials produce the results companies want

You may be surprised at the way the regulation of clinical trials works, but
the tentacles of drug-company influence are even more all-embracing.
Until about 15 years ago, most drug trials were run by universities
independently of the drug companies. Since then, that work has
increasingly been taken over by private firms.

According to an investigation a few years ago, many of these private
research firms are actually owned by the same major advertising
companies, such as Omnicom, Interpublic and WPP, that handle the
drug companies' multi-million dollar advertising accounts. The results
of these trials are then used to promote drugs in the UK and the rest of
the world.[106]

Executives of these agencies deny that they do anything to distort the
findings. Studies of the testing scene suggest otherwise. 'The evidence is
strong that drug companies are getting the results they want,' writes Dr
Richard Smith, long-time editor of the *British Medical Journal*. 'This is
especially worrisome because between two-thirds and three-quarters of
the trials published in the major journals are funded by the industry.'[107]

So what is the evidence? These are the kind of practices Smith is
referring to:

- A study in the 1990s found that out of all 56 of the studies conducted
  by drug companies themselves into painkilling drugs, not a single one
  was unfavourable to the company that sponsored the trial.[108]

- Trials funded by a drug company were four times more likely to have
  results favourable to the company than studies funded from other
  sources.[109]

- At the annual meeting of professionals in one medical speciality, six in
  ten of the papers had been sponsored by the drug industry, and every
  single one of them 'supported the product use.'[110]

In the UK, the extent to which drug companies finance trials is even greater than in the US. According to the Parliamentary health committee report, the pharmaceutical industry spends £3.3 billion a year on research in the UK, financing about 90 per cent of all clinical drug trials.

How the medical journals are bought on board

Once a favourable trial has been completed, it needs to be published in one of the reputable journals that doctors, right from the start of their training, are taught to rely on. In theory, the results of trials and studies, once written up and properly presented in these journals, is what distinguishes scientific medicine from the traditional or 'folk' medicine that preceded it. In reality, the relationship between the journals and the drug industry is, according to *The Lancet* editor Richard Horton, 'somewhere between symbiotic and parasitic'.

In giving evidence to the Parliamentary health committee, Horton described how drug companies 'regularly try to exert pressure on a journal to run a research paper'. When a favourable research paper is printed, it is often reprinted and bought in bulk by the company involved, which gives them leverage. For example, on one occasion, after Horton had been querying a lot of points in a paper on a COX-2 inhibitor drug such as Vioxx, he was contacted by an executive of the drug company involved and asked to 'stop being so critical'. Otherwise, warned the executive, they would pull the paper and *The Lancet* would lose lucrative reprint rights.[111]

This is not to suggest that journals are all in the pay of the drug companies. Far from it. Most of the revelations about the extent to which drug-company money buys influence has come from papers published in top medical journals. But the potential for distortion is obviously enormous.

The Influence of the Pharmaceutical Industry found that the British industry 'influences the interpretation and reporting of results of trials'. Negative results can be dismissed as erroneous ('failed trials'), whereas positive ones can be published repeatedly in different guises. Some astoundingly misleading articles have appeared in reputable journals (see the 'When hospitalisation isn't an ADR' box opposite).

WHEN HOSPITALISATION ISN'T AN ADR

What happens when a company-sponsored trial doesn't produce favourable results? Sometimes, as a team of independent scientists found with a paper on the anti-depressant Seroxat, the summary says otherwise.

Summaries or abstracts of trials are usually all that gets quoted in the marketing literature. In the case we're looking at here, drug-company researchers compared the effects of Seroxat with a placebo on adolescents. The summary said the drug was 'generally well tolerated' and that 'most adverse effects were not serious'.

But when a team of independent scientists looked at the whole paper, they found this: 'Out of 93 children given Seroxat, 11 had serious ADRs compared with 2 in the placebo group'. Just how serious? 'Seven of these children were admitted to hospital during treatment.' How many hospitalisations would it take for the drug not to count as 'well tolerated'?

The researchers also found that the drug was only 2.7 points more effective than a placebo on a 113-point scale.[112] How effective is that?

How academics are encouraged to do what the companies want

With favourable results published in a top-line journal, the next step in establishing full spectrum dominance is to recruit academics who will give talks and lectures supporting the use of the drug in question. Details of how the system works emerged in a major investigation by the *Los Angeles Times* into the relationship between the prestigious National Institutes of Health (NIH) in the US and the drug companies.[113] Many Americans assumed that the NIH were bastions of independence, staffed by independent academics, who impartially advised the US government on medical matters and contributed to major journals.

But the investigation showed some had extensive financial links with drug companies and supported them in return. For instance:

- Between 2000 and 2004, at least 530 NIH scientists received fees and stocks from biomedical companies. They did not break the law because there was no requirement to reveal such links.

- One of them, Dr Bryan Brewer, received over $100,000 dollars from the manufacturers of the statin drug Crestor. Brewer wrote an article in a leading heart journal dismissing concerns over the links between the Crestor and a serious muscle-wasting ADR.

- Just two months later an editorial in *The Lancet* said: 'Physicians must tell the truth about Crestor ... [which] has an inferior evidence base supporting its safe use.'

- Brewer was one of the nine authors of the guidelines that lowered the recommended safe levels of cholesterol so sharply that 23 million more Americans became eligible to take them. Seven other members of that committee also had financial links with the makers of statin drugs.

But this is not just an American oddity. Not only do these practices directly affect most other countries – many follow American statin guidelines, for instance – but in the UK, evidence has recently emerged that some pharmaceutical companies offer bribes to consultants not to publish inconvenient findings.

Giving evidence at a Parliamentary health committee hearing, Dr Peter Wilmshurst, a consultant cardiologist at Royal Shrewsbury Hospital, told how he has been offered bribes by a pharmaceutical company not to publish unfavourable research results. He also claims that he knew of three professors of cardiology who were told their results were aberrant and were persuaded by the pharmaceutical company who had sponsored the study not to publish. 'I suspect this is as common now as it ever was,' said Dr Wilmshurst.

He also told the committee that key opinion leaders can be paid in the region of £5,000 for an hour's talk about a drug they have no experience of using, and that their influence can have a big impact on practice. (For an example of the way academics can support a drug launch, see the following box 'Building a bestseller').

BUILDING A BESTSELLER

A vivid example of how much an obliging academic and some free entertainment can contribute to the building of a blockbuster comes from a *New York Times* investigation into what happened when a drug company called Forest was threatened with a dramatic drop in revenue because the patent on one of its bestsellers was about to run out.

Forest's patented drug was an anti-depressant called Celexa and its replacement – Lexapro (known as Cipralex in Europe) – contained an only slightly modified version of the drug molecule, escitalopram. The problem lay in persuading doctors to switch to the new (and far more expensive) version.

According to the *New York Times* investigation,[114] the key piece of evidence in Lexapro's favour was a review of three earlier studies that had found it acted more quickly – the work of academic Dr Jack M. Gorman. But it was hardly objective science. Not only was the author a paid consultant for Forest. He was also the editor of the journal that had published it, in a special supplement paid for by Forest.

Undaunted, Forest organised a two-day conference in New York and flew in one student from nearly every medical school in the country as attendees, saying it was to 'get medical students interested in psychiatric research'. Dr Gorman gave a talk on anti-depressants and the students stayed in the Plaza Hotel and went to a Broadway show. Meanwhile, a not-for-profit newsletter – *The Medical Letter* – with no pharmaceutical links had analysed the same three studies on Lexapro and found no advantages. It's not recorded whether the newsletter's findings were presented in New York.

Forest held a whole series of sessions to educate doctors about psychiatry and the use of anti-depressants, and the value of Lexapro's sales reached $1.1 billion in 2004. Subsequent trials have reported it was effective in 'treating panic disorder and generalised and social anxiety disorders'. Sales are estimated to reach over $2 billion a year before the patent runs out.

How doctors are encouraged to do what the companies want

The ultimate aim of this chain of influence is to affect the behaviour of the doctors who are at the sharp end: unless they actually prescribe a new drug in favour of the old one going off patent, the whole project has failed. Doctors are targeted in two main ways: through continuing medical education and directly by visits from drug sales teams.

Lifelong learning?

Medical research advances at such a fantastic rate that it is impossible for individual doctors to keep up, so every doctor in the UK is required to attend about 50 hours of 'medical education' a year.[115] Very sensible, you might think, and so do the drug companies. Currently in the US, over $1.5 billion goes on 'continuing medical education'. As a result, American third-year medical students receive on average one gift or attend one activity sponsored by a pharmaceutical company per week.[116]

In the UK, the industry funds over half of all postgraduate medical education, and much of the education of nurses, from its annual marketing budget of £1.65 billion.[117] By way of contrast, the UK Department of Health spends just 0.3 per cent of this on publishing independent information on drugs.[118]

If ever you have wondered just why doctors seem so sceptical about non-drug treatments, even when you tell them how well a change of diet or some supplements have been working for you, it's worth bearing in mind the source of the information they are relying on when making decisions. Not only will any new positive findings about non-drug treatments have been ignored as part of this ongoing education – but so will any new evidence that a particular drug is causing problems. (For an example of how doctors on educational trips were kept in the dark about HRT problems, see the following box 'Don't mention the heart attacks'.)

DON'T MENTION THE HEART ATTACKS

In 2000, doctors across the US received a letter from the pharmaceutical company Wyeth telling them about a new campaign to educate consumers about the menopause. It featured the actress Lauren Hutton and warned of the horrifying consequences of 'oestrogen loss'. These included heart attacks, Alzheimer's disease, night sweats, vaginal dryness and bone fracture. The solution to these dangers was, of course, to take HRT.

It was a particularly one-sided sort of education, however, that made no mention of the finding from the first properly randomised controlled trial of HRT, published two years earlier. This found that if you'd had a heart attack, HRT actually made another slightly more likely.[119] It also kept mum about an independent analysis of trials that detected a raised risk of heart attack with HRT.[120] Most misleadingly, it ignored the fact that the organisers of the huge Women's Health Initiative trial of HRT and healthy women had just taken the highly unusual step of writing to the thousands of women involved to warn them of a slightly raised risk of strokes and heart attacks on the treatment.

The information in this letter, 'WHI HRT update from the Women's Health Initiative', was based on the results of ongoing research, later published as an article in the *Journal of the American Medical Association*.[121] The full story is told in Chapter 3 of the excellent book *Selling Sickness: How Drug Companies are Turning Us All into Patients* by Ray Moynihan and Alan Cassels (see Recommended Reading, page 400).

This situation represents the kind of one-sided information about drugs your doctor is likely to be getting from the drug companies, and it directly affects the advice you are going to get in your doctor's surgery. Drugs become the obvious choice because all the problems have been airbrushed out. No wonder nutrition and other non-drug approaches barely register on their radar.

Selling the product

But by far the largest chunk of the marketing budget goes on targeting doctors directly. Currently, the spend in the US alone is $12 billion to $18 billion dollars (precise figures are hard to come by), according to the same study that gave the figures for the cost of educating doctors. 'All this,' commented the authors delicately 'may be inconsistent with evidence-based guidelines.' [122]

In the UK, we know that some drug companies can spend up to £10,000 a year targeting an individual doctor with drug reps or sales-people who provide information about the latest drug developments. In the past some doctors have been rather cavalier about all this. They were trained, they said, they could handle it; they knew how to separate the hype from the hard evidence. Unfortunately for them and their patients, there's considerable evidence that that is just a comforting delusion.

What happened with Vioxx, for instance, is not reassuring, as an article in *The Lancet* shows. 'The COX-2 drugs were adopted as the preferred NSAID by 55 per cent of physicians within 6 months of their being marketed,' it declared. 'This was due not to what the patient needed but was based on "physician preference".' [123–124] We have already seen that a close reading of the research data would have told any doctor that there were potential problems with Vioxx, so they must have been persuaded not by the journal evidence but by the education and marketing material they received from the company.

Certainly the Parliamentary health committee felt there was a problem. In *The Influence of the Pharmaceutical Industry* it commented in general on the 'aggressive promotion of medicines shortly after [their] launch' as well as the 'absence of effective countervailing forces', and con-cluded that 'all contribute to the inappropriate prescription of medicine'.

Its recommendation, which the government rejected, was that there should be a limit to the amount of information doctors receive in the first six months of a launch, and stricter control on the promotions by the drug reps. The reason was blunt and to the point. '[Doctors] do not keep abreast of medicines' information and are sometimes too willing to accept hospitality from industry and act uncritically on the information supplied by the drug companies.'

New doesn't mean better – just more expensive

In the end, full spectrum dominance has one simple aim – to ensure that you get prescribed the latest drugs because they are the ones covered by a patent and so highly profitable. That would be fine if they represented a big improvement on the older ones. But do they? Not according to a recent Canadian study, which found that during the 13 years between 1990 and 2003, out of 1,147 newly patented drugs classified by the Canadian Patented Medicines Prices Review Board, only 5.9 per cent were considered to be 'breakthrough drugs', that is, those providing a 'substantial improvement over existing drug products.'[125]

And yet according to the same research, spending on prescription drugs in Canada doubled between 1996 and 2003, and 80 per cent of that was accounted for by new drugs 'that did not offer substantial improvements on less expensive alternatives available before 1990'. The shift from Prilosec to Nexium described in Chapter 2 is a good example of the process at work. And it's not just Canada that is affected. The report concludes that 'me-too drugs probably dominate spending trends in most developed countries'.

Just how important protecting and extending patents is in comparison to developing genuinely innovative drugs is dramatically illustrated by another set of figures. According to these, the number of patent lawyers retained by drug firms is rising faster than the spend on drug research and development. In 1987, 46 lawyers were employed for every billion spent on R&D, whereas ten years later it was 75 per billion.[126]

It is this concentration on patents and copycat drugs offering minimal improvements that explains why there has to be so much tweaking of results and wining and dining of doctors. You wouldn't need to spend £10,000 pounds on each doctor to get them to prescribe a drug that cured 90 per cent of cases of people infected by the antibiotic-resistant bug MRSA. The trouble with this approach is not just that it doubles our drug bills for very little return, but that it actively denies funds to non-drug treatments.

For instance, the authors of the Canadian study estimate that a saving of just half its copycat drug bill could have paid for 1,000 new doctors.

Alternatively, it could have been spent on researching the best ways to help people switch to a healthy diet combined with nutritional medicine and an exercise regime.

The watchdog that didn't bark

Every country has a drug regulatory agency that, in theory, could counterbalance or at least restrain the drug companies' full spectrum dominance. Bodies like the UK's MHRA and the FDA in the US are charged with first licensing drugs – reviewing the evidence to make sure that they are safe and effective – and then monitoring what happens to patients once they are being widely used. But the FDA has been heavily criticised for its failings over Vioxx, and the far more secretive MHRA doesn't seem to be doing either job very effectively. Not only is it almost entirely funded by the drug companies to the tune of £65 million,[127] but it's also very poor at picking up problems once they appear.

A little too cosy?

It wasn't until the beginning of 2005 that MHRA members were banned from having shares and financial links with drug companies.[128] The MHRA is currently headed by Sir Alasdair Breckenridge, previously on the scientific advisory committee of the pharmaceutical giant GlaxoSmithKline. Documents obtained recently via the UK's Freedom of Information Act showed that the industry privately drew up its own detailed blueprint of how the MHRA should be run, proposing to 'build on the excellent working relationship between the industry and the regulator'. They also revealed that the industry was 'agitated about the ministers' unrealistic plans to tighten the rules on conflicts of interest'.[129]

The sense that drug companies' interests were the agency's first priority and patients' a distant second was reinforced by Richard Brook, director of the mental health charity Mind and the first patient's representative to sit on an MHRA review committee. He declared himself 'horrified' to find that the agency had kept quiet about the possible dangers of higher doses of SSRIs for at least a decade. When he resigned, he declared that the MHRA was either guilty of 'extreme negligence or worse dishonesty'.[130]

Are they experimenting with you?

Although properly run clinical trials can tell if a drug is more effective than a placebo or another drug, they are poor at spotting if it is likely to cause damaging side effects once it is being widely used. This may be because the type of people in the trial – younger males, for instance – are not the ones most likely to get the drug (who may be elderly women). Or it may simply be a question of numbers – a few thousand people at most will get the drug in a trial, while millions may get it on prescription. What this means, however, is that when you are prescribed a newly licensed drug you are, and people are rarely told this, effectively taking part in a huge experiment to discover whether it has rare (usually) but possibly deadly complications.

You could also easily be prescribed a drug that hasn't gone through any trials at all to target the problem you've got. That's because many drugs – 21 per cent, according to a recent study – are prescribed off-label (see also page 66). The idea is that doctors are able to use their skill and judgement to work out that a certain drug licensed for one thing might help with another. That may well be appropriate at times, but it is certainly open to abuse. Drug companies heavily push off-label prescribing to increase sales.

One example is the drug Neurontin. In a court case it emerged that it was being promoted by the manufacturer for 11 conditions it wasn't actually licensed for.[131] An even worse case of off-label prescribing, actively encouraged by the company, was Propulsid for children (see Chapter 2, page 48), even though unpublished trials showed it was neither effective nor safe.

Children are, in fact, particularly at risk from this practice because few drugs are actually tested on them. The 60,000 children who got SSRIs for depression were treated off-label. Recently, the journal *Science* reported that 'between 50 per cent and 90 per cent of drugs used on adults have never been tested or licensed for use on children, as a result 100 million children in the European Union are often prescribed off-label products or unauthorised drugs'.[132]

But it's not only children who are affected. Until very recently, hard data about just how many prescriptions in general are written for drugs used off-label was hard to come by. But last May a major study reported that on average, 21 per cent of the 160 most commonly prescribed drugs in the US were given to people on an off-label basis. What's more, the evidence for using nearly three-quarters of them had, wrote the authors, 'little or no scientific support'.

In other words, rather than being backed up by clinical trials, their use was based on observational studies, case reports or no discernible evidence at all. In some specialities, the level of off-label prescribing was higher than others. In psychiatry, for example, a staggering 96 per cent of off-label prescriptions lacked strong scientific support.[133]

This is precisely the sort of charge levelled at non-drug therapies and used as grounds for dismissing them. This wasn't a small-scale study either, being based on an analysis of an American national database that tracks the prescribing habits of a representative 3,700 doctors around the country. Whether the pattern is the same in other countries is impossible to say – in the UK, for instance, no central record is kept of what drugs are actually prescribed for what conditions – but it would be surprising if the pattern was very different.

The agency that polices itself

In the light of all this, you might reasonably expect that systems would be in place to actively check for such problems and respond quickly. And because such a system would essentially involve policing how well the licensing experts had done their job, you might expect it to be done by a separate and independent agency. In fact, both the UK and the US agencies do both jobs, effectively policing themselves. The system the MHRA uses to check for problems post-licensing was described by the Parliamentary health committee in *The Influence of the Pharmaceutical Industry* as 'extremely passive'.[134] It relies on the 'Yellow Card scheme', which depends on doctors voluntarily filling in reports of ADRs.

One witness giving evidence to the committee commented: 'We track the fate of the parcels though the post 100 times more accurately than we track the fate of the people who have been killed by SSRIs or other drugs.'

Only between one and ten per cent of adverse reactions are ever reported, and even those 'are not always investigated or pursued with sufficient robustness'.[135]

However, recommendations that the system should be beefed up and made independent[136] were ignored by the UK government. Exactly the same recommendation has been made by American and Canadian safety experts about the drug regulation agencies in their countries – and also ignored.[137–138]

Such governmental stonewalling is perhaps the ultimate triumph of full spectrum dominance. But while this system can, and possibly should, be an embarrassment to doctors who have to live with it, you don't have to. Now you are armed with a much better sense of what actually lies behind the drug companies' façade of scientific healing, you can start to ask the questions about any drug you are prescribed that should give you a clearer and more truthful idea of what you are getting. This is what is covered in Chapter 4.

4.

On Guard
How to tell good medicine from bad

IN OCTOBER 2005 Nancy Yost, a 73-year-old New Yorker, did something rather remarkable. She sued a drug company. Now in America that in itself is not remarkable – it happens all the time. But what made Nancy Yost's case so unusual was that she hasn't actually suffered any harm. However, for the last eight years she has been taking the bestselling statin, Lipitor, and she doesn't have heart disease. Therein lies the crux.

Yost is now the figurehead of a class action against the manufacturer Pfizer that alleges the drug was prescribed under false pretences. The action claims that the company aggressively promoted the drug to patients like Nancy, even though 'there is no proof that statins prevent heart attacks in women and seniors who aren't already suffering from heart disease or diabetes'.[139]

The coming revolution

Nancy Yost is part of a revolution in the way we take our medicine. If you've read this far, you may be part of it too. All that is needed to join is a change in attitude. You don't need to regard a prescription as an instruction, but instead, as more of a suggestion. And if you are going to put a chemical into your body for months, if not years, you want to know far more about it than was normal in the past. For Nancy Yost, the issue was that the revolution wasn't really underway eight years ago, when she started on the drugs.

One of the triggers for this revolution has been the failures, damage and cover-ups described in the last three chapters. The story they tell is how an earlier revolution, the arrival of drug-based scientific medicine that kicks off Chapter 1, has gradually gone sour. Its big promise had been that all the somewhat messy, human elements of medicine – herbal remedies, good food, fresh air, the personality of the doctor, exercise – could be swept away and replaced with single chemical molecules, measured and tested.

This 'appliance of science' approach was one of the defining faiths of the 1950s. Modernist architects tried to do something similar with their severe, unadorned buildings, described as 'machines for living'. But just as few people actually wanted to live in modernist machines, so the older forms of medicine gradually began creeping back, often with impressive support from the scientific system that was supposed to outlaw them. Plain geometric blocks of flats proved a bad fit for our complex lifestyles and complicated social networks, and now modernist pharmaceutical medicine seems similarly narrow-minded and inhumane compared with the range the non-drug approach has to offer. They are also out of step with the 'networked' design of our body, a complex adaptive organism, which we explore in Chapter 5.

However, the second revolution wouldn't have grown up organically without the internet. This not only allows you to examine just how strong or weak the evidence for the claims of modernist medicine are, but also to swap your experiences and what you've learnt with others. The web is now full of sites where you can learn what it's like taking a particular drug and where warnings of dangerous but still largely hidden side effects can be swapped. (See Resources, page 401, for more details.)

Manifesto for the new medicine

All this has given rise to a new breed of informed health consumers, net-worked via the web. This is a revolution anyone can join. And networks have another effect: they are great levellers. The first modern medical revolution set up a classic hierarchy. Pharmaceutical companies produced the drugs according to commercial potential rather than patients' needs, and doctors doled them out. In the second revolution it is patients who are becoming involved in setting the agenda and demanding treatments from our doctors that better fit with some of medicine's more ancient values.

If there was a manifesto setting out what the second revolution means by good medicine it might look something like this:

Treatments target the underlying problem rather than just the symptoms.
For example, you and your doctor could focus on finding out whether your child's ear infections are triggered by allergy rather than just relying on antibiotics every time.

Treatments cure the underlying disorder or ensure it considerably improves.
For example, a diet designed to control blood-sugar levels, plus exercise, could be used to help control diabetes rather than just relying on drugs.

Treatments are safe and don't cause further problems which then have to treated.

Treatments don't have to repackaged to be launched in new and more expensive versions every few years.

Treatments are researched and developed because they work regardless of whether or not they can be patented.

Treatments may be safely used in combination.

Treatments for the same condition may be different for different patients depending on the underlying cause.
For example, you may work out your own personal nutrition programme, tailored to specific health needs.

Like all manifestos, there is a lot of hope in there, but that's no reason why you shouldn't try to ensure that, as far as your own treatment is concerned, it's followed as closely as possible. One of the things you certainly can do is to take reasonable steps to protect yourself from the damaging effects of drugs.

We are not talking here about emergencies or a serious health crisis, where drugs have their place. The main area in which to be wary is when one of the blockbuster drugs is being offered. They may be just what you need, perhaps in the short term; but it's worth finding out more about it if you feel you're not getting the full story on possible side effects or efficacy. Before we get on to a list of the top ten questions to ask your doctor about a drug, let's just look at the major issues it's worth keeping in mind when deciding whether to go on one.

Prescription drugs: the biggest issues

Is it a new drug?

New drugs come in two forms, both of which have their drawbacks. Some, as we've seen, are designed to overcome a known problem with an earlier version. Vioxx, for example, was promoted as the solution to the gut damage that older painkillers cause. Very often the old problem still lingers, though: the new range of sleeping pills has turned out to be no better than the old ones, for instance.

Others do work in a new way, and always promise to be a great improvement. But the very fact that they are focusing on a new pathway means that, inevitably, not all possible side effects will have shown up in the trials. Combine that with the fact that we don't have a dynamic or independent system for picking up problems – as we saw in Chapter 2 – and the reality is that you are essentially going to be taking part in a huge experiment.

As we saw in Chapter 3, new drugs are also heavily marketed, so you will need to bear in mind that your doctor's practice will probably have been the target for some skilful promotion.

Is it a blockbuster?

If it is (see page 35), then it is worth asking whether it is really right for you and why your doctor thinks you need it. For instance, even if your cholesterol is high, that may not be a problem for you. As you'll see in Chapter 15, having a slightly raised cholesterol level isn't a problem if your 'good' HDL (High Density Lipoprotein) cholesterol is high. Statins do next to nothing to raise HDL. And even the best-run clinical trials only tell you what happens to people on average. The assumption behind all the drugs prescribed for prevention is that there's a norm that is best for everyone, but maybe you don't fit it. Relief from symptoms may be worth having for a while but it's not good as a sole, long-term strategy.

The trials of drugs given to millions probably weren't tested on lots of different types of people. You need to ask yourself whether they were conducted with participants like you. Indeed, given the problems with off-label prescribing (see page 65), there may not have been any trials of the drug at all for the conditions you've got. Ask your doctor about this.

Remember the relatives

This refers to statistics rather than your family. Presentation plays a big part in drug promotion: new drugs often claim they can produce a 25 or 30 per cent drop in, say, your chances of having a heart attack. But, as covered in the section on statins (page 43), you need to know if that is a relative or absolute drop. If only four per cent of people on the placebo have a heart attack, compared with three per cent on the drug, that is certainly a *relative* drop of 25 per cent. However, the *absolute* improvement is just one per cent, and that simply doesn't sound as impressive. Ask your doctor what the real benefit of the drug is likely to be.

'Numbers needed to treat' or NNT

This is another set of numbers not often bandied about in drug-company promotions. It refers to how many people have to receive this drug over a certain period of time to achieve one successful treatment. An NNT of one means that everyone who is treated benefits – this would be the result you'd get with a treatment for head lice. Aspirin scores two for 'reducing the pain of severe sprain by 50 per cent within minutes', and glucosamine is not bad, with an NNT five, for improving arthritis over three to eight weeks. It's certainly better than the flu vaccine, which scores 23.

Ironically, the point where NNTs start to go off the scale is precisely with those drugs that head the bestseller list – the ones for cholesterol lowering and hypertension. According to the website Bandolier (www.jr2.ox.ac.uk/bandolier), which is devoted to evidence-based medicine,[140] you have to give the drug Privastatin to 641 people for 4.9 years to prevent one stroke a year. Giving a diuretic drug and a beta-blocker to 70 patients with high blood pressure for 5.8 years will prevent one stroke a year. Is it worth it? The choice is yours.

LEARNING FROM THE PAST

The history of drug disasters is a very good example of the old adage about being doomed to repeat things if you keep forgetting them. Below we list some conditions that have been linked with problem drugs in the past. Use it to help decide if a similar treatment might or might not be right for you.

Weight loss: An SSRI-type drug called Pondimin plus an amphetamine, phentermine, formed a popular combo known as 'fen-phen'. However, it caused heart disease and hypertension and was withdrawn in 1997. The manufacturers, Wyeth, have set aside $22 billion to pay damages to 600,000 people.[141]

Cholesterol lowering: The statin Baycol was banned in 2001 after being linked with 31 deaths in the US and at least nine more elsewhere. So far, the company Bayer has paid out $1.1 billion in 3,000 cases.[142]

Diabetes: Rezulin resensitises the body to insulin, but it has been officially linked to 90 cases of liver injury – with some people needing transplants – and 63 deaths. Settlements by Pfizer are reckoned to have reached $1 billion.

Heartburn: As we have seen, Propulsid was withdrawn in 2000 after it was linked to 300 deaths, some of them of children, from heart problems. Estimate of cost run at $1 billion.[143]

Often the warning signs later turn out to have been there early on. For example, in the case of Redux – a drug very similar to Pondimin and also used in the same combination – 20 academics wrote to the FDA at the time of its licensing warning about the possibility that it might cause brain damage that appeared later.[144]

Questions to ask your doctor

If you join the second medical revolution, it's going to have a major effect on your relationship with your doctor. Not only will you be treading on their professional toes – as, after all, they're supposed to be the knowledgeable ones asking questions – but you will also be pushing them into areas not covered at medical school, such as nutrition. Some may welcome your input, especially if you are involved in managing a chronic disorder. But others will find it threatening.

You may find yourself tempted to abandon doctors altogether. But that would be giving up a valuable resource. Not only have they had years of training, especially in diagnosis; remember that not all are hidebound by convention, some are eager to learn more, and if they sympathise with what you are doing, they can be a valuable ally. So treat them with respect and sensitivity rather than just bombarding them with your 'informed consumer' questions.

In an ideal world, your doctor would give you reliable and up-to-date information about the drugs you were getting and your other options. But given all the ways that we've seen the truth about drugs can be spun, and until we have a drug-regulation system that is independent and proactive, you are going to have to be rather more proactive yourself.

Note that the 'you' in all the questions below refers to your doctor, and the 'me' to you, the patient.

Prescription drugs

Here are the crucial questions to ask if your doctor is about to prescribe a drug.

- Is this a drug that has only recently been licensed, and if so have you received a lot of promotional material from the manufacturer about it?

- Is this a replacement for a drug that has just run out of patent (in which case it is likely to be very similar but a lot more expensive)? What are the figures for absolute vs relative risk and the NNT?

- Is this being prescribed off-label – in other words, has it been specifically licensed for the condition it's treating or is there no actual evidence that it is effective?

- Have there been any trials of the drug run by researchers who are not financed by the manufacturers?

- Was the drug tested on people like me, who belong to the group most likely to use it? In other words, if older people were most likely to take it, was it tested on them or on younger, fitter people?

- Has the drug been tested against any other drugs already in use, and if so how did it perform?

- Are there any non-drug treatments that are more effective than drugs for this condition?

- Have all the trials that have been done on the drug been registered anywhere so I will know what all the results were? Did any trials show no effect or signs of problems?

- Do you think it is worth filling in Yellow Cards (see page 66) reporting side effects? Did you fill in any cards for any of your patients taking SSRIs, Vioxx or any earlier problem drugs?

- Is this drug likely to cause any vitamin or mineral deficiencies such as statins do with co-enzyme Q10?

Your doctor's relationship with drug companies

Given what we have learnt about the way drug companies keep control, it is also useful to ask your doctor about drug PR. Here's a list of good questions to ask if you are in the process of finding or changing a doctor.

- How often to drug reps visit you every month? Do you see them or send them away?

- How many further-education sessions do you go to a year?

- How many of them were funded by drug companies?

- How much promotional literature have you received about the drug you are about to prescribe me?

- How many seminars have you attended on it?

- How many independent sources have you consulted about it?

- How much do you believe drug-company promotion influences your judgement?

Non-drug alternatives

Assuming you have a good relationship with your doctor, it makes sense to discuss non-drug therapies and nutritional changes. Doctors almost certainly have a better knowledge of biochemistry than you do, and yours may be able to talk to you about the pathways a drug is targeting so you can check if non-drug treatments are acting in a similar way. However, it is worth reading this book first as there are some common misconceptions about the safety and effectiveness of vitamins which are covered in Chapter 18.

A medical system where all this isn't necessary

What we all want is a medical system that is responsive to what patients actually need and doesn't threaten to do them any damage while treating them. In the next chapter we explore what such a system might look like, and why drug-based medicine can't ever deliver that. Part 3 looks in detail at how you can treat the top nine chronic diseases with non-drug approaches, while Part 4 deals with some of the ways that this revolution is going to have to change the existing system if it is to have any realistic chance of delivering good medicine rather than a brand that is simply profitable.

Part 2

A Different Way of Looking

5.

How to Regain Your Health
Getting to the true causes of disease

Einstein once said that 'the problems we have created cannot be solved at the same level of thinking we were at when we created the problems'. In relation to most of today's major health problems, the fundamental underlying causes relate to a combination of lifestyle factors, including sub-optimum nutrition, psychological factors such as stress, physical factors such as a lack of exercise, other environmental factors such as smoking, pollution or poverty and, to a very small extent, as we'll show you, genetic predispositions. None of the major diseases is caused by a lack of drugs.

So even if a drug can suppress a symptom, it makes little sense to keep doing what you are doing in terms of diet and lifestyle and expect better health in the long term. Many drug-based approaches allow the patient to do just that. For instance, instead of eating a diet that restores blood-sugar balance, diabetic drugs allow you to keep eating the wrong stuff and get away with it – at least for a while.

It makes a lot more sense to find a way of living that really does resolve your health issues. And this is not just a nice idea, but a reality that you could achieve. A simple illustration of this is the fact that for almost every disease, there's a country that doesn't have it.

For example, Chinese women rarely get menopausal symptoms or breast cancer, and Chinese men rarely get prostate cancer. In rural China, the lifetime risk of developing prostate cancer is less than one in 20,000, whereas in the UK the risk is more than one in ten. The Japanese, at least those on the traditional diet, don't get heart disease. Pacific island children have a fraction of the diabetes incidence of European children. Cases of depression are the lowest in regions of the world where fish-eating is the norm. So the question is – what are you doing that's different from what people are doing in countries where your disease is extremely rare?

Throughout Part 2, you will discover the factors that tip you over into less than perfect health, and in Part 3 you'll discover what to do about it. There is hardly ever a single cause, and the causes aren't usually immediately obvious. You don't, for example, smoke a cigarette and instantly develop asthma or lung cancer, or eat a bag of sweets and develop diabetes. Most diseases develop over years, as a result of a number of factors that eventually push your complex biology over the edge. The fact that most diseases are multi-factorial explains why food and lifestyle changes have to be better medicine than drugs – although at first sight, that could seem like a ridiculously ambitious claim.

Your body as an ecosystem

To understand why this claim is not unrealistic, consider this scenario. Imagine that it is possible to identify your level of health with the ultimate body scanner. This would be a super machine that combines brain scanners with thermography (warmer and cooler areas show up as different colours) and some not-yet-invented devices that show genes being turned on and off in every cell, the activity of your immune system, the flow of blood around the body, the levels of various fats and the changes in blood pressure.

If you were to watch yourself being scanned by this sci-fi device, several things would soon become obvious. The first would be that your body is in a state of constant dynamic flux, changing from moment to moment. Not only would your brain cells be flicking on and off as thoughts and feelings coursed through the brain, but your heart rate, blood pressure, and balance of hormones in your blood would all be fluctuating in interconnected, complex and seemingly chaotic patterns. But if you analysed the data with a sophisticated computer, you'd see that the changes, at least in a healthy person, all stayed within a certain range.

As you watched for longer – and let's assume the scanner was so advanced that it allowed you to move about, walk, talk, eat – you'd see that this astonishingly complex network also changed moment by moment as you reacted to the environment. If you started exercising, you would immediately see changes in blood pressure and blood flow, as well as new patterns of activity in the brain and in individual cells.

Now let's suppose that someone came in and stressed you by being angry with you or very critical. You'd see a very different pattern activated, at first in the brain but then almost instantly, the new rhythms would flow around the rest of your body, changing what was happening in the blood, guts, stomach and immune system. Eating would provoke changes in the levels of hormones, fresh activity in the brain, a shift in blood-sugar level and, if the meal came after the stress, the patterns would be different again.

What you would be seeing in this scanner would be a sort of eco-system at work, a web of life with all the parts interacting and affecting one another, constantly changing but also programmed to stay within certain limits for optimum health.

It's a way of looking at the body that is becoming increasingly common in cutting-edge medical research (see 'The body as an ecology' box opposite), but it's also very useful in explaining why food is better medicine than drugs.

Let's suppose that you are on the brink of becoming chronically ill. You've been under a lot of pressure, you haven't been taking care of your-self and your personal ecosystem is shifting out of the optimum range and settling into a series of less efficient patterns. It's a state you might experience as being tired all the time, rather depressed and irritable, possibly with raised blood pressure and an overactive immune response. In short, precisely the kind of poor functioning that is the target of blockbuster drugs.

THE BODY AS AN ECOLOGY

While nutritional and other non-drug practitioners have always treated the body as a whole system, mainstream medical researchers have tended to look at its parts in isolation. They are only now edging towards the notion that they should perhaps consider some of the elements of the body as part of a wider system.

'It's the ecology, stupid!', was the headline of a recent *Nature* article on stem cells (the basic cells which can develop into different types of more specialised cells), reported that trying to understand them by looking at the way they behave in a Petri dish doesn't work. The latest model describes them as inhabiting a 'niche', a term borrowed from ecology. The article points out that stem cells, like other cells, depend on support cells, protein scaffolds, blood vessels and biochemicals – a network which 'may be every bit as complex as a forest ecosystem'.[1]

Even the hallowed 'magic bullet' – the goal of drug design for half a century – is being rethought because of problems with the new generation of cancer drugs like Gleevec or Iressa, which are designed to precisely target molecules involved in carcinogenesis – the process whereby normal cells become cancerous. (Many tumours were found to develop resistance to Gleevec, for instance, while Iressa was very effective in only a few patients.) 'Common disorders tend to result from multiple molecular abnormalities, not from a single defect,' observes another *Nature* article.[2] So the latest idea is for the 'magic shotgun' that will hit multiple targets in the system. There is now an 'emerging field of network biology' aiming to 'model all the complex interactions between all the molecular constituents of a cell'.

This could take some time. In the meantime, for some chronic disorders, something as simple as vitamins, minerals and omega-3 essential fats are a pretty good magic shotgun: after all, our bodies have evolved to use them in myriad ways, affecting almost every element of the overall network.

Why drugs fail to fit the new paradigm

So are drugs the best way of shifting your body network back into a healthier pattern? To see why not, consider this simple question. If the UK's National Health Service could dispense an unlimited amount of drugs, and had no waiting lists for surgical procedures, would we be healthier? Would this free us from the major chronic diseases – Alzheimer's, arthritis, cancer, cardiovascular disease, depression, diabetes and obesity? One reason it wouldn't is because we know that there is no relationship between the amount spent on medical treatment and overall health (see the 'More money doesn't add up to better health' box below).

MORE MONEY DOESN'T ADD UP TO BETTER HEALTH

When trying to estimate the benefit of the money a country spends on medical services, researchers use a measurement known as DALE (disability adjusted life expectancy) – in other words, the average number of years people can expect 'to live in full health'.

The people of Greece, for example, can expect a DALE score of 72.5 years, which is among the highest in the developed countries. But in 2000 they spent the least on health services of any developed country – $964 per head per year. At the other end of the scale, Americans got the fewest years (70) for the most money – $3,724. The UK spent a hundred dollars more than Greece – $1,193 – but only got 71.7 years.[3] The reasons for these big gaps are disputed, but lifestyle factors such as stress and diet play a part; they affect the entire body 'ecosystem' and drugs can't influence them.

Similarly, you might think that countries with more doctors per population would live longer, but they don't. Take the US. There are more than 300 doctors per 100,000 and people live to be 71.5, on average. Yet England, with a slightly longer life expectancy of 72, has nearly half that number – a mere 160 doctors per 100,000. Italy has even more doctors than the US – 550 – but an identical lifespan to the English. Whichever way you cut it, there's no statistical link between

---

numbers of doctors and lifespan, according to economics professor Andrew Oswald of Warwick University in the UK.[4]

The reason there's no correlation between the amount spent on so-called healthcare, or the numbers of doctors in a country, is likely to be because neither the health-care system, nor doctors, are making much impact on the true causes of disease.

The high cost of health services

But there is a more fundamental reason why unlimited medical treatments wouldn't make us all healthy. Not only are most drugs not designed to remove the causes of sickness but, taken for any length of time to relieve symptoms, they very often create new problems. And that costs, in health and cash alike.

We are spending more and more on health. British taxpayers, for example, according to another set of calculations, spend over £2,500 per year each,[5] a figure echoed in other developed countries – and 70 per cent of the UK population is taking medicines to treat or prevent ill health.[6] One professor of medicine described the health service as 'the fastest-growing failing business'.

If you are one of the people on this kind of treatment, you are likely to be taking at least one or more of the three most widely prescribed drugs – aspirins, statins and anti-depressant SSRIs. We've already seen some of the problems with each of these classes of drugs, but recent research suggests they may well be disrupting your body's biological balance, and damaging your body in other ways. Let's look at these three.

If you take aspirin to help ease the pain of a broken bone, the healing process in the bone will slow. A COX-2 inhibitor painkiller like Vioxx or Celexib will slow down soft-tissue healing as well.[7] NSAIDs such as aspirin damage stomach and gut linings, as we've seen, and cause around 2,300 deaths a year in the UK from gastrointestinal bleeding – and now it turns out that if you combine aspirin with an SSRI, your risk of such bleeding goes up 2.5 times.[8] Although many people over 70 will be taking low-dose aspirin to cut the risk of a heart attack, the benefit may well be cancelled out by the gastrointestinal risk.[9]

Statins don't seem to cause so many ADRs as aspirins, but they account for the largest chunk of the NHS drugs bill – so are they a good way of bringing your body's ecosystem back into health? Recently, the manager of an NHS primary care trust reported on their cost-effectiveness.[10] He pointed out that 71 patients with cardiovascular risk factors have to be treated with a statin for five years to prevent one heart attack or stroke.[11] That leaves 70 people taking a drug for five years and gaining no benefit from it. So the cost of preventing that one heart attack would run at between £33,000 and £55,000.

SSRIs, as we've seen (see page 36), have been shown to increase the risk of suicide and to be little more effective than a placebo, but according to a report from the International Center for the Study of Psychiatry and Psychology, based in the US, they could also actually be increasing the rate of mental illness. It says, 'Selective serotonin reuptake inhibitors commonly cause or exacerbate a wide range of abnormal mental and behavioral conditions.' Since the massive increase in prescribing these drugs, rates of mental health problems have soared: 'The number of mentally disabled people in the US has been increasing at a rate of 150,000 people per year since 1987.'[12]

Similarly, since the introduction of anti-psychotic drugs for the treatment of schizophrenia, the rate of suicide has gone up twentyfold.[13] The fact is that most drugs work against the body's design, not with it, and consequently run the very real danger of making matters worse in the long run. Peter Smith discovered the hard way that SSRIs were not for him.

Peter was a civil engineer who for years had been working on contracts in developing countries. The hours were long, he was endlessly juggling competing interests, and sometimes there was danger from terrorists.

The workload took an increasingly heavy toll on his health, and he began having chronic and persistent headaches, stomach disorders, problems with sleeping and nightmares, and low energy. Here was a clear example of the way that stress and psychological pressures can have a very definite system-wide effect, loading the body's ecology with more disruption than it can cope with.

So Peter took some leave in the hope that a rest would allow him to recover. A year later, however, he was worse – depressed, with a failing short-term memory and poor concentration. He often felt lethargic and nauseated during the day – feeling unwell, but unable to pin it down to a specific local problem. The only solution that drug-based medicine had to offer was increasingly powerful pills to target some of the symptoms.

Peter's doctor tried three different anti-depressants, including Seroxat. A headache consultant handed out migraine pills, painkillers and the original heavyweight anti-psychotic drug, chlorpromazine. None of them helped and all had unpleasant side effects. Then a psychiatrist prescribed two more anti-depressants plus an anti-epileptic drug that is also used in bipolar disorder, or manic depression.

In the end, it wasn't the cascade of pills that helped restore Peter's system-wide imbalance. It was something much more basic and decidedly drug-free: learning how to breathe properly. A well-known effect of chronic stress is that it causes people to breathe too quickly and too shallowly. The result is a drop in the amount of carbon dioxide (CO_2) in the bloodstream – and that has wide-ranging and largely unappreciated effects.

This may come as a surprise because as we all know, we breathe in life-giving oxygen, while CO_2 is the waste product we breathe out. But it's standard textbook knowledge that the body needs a tightly controlled amount of CO_2 to function properly. Too little and you can develop hypocapnia, which can trigger all sorts of harmful changes in your metabolism because CO_2 plays a crucial role in maintaining the acid/alkaline balance in the body.[14]

Remember the sci-fi scanner? If you were go into it after breathing too quickly and shallowly for some time, a whole range of changes would show up, flashing across the entire network. Your blood pressure would drop, as would the amount of oxygen getting to cells in both the brain and the muscles. You would also be making less of the 'feel-good' neuro-transmitter (or 'messenger' chemical in the brain) serotonin.

How people experience this varies, but you might suffer from a lack of energy, tingling in hands and feet, and headaches and depression, and you might also have trouble sleeping – all symptoms that were immediately recognisable to Peter and all of which began to clear up as his breathing became better regulated and his ability to relax improved. (We've provided a simple breathing exercise that you can do on page 394 in Appendix 2.)

Drugs for chronic disorders are always going to cause complications and the medical solution if they get too bad is another drug to deal with the side effects. If you are on aspirin long-term, the add-on drug could be an acid suppressant to help with gastrointestinal bleeding. It's rather like the remedy followed by the old lady in the nursery rhyme beginning, 'I know an old lady who swallowed a fly . . .' And if you go down the drug route, it's one you are likely to become familiar with as you get older.

How to work with the body's design

There is a basic reason why food is better medicine than drugs. Drugs are designed to work in such a way that they are almost guaranteed *not* to push the system back into a state of optimum health. What showed up very clearly on our 'super-scanner' was that when something happens at one point in the network – when you're made to feel stressed and under attack, for instance – the effect is felt all over the system.

But what would show up on the scanner if you took a painkiller? Like nearly all drugs, it's designed to target a single protein, in this case one involved in inflammation. So you'd see a very limited and precise flicker of action. Any extra activity would likely be a sign of an ADR – perhaps a protein involved in blood clotting would be turned off, or the protective lining of the gut would be disrupted.

You'd see something very different, however, if the substance you took was an omega-3 fish oil. Responses would be seen lighting up all over the body. There would be activity in the brain because omega-3 fatty acids are an essential part of cell walls, including those of neurons. These special fats would also home in on the same protein involved in inflammation that Vioxx was going for – but rather than turning off a pathway in the blood that made clotting more likely, it would boost one that kept clotting within healthy limits. (And its actions wouldn't end there, as you'll see in Part 3.)

Food works in a way drugs can't because the body's ecosystem has been designed to work with it. It's obvious: we have evolved to depend on nutrients. That's why they are called nutrients – because they feed us and keep us healthy and functional. It's also obvious, when we stop to think, that the most highly nutritious foods would have this beneficial, system-wide effect. Omega-3s are hardly alone in this – all nutrient-rich foods and supplements have this systemic capability. Vitamin C, zinc, magnesium, or carrots, broccoli, garlic – all trigger many positive responses all over the body. Not only that, these nutrients work synergistically, and to isolate each one and study it as if it were a drug is to miss the point that we humans are a complex ecosystem that interacts with the complex natural chemistry of a varied wholefood diet.

And the same is true of a range of other non-drug treatments, such as psychotherapy, meditation, relaxation, exercise and learning how to breathe properly. If you combine these treatments, they work together to reinforce one another rather than interacting in potentially dangerous ways, as drug combinations can do. The reason, again, is simply that our biological interaction with the world involves our entire body 'eco-system'. Beneficial interactions such as learning a relaxation exercise or taking a long walk in the countryside will engage that complex biological system completely, and the more such activities we engage in, the richer the response from the system – in other words, the healthier (calmer, more focused, fitter and so on) we will get. This is literally how we are designed. We are a complex adaptive system.

You can see that clearly if you look at why we get sick. As we saw at the start of this chapter, environment is the overall causative factor: the major disorders that afflict us are caused by faulty nutrition, lack of exercise, excess drinking, smoking and drugs (both 'recreational' and prescribed), too much stress and simply being poor. None of these has an isolated effect on us. If you were watching yourself in the super-scanner as you indulged in any one of them for a month or two, patterns of reduced functioning would begin to show up right across your network.

One big piece of evidence for this comes from a major study by the US Centers for Disease Control and Prevention, which found that over a third of the deaths that occurred in the US in 2000 were the result of smoking, poor diet, drinking alcohol and a lack of exercise.[15] So under a rational health system, a large portion of spending would target these environmental factors.

Not so. Another big study by the American Institute of Medicine estimated that 95 per cent of health costs go on medical care and bio-medical research – leaving just five per cent for everything else, including prevention. This study also put the contribution to avoidable deaths achieved by changes in behaviour and environment, including diet, at 70 per cent.[16] So we know what makes people ill; we just have a system of 'scientific medicine' that largely ignores this, and spends 95 per cent of the money elsewhere.

Going for what's safe and effective

Nutritional medicine and the other non-drug therapies offer a much more sophisticated way of taking responsibility for your own health. At the moment, as we've seen from those big American studies, there is a huge gap between what is actually making us ill and the mainstream remedies for healing. Large-scale public health programmes, such as banning smoking in public places, improving food in schools and so on, could well improve the national health in the long run. But where does that leave you now?

If you opt for drugs, you have very few options if your system shifts out of optimum functioning – perhaps because you've gone through a period of being very stressed. But if you follow the nutritional and non-drug approach, all sorts of possibilities are open to you. Just as different harm-ful influences in the environment can cause similar network problems, so different non-drug treatments can target the same problems, giving you much more of a choice.

For example, if you are mentally stressed, it's known that your ability to think clearly becomes poorer. But recently it has also been found that a bad junk-food diet and lack of exercise gives rats a much poorer memory.[17] Exercise, however, can reverse that. In humans, regular meditation on compassion, for instance, increases activity in an area of the brain that integrates emotions, thoughts and senses.[18]

Perhaps even more surprising is that not only can taking vitamins reduce the harmful effect of certain inflammatory chemicals in your body, but so can just getting some additional social support. The inflam-mation is caused by the immune system chemical IL-6, which has been linked with a number of chronic disorders such as arthritis, heart disease, cancer and Alzheimer's. It's pushed up by stress and a study has found that older women can bring it down simply by sleeping well and having good social support.[19] But you can also bring down IL-6 with a combination of vitamins C and E.[20]

Of course, one of the best examples of a non-drug way of shifting your whole system in a healthier direction is with exercise.

Mavis was a nurse. In her mid-sixties she began suffering from severe asthma and frequent pneumonia and was hospitalised twice a year. She was given antibiotics to clear her lung infections, but with each bout her lung function deteriorated. She seemed to be losing ground, and in the face of a bleak, short future, she became depressed.

However, Mavis roused herself to go a lecture by an exercise physiologist, who recommended running for people with problems similar to hers. He suggested they start with simple walking, then fast walking, then jogging. Despite never really having been interested in exercise, she was convinced and decided to go for it.

Mavis is now in her eighties and has run more than 20 marathons. She completed her latest one in a little over four hours – not bad for an 82-year-old. She no longer has lung problems and is a model of fitness. Simply by changing her lifestyle, she knocked 25 years off her biological age. (Case supplied by Dr Jeffrey Bland.)

All sorts of non-drug approaches allow you to improve your body's intricate biological balance – a balance we've seen drugs do little about. One of the most reliable signs that any one part of your body's ecosystem is in good health is that its rhythms are changing all the time, usually in unpredictable ways. In a healthy heart, for instance, the time between beats is constantly changing, and when this gap (known as 'heart rate variability' or HRV) starts to become regular and predictable, it's a sign that all is not well. Among the non-drug treatments that can raise your HRV and push you back towards health are omega-3 oils[21] – and even reciting religious mantras such as the 'Ave Maria', which synchronises the blood pressure and breathing rhythms that in turn raises HRV.[22] Another study has found that just losing weight can lead to an improved HRV.[23]

So this approach offers safer treatments and much more flexibility and precision. But there is yet another benefit. All the methods require you to become actively involved. They give you something specific to do. You can decide to improve your breathing, practise meditation or biofeedback, start up a new exercise regime and make healthier choices about the kind of food you eat. This kind of active participation and increased awareness also helps improve your health through biofeedback. By becoming aware of your thoughts in meditation, your pattern of thinking changes; by becoming aware of your breathing patterns, your breathing changes; by becoming aware of the effect food has on your health, your diet changes; and by becoming aware of your body through exercise, your relationship with your body changes. Drug-based medicine, on the other hand, leaves you ignorant and unempowered.

Ill health is frightening, not least because your body is functioning in a faulty way and you don't know why or what to do about it. Taking a pill, quite apart from the risks, leaves you in a passive state, but being able to do something that will benefit the whole system gives you back some power – and just feeling you are more in control has further health benefits in and of itself.[24]

Genes or environment?

It may come as a surprise to learn that genes – as we saw in our sci-fi scanner – can be switched on and off in our cells. The popular view is that genes are immortal, unchanging strings of code that pass down the generations. We also, quite mistakenly, believe there's an absolute quality to them – so if you've got the gene for some disease, that's it. It's a life sentence.

However, because of the ability of genes to switch on and off, you can change the way your genes behave. And one of those ways is with nutrition and supplements. This constitutes an entirely new approach to genetics that fits very well with the network approach to health we've looked at above. We'll explain how the 'new genetics' works in a minute. But first, let's get rid of the notion that genes predict disease in any significant way. Even though biotech companies have spent billions trying to find the gene for asthma or the gene for heart disease, our bodies simply don't work like that.

One major study, for instance, looked at the medical records of 44,788 pairs of identical twins (who have identical genes) and found the risk of both getting any one of 28 different kinds of cancer was very small – between 11 and 18 per cent. The researchers concluded that 'the over-whelming contributor to the causation of cancer was the environment',[25] meaning what you eat and how you live. The influence of our genetic makeup only goes so far, it seems.

The same holds for Alzheimer's. 'A mere fraction of people with Alzheimer's disease, perhaps only 1 per cent, develop the condition because of mutations in certain genes,' says David Smith, Emeritus Professor of Pharmacology at the University of Oxford and one of the world's top experts on this devastating condition.

Reprogramming your genes

Even if you do have genes that predispose you to certain diseases, the good news is that you can reprogramme your genes for health by improving your nutrition. This field of study, and associated treatments and therapies, is called epigenetics.

The key point here is methylation – a way some of the genes in every cell can be turned on and off (see the 'Inside epigenetics' box overleaf for the details). This is another of those network-wide, flexible systems, like breathing, that allows your cells to respond moment by moment to what's happening in the environment. In fact, there's a billion of these methylation adjustments every second! Methylation can be directly affected by food supplements such as vitamins and amino acids as well as by good early parenting. So, what you eat and how you live literally changes your genes.

Clear evidence that genes can be affected so simply and directly came a few years ago from Professor Randy Jirtle of Duke University Medical Center.[26] Jirtle worked with pregnant mice that had a gene mutation giving them yellow coats and a tendency to put on weight. After giving these mice a basic over-the-counter vitamin supplement, they gave birth to lean pups with normal brown coats. Thus, the supplement had effectively switched the so-called 'agouti' gene off, thereby changing the gene expression – the process whereby instructions in genes are activated. They still had the same programming; it's just that the program wasn't running.

More recently, Professor Moshe Szyf at McGill University in Montreal, Canada, found that in deprived baby rats that hadn't been properly licked and groomed after birth, the programming of a gene that controls the level of a stress hormone changed. So as adults, these rats produced more stress hormones and responded badly to being put under pressure.[27] This is evidence that simple behaviours can also affect the way genes work – and, more, that nothing is set in stone.

INSIDE EPIGENETICS

Most people know that our genes are carried in DNA, the 'double helix' or twisted, chain-like molecule that sits in the centre of nearly every cell of the body and contains instructions for the cell's activities. What's often not appreciated is that much of the DNA in any one cell is turned off for much of the time. You don't want liver cells producing teeth, for instance, and all women have one of the two X chromosomes 'silenced' or switched off in each cell – two would cause a deadly overproduction of proteins.

So how is this done? When you see pictures of DNA, the double helix looks all smooth and pure. Inside a cell, however, its look might be described as hairy, because each gene has a sort of tail that sticks out into the surrounding cell, known as a histone. It's histones that allow genes to be silenced or switched off, and they are crucial to epigenetics.

The cell can put certain molecules known as 'methyl tags' on to these histone tails, which can affect how active a particular gene is. It may be switched off completely – silenced – or it may be just toned down. The methyl tags can also be taken off, which means the gene becomes activated or expressed again. Methylation, doesn't actually change the gene itself but it does change the way genes behave. Nutrients that help boost methylation are vitamins B2, B6, B12, folic acid, zinc, magnesium and TMG (Trimethylglycine). Ensuring you have an optimal intake of these effectively raises your 'biological IQ', with amazing health benefits – as we'll see in more detail in Part 3.

The new model of health

So finally it looks as if we are ready to answer our original question – how can we justify the claim that food is better medicine than drugs and, most importantly, how can we regain our health? The answer is, by finding our personal 'optimum' nutrition and lifestyle that literally reprogrammes our complex biological network or ecosystem for health.

Far from being non-scientific, the fact that the changes we'll be recommending affect many body systems simultaneously, without causing more damage, is not only highly scientific, but much safer and usually more effective. Be aware that even if the drug model was cleaned up, properly regulated and freed of all the spin and cover-up that comes with being dominated by marketing, it would still be a very narrow and limited approach that can't tackle the underlying causes of disease or restore people to health.

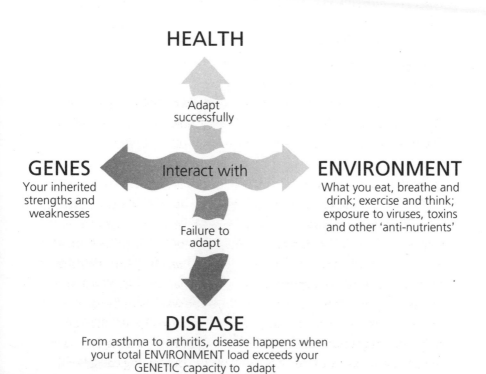

HEALTH

Adapt
successfully

GENES — Interact with — ENVIRONMENT

Your inherited
strengths and
weaknesses

What you eat, breathe and
drink; exercise and think;
exposure to viruses, toxins
and other 'anti-nutrients'

Failure to
adapt

DISEASE

From asthma to arthritis, disease happens when
your total ENVIRONMENT load exceeds your
GENETIC capacity to adapt

The new model of health

So we are evolving a new model of health. As you can see in the figure on the previous page, in this 'network' model your state of health is a result of the interaction between your inherited adaptive capacity (your genes) and your environment. If your environment is problematic – say, you eat badly and live in a heavily polluted place rife with viruses and toxins – and you take little exercise and suffer from stress, you are highly likely to exceed your ability to adapt and you may eventually develop disease.

Whatever disorder you have – allergies, angina, arthritis or atherosclerosis – in this model, each is seen as what happens when your total environmental load (meaning everything you eat, drink, breathe and think) exceeds your particular capacity to adapt.

Instead of having only one possible genetic program running, you have thousands, if not millions of possible genetic expressions, determined by a huge range of epigenetic factors. As medical biochemist Dr Jeffrey Bland, founder of the Institute for Functional Medicine in Gig Harbor, Washington, author of *Genetic Nutritioneering* says,

> Those codes, and the expression of the individual's genes, are modifiable. The person you are right now is the result of the uncontrolled experiment called 'your life' in which you have been bathing your genes with experience to give rise to the outcome of that experiment. If you don't like the result of the experiment that makes up your life thus far, you can change it at any moment, whether you are 15 or 75 or 90.[28]

And the way you can change it is by changing the chemical environment that your genes bathe in and by changing their expression, either by putting those methyl tags on or by taking them off.

One cause of faulty methylation is damage caused by free radicals or oxidants – molecules that are being constantly created in our bodies as well as being generated in the environment by sources such sunlight, pollution, radiation, fried food, poor diet and smoking. According to geneticist Bruce Ames at the University of California, Berkeley, 'By the time you're old, we'll find a few million oxygen lesions per cell.' As an antidote to this damage caused by oxidation, our bodies create antioxidants to neutralise them, and of course we also get antioxidants such as vitamins A, C and E from our foods.

An imbalance between our oxidant exposure and our antioxidant supply can disrupt the methylation process, sometimes triggering cancer. 'One in four gene changes that cause human disease can be attributed to methyl groups on our genes,' says genetic scientist Dr Adrian Bird from Edinburgh University. So it is vital to know about another way of keeping your methylation on track. That involves boosting your intake of vitamins B6, B12, folic acid and other key nutrients (all of which are described at greater length in Chapter 15).

Chemical cocktails

Some of the most damaging factors in the environment are pesticides and other toxic chemicals that we are now constantly exposed to from birth. Just how extensively they have colonised our bodies was vividly illustrated by a report from the conservation charity the World Wildlife Fund (WWF), published in 2004.[29] The WWF tested 47 members of the

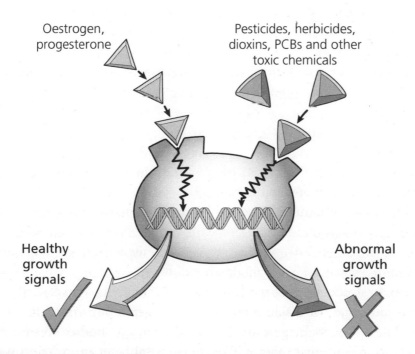

How hormones and chemicals affect genes

European parliament and found that on average they each carried 41 synthetic chemicals in their blood, including, in many cases, the banned pesticide DDT – a suspected cause of breast cancer. Another WWF report found 350 contaminants in breast milk, including flame retardants, DDT and dioxins. Some of these highly carcinogenic chemicals are still in widespread use.

Many of them, such nonylphenol – found in paints, detergents, lubricating oils, toiletries, spermicide foams and agrochemicals among other substances – have an effect similar to that of oestrogen, a hormone that encourages growth.

Such hormone-disrupting chemicals can activate genes, but not necessarily in the right ways; so eventually they can change the way our biology works, depending on how much of them you are exposed to, and how 'receptive' your cells are to them. The oestreogen-mimicking chemicals, for example, can trigger an overgrowth of breast or prostate cells, leading to cancer. But as with harm from oxidants, certain foods provide a way to reduce the damaging effects. Soya beans also contain an oestrogen-like molecule known as a phyto-estrogen ('phyto' meaning plant), and because it can also occupy the same 'receptors' on cell surfaces that the hormone-disrupting chemicals attach themselves to, it can colonise them instead and so help maintain hormonal balance.

Find the 'wobble' – and fix it

The network approach makes it obvious that the way to stay healthy is to focus on changing the circumstances that lead to a disease like diabetes or heart disease, rather than simply trying to fix the damage once it has happened. After all, if you've been driving your car too hard, without enough oil, there's not much point fixing the damage if you don't also replace the oil and start driving more carefully.

Contrast the difference between the network approach and the pharmaceutical approach in treating Alzheimer's. If you're diagnosed, you are likely to be offered a drug like Aricept, which works by temporarily increasing levels of the neurotransmitter acetylcholine, which is a crucial player in memory. Taking Aricept does nothing to deal with the underlying cause or the progression of the disease, however. In fact, one recent study found it had 'no significant benefits' over a placebo.[30] Some patients do feel better for a couple of years, but then rapidly degenerate and soon are no better off than those who never took the drug. Few people with dementia, or their families and carers, are told there is another way – that increasing fish oils, B vitamins, and vitamin E and other antioxidant nutrients in food can make a big difference, as we'll see in Chapter 11.

The network approach makes life an awful lot easier and more enjoyable for the patients, and it can also be far more cost-effective. A recent computer simulation compared the cost of saving the life of a diabetic with drugs or with lifestyle changes, and found that while a lifestyle programme costs about $8,800 per year of healthy life saved, the cost with drugs was $29,000.[31] And while diet and exercise delayed the onset of diabetes by 11 years, the drug only held it off for three.

So the goal is to find out where the wobble is in your biological eco-system and what adjustments to your diet and lifestyle will most rapidly restore balance and reverse the disease process. While our super-scanner is still only sci-fi, an emerging science of health – as you'll see in the next chapter – will allow you to find your own prescription for drug-free health.

6.

The Road to Health
Six key steps to recapture well-being

MODERN MEDICINE MIGHT know a lot about disease, but it doesn't know that much about health. Many doctors, in fact, are liable to call a person 'healthy' when they can't find any obvious signs of identifiable disease, even though that person may be very far from the glowing, energetic reality of true health.

Consider Joan. She suffered from chronic tiredness and headaches; painkillers eased them somewhat but, if anything, the symptoms were getting worse. Her doctor gave her a physical and ran a blood test. There was no obvious cause of disease – no diabetes, no high blood pressure, no musculoskeletal problem. 'You're completely healthy,' he said. 'No, I'm not,' said Joan, repeatedly, each time leaving with a new prescription for a different painkiller.

Ask yourself this question: if you woke up 100 per cent healthy tomorrow, how would you know? Take a piece of paper and a pen and write down at least six concrete signs that would tell you something had improved.

Once you've finished, your list might include some of these:

- More energy
- More motivation

- Better mood

- No PMS or hot flushes

- No aches and pains

- More focused concentration

- Better skin, hair and nails

- Less fat

- Normal blood pressure, cholesterol or homocysteine

- Better digestion

- Deeper, more even breathing patterns

- Better sleep patterns

- Better sex drive.

Most people have a pretty good idea of what it would feel like to be healthier. But all too few achieve it or, in our experience, have fully experienced how good it can feel. Essentially, as we'll see in a moment, it's all down to six key factors. Just now let's look at an unusual survey that pinned down how tens of thousands of UK residents actually feel.

This – the 'Optimum Nutrition UK' (ONUK) survey published in 2004 by the Institute for Optimum Nutrition – was Britain's biggest ever. Over 37,000 people filled in an online questionnaire asking how they felt. Here's what they told us. (You might like to compare yourself by answering this small selection of the 170 questions and scoring your 'yes' answers.)

As one child said in an exam howler, 'Modern man is a knackered ape' – and judging by the results of this survey, they weren't far wrong. In fact, the average health score was 55 per cent, where 100 per cent means effectively no symptoms of ill health at all. At the Institute for Optimum Nutrition we've treated close to 100,000 people and know that, by changing a person's diet, giving appropriate supplements and recommending simple lifestyle changes, most people achieve a health score of above 80 per cent, which we call 'optimum health', within three months. In the

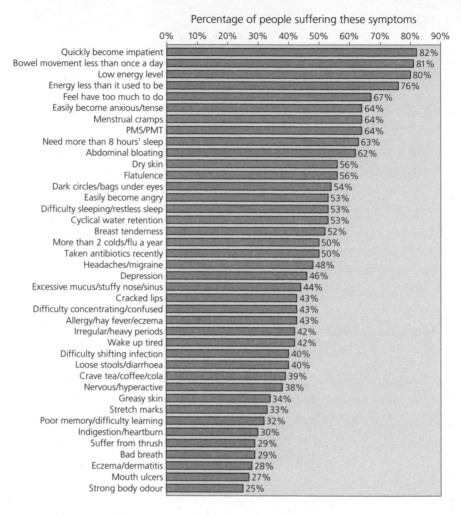

Percentage of people suffering these symptoms

Symptom	Percentage
Quickly become impatient	82%
Bowel movement less than once a day	81%
Low energy level	80%
Energy less than it used to be	76%
Feel have too much to do	67%
Easily become anxious/tense	64%
Menstrual cramps	64%
PMS/PMT	64%
Need more than 8 hours' sleep	63%
Abdominal bloating	62%
Dry skin	56%
Flatulence	56%
Dark circles/bags under eyes	54%
Easily become angry	53%
Difficulty sleeping/restless sleep	53%
Cyclical water retention	53%
Breast tenderness	52%
More than 2 colds/flu a year	50%
Taken antibiotics recently	50%
Headaches/migraine	48%
Depression	46%
Excessive mucus/stuffy nose/sinus	44%
Cracked lips	43%
Difficulty concentrating/confused	43%
Allergy/hay fever/eczema	43%
Irregular/heavy periods	42%
Wake up tired	42%
Difficulty shifting infection	40%
Loose stools/diarrhoea	40%
Crave tea/coffee/cola	39%
Nervous/hyperactive	38%
Greasy skin	34%
Stretch marks	33%
Poor memory/difficulty learning	32%
Indigestion/heartburn	30%
Suffer from thrush	29%
Bad breath	29%
Eczema/dermatitis	28%
Mouth ulcers	27%
Strong body odour	25%

Results of Optimum Nutrition UK (ONUK) survey 2004

ONUK survey, only six per cent of people were in this optimum health category, while 44 per cent were in the poor or very poor health category.

If you too are in what could be described as 'average poor health', probably eating what you might describe as a 'reasonably well-balanced diet', you are what we call one of the 'vertically ill' – upright, certainly, but not feeling great. Feeling just 'all right' isn't all right.

Either you get better and attain optimum health, or you could get worse and join the horizontally ill (that is, too ill to function) by develop-

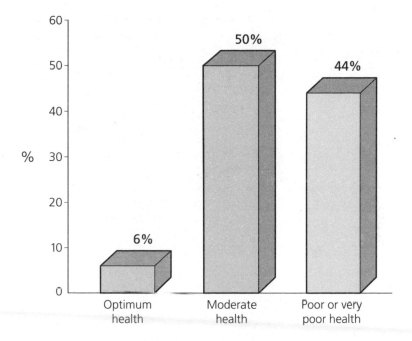

Overall health – ONUK survey 2004

ing diabetes, becoming obese, chronically tired, or experiencing chronic pain, perhaps from joint aches, headaches or indigestion – or, even worse, developing cardiovascular disease or cancer. Most of mainstream medicine deals with the horizontally ill. Your doctor's job is to get you back into action, often by prescribing a drug. But a much greater proportion of people are walking around vertically ill.

The point is that the horizontally ill start off as vertically ill. In Chapter 7, you'll find an overall health check that will help you take action sooner rather than later. Or you may decide you'd like to take Patrick's 100% Health Profile (see Appendix 1, page 392).

Elaine was a case in point. After having a 100% Health Profile, she found that her health was rated at a mere 33.6 per cent, which we can say was poor. Here's how she described herself: 'I have been suffering with PMS for as long as I can remember. As my period approaches my moods are terrible, my stomach is churning, my breasts are sore and I go nuts. It is so bad that my family leave the house!' In fact, her PMS was so severe that, on one occasion, the neighbours were so concerned by the screaming, shouting, and smashing that they called the police, who assumed the worst and wrongfully arrested her husband!

Concerned about her terrible PMS, Elaine then embarked on a new diet and supplement programme. She had an allergy test and eliminated her food allergies, cut the sugar and caffeine from her diet, started eating more fish and seeds – high in essential fats and minerals – and also took supplements of essential fats, vitamin B6, zinc and magnesium and some herbs (dong quai and *Vitex agnus-castus*). Her 'prescription' was very similar to that in Chapter 9 ('Balancing Hormones in the Menopause'), based on the evidence of what actually works. Within four weeks she was feeling almost completely better. All her symptoms have improved.

Elaine H – before

Overall health score – 33.6% Level D

Key health factors

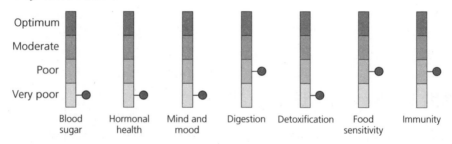

Elaine H – after

Overall health score – 85.7% Level A

Key health factors

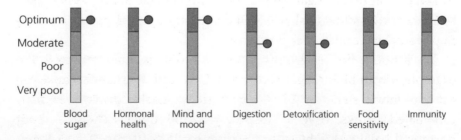

Elaine's 100% Health profile: before and after

In her own words,

'I haven't had any PMT – it should be really bad right now. I've had none of my outbursts. I've stuck to the diet completely. My energy has gone through the roof. I just feel like a completely different person. I can't believe it's happened so quickly. My husband can't believe the change. No breast tenderness. My middle daughter said, "What have you been doing to your skin? You look so much younger." I explained to my doctor, who said he should have considered this approach. He's so relieved. I'm really enjoying the diet. I'm trying new foods and they taste great. This is the best week my husband has had in years.'

Elaine retested herself on the questionnaire and, as you can see, the improvement was dramatic. She is delighted, and her doctor is delighted – but why isn't this kind of medicine the first rather than the last resort? Why aren't doctors trained to think in this way? After all, as you'll see in Part 3, it's not because there isn't good science to back up the 'new medicine' approach. The evidence is there: it does the job, it's safe and it's cost-effective.

The six key health factors

Our health profile is based on a 'systems' way of thinking – an understanding that there are six key functions going on inside us that, once out of balance, inevitably lead to ill health. These six are shown in the figure overleaf.

Elaine's profile assessed how each of these six core processes was working – her blood sugar (16 per cent), hormonal balance (14 per cent) and neurotransmitters balance (mind and mood in the profile report – 14 per cent) were all at rock bottom.

You'll notice how each process in the profile is interconnected. For example, if your blood sugar becomes unbalanced – perhaps because you eat too much sugar or too many starchy snacks, drink too many caffeinated drinks, have a stressful job and don't exercise – your hormonal balance might suffer, leading to PMS (if you're a woman). That has a knock-on effect on the brain's neurotransmitter balance. Your

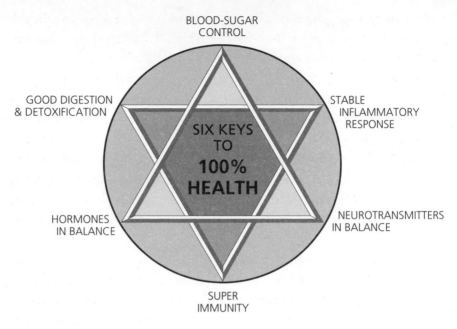

Six keys to 100 per cent health

level of serotonin, the 'happy' neurotransmitter, might be too low, making you depressed, while your adrenalin levels from all that stress, sugar and caffeine, might be too high.

This kind of dynamic isn't just a theory – it's exactly what happens. For example, researchers at Yale University in the US gave 25 healthy children a drink containing the equivalent amount of glucose found in a can of cola. The body overeacts to this flood of glucose by producing loads of insulin, which causes a rebound low blood sugar. The rebound blood-sugar drop boosted their adrenalin to over five times the normal level for up to five hours after consuming the sugar. Most of the children had difficulty concentrating and were irritable and anxious, which are normal reactions to too much adrenalin in the bloodstream.[32] Meanwhile, stress is known to lead to low serotonin, more so in women than men.[33] PMS is also now known to cause specific changes in the brain,[34] and to lead to increased cravings for sugar and stimulants, and many of the symptoms of blood-sugar imbalances – low energy, irritability, depression, anxiety and cravings for sugar and stimulants.

As you can see, there can be a circularity to all this – with health problems leading on to poor lifestyle habits and vice versa – that can eventually build up to a classic vicious circle.

Going back to Elaine's original profile, you can see she also had a poor digestion score (51 per cent) and plenty of symptoms of food sensitivity (39 per cent). These two imbalances often go together. The reason is that if you eat foods you are unknowingly allergic to or that you don't digest very well – for example gluten in wheat – or drink alcohol or take painkillers frequently, all these things can end up irritating your digestive tract. This can add up to a pretty hefty problem, as its surface area is the size of a small football pitch. Gradually, if you continue to consume the irritants, your gut will become less healthy and more 'leaky'.

This condition, known as gastrointestinal permeability, has been the focus of some 1,500 studies. What it means is that undigested foods, such as whole proteins, get into the bloodstream, triggering a reaction in the immune system. This is the source of most food allergies. Over time the leakiness leads to more inflammation and, eventually, weaker immunity. So you might develop irritable bowel syndrome, asthma, eczema or arthritis (all of which are inflammatory diseases that have been strongly linked to food allergy), or become more prone to infections. If you are given a non-steroidal painkiller, such as aspirin or ibuprofen, or a course of antibiotics, this further irritates the gut and makes it more permeable. You can see this cycle in the diagram overleaf.

This shows just how most states of ill health develop – they knock your body's ecosystem out of balance. It also explains a key dynamic of many drugs. They may make you instantly feel better, but don't solve the underlying disease. And in this case they make matters worse. So you've got to keep taking the drug, but the longer you take it, the more side effects you get. In the case of NSAIDs in the US it amounts to an $8.5 billion dollar industry – $6.5 billion for the drugs[35] and $2 billion for treating the side effects.[36]

The alternative to all this is an approach that aims to restore health to your physical ecosystem. These days, if you go and see a nutritional therapist, each element of the cycle can be tested, from 'leaky-gut syndrome' to whether or not your body is reacting allergically to foods by

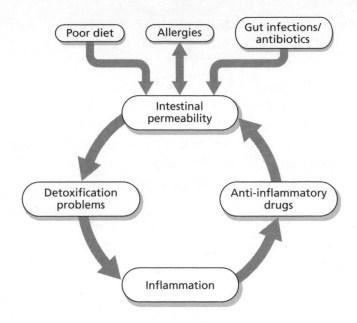

The cycle of inflammation

producing antibodies. It's hard science rather than throwing pills at symptoms.

The tests a nutritional therapist might give you aren't for disease. They don't diagnose cancer or colitis. They are tests of function. They measure how well you are functioning in relation to the six vital key steps to 100 per cent health we outlined above. They pick up functional imbalances while you're still 'vertically ill' and, with the right action, stop you ever becoming horizontally ill. Some of the tests nutritional therapists and doctors commonly use are shown in the table below.

Key function	Test and what it shows
Blood sugar	Blood glucose
	Glycosylated haemoglobin
	Insulin sensitivity
	These blood tests don't just show if you have diabetes, they show if you are losing your blood-sugar control and need to take action to prevent diabetes.

Key function	Test and what it shows
Hormone balance	Oestradiol, progesterone, testosterone Cortisol, DHEA *These hormone tests, often measured in saliva, show if your hormonal system is out of balance and the action you need to take to bring it back into line.*
Mind and mood	Homocysteine Platelet serotonin, adrenalin, noradrenalin, dopamine and acetylcholine *Homocysteine is an indicator of how good you are at methylation reactions, which help to keep neurotransmitters in balance, while platelet levels of serotonin, for example, indicate deficiency and the need for amino acids that help restore health and mood.*
Digestion	Gastrointestinal permeability *This test involves drinking a solution, then taking a urine sample to find out if your digestive tract is working properly. If not, you're more likely to develop allergies.*
Immunity	IgE and IgE 'ELISA' allergy tests *These blood tests, which can be done using a pinprick of blood from a home-test allergy kit, identify if your body is producing antibodies that attack the food you eat, identifying food sensitivities.*
Inflammation	Erythrocyte Sedimentation Rate C-Reactive protein *If raised, these indicate your body is in a state of inflammation. Rather than just suppress the resulting pain, the ultimate goal is to find out why.*

Gut feelings

Zoe, for instance, had suffered for six years with irritable bowel syndrome, an unpleasant condition characterised by bloating, extreme pain, urgency and wind. She also suffered from PMS. She'd seen her doctor many times and tried Fybogel, a kind of fibre, but it didn't work, and her condition got steadily worse. IBS was ruining her nights out and other social occasions. She noticed it was worse when she ate late at night, and that bread and stress seemed to exacerbate it too. So she eliminated wheat from her diet, which made a little difference, but she was struggling and still getting worse – effectively slipping towards a 'horizontal' state.

Zoe's 100% Health Profile, shown opposite, identified that her digestion, blood sugar and hormonal balance were all well below par, while her food sensitivity was heightened. She decided to have a food allergy test and sent off for a home-test kit. This involved a tiny pinprick to obtain a small blood sample, which Zoe then sent off to a laboratory. The sample was tested for the presence of what are called IgG antibodies, a kind tailor-made to attack certain food proteins. (Conventional allergy tests measure IgE antibodies, but these are less frequently the cause of food intolerances associated with IBS.)[37] The results showed that her immune system was reacting to cow's milk and egg white.

Zoe eliminated these foods, improved her diet and supplemented digestive enzymes to boost her digestion. She also took probiotics, which are beneficial bacteria to restore digestive health, and every night had a heaped teaspoon of glutamine powder in water. This amino acid helps to heal the digestive tract and make it less permeable. She also supplemented chromium, a mineral that reduces sugar cravings (see Chapter 8, page 150).

Within three days, Zoe was better. Within a month, she was much better. Here's what she said at that point:

'I'm enjoying the change of foods. No IBS (I had it once only – I had fajitas and sour cream, and I got it bad that night). I've had one headache. I have much more energy. I'm not tired in the afternoons. Occasionally I have a craving for sweet foods. I have my porridge every morning. Then I have a banana or oat cakes as a snack. I'm very happy with the results and I've lost a couple of pounds.'

Zoe M – before

Overall health score – 64.4% Level C

Key health factors

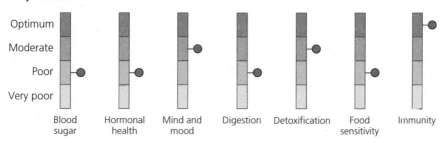

Zoe M – after

Overall health score 81.3% Level B

Key health factors

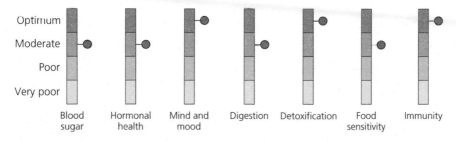

Zoe's 100% Health profile: before and after

When Zoe retested herself, her overall health score had gone from 64 per cent health to 81 per cent health. That put her into the 'optimum' health category, and showed she was making rapid improvement.

Prevention is a better cure

This kind of approach is highly effective partly because the earlier you take action the better. It is much safer than popping a pill, as it's based on healthy changes in diet and a judicious use of non-toxic food supplements. It works fast – most people start to feel better within a week and certainly within a month. It's relatively inexpensive, although supplement programmes can cost from 30p to £1 a day if you're out of balance and need quite a few to get your system back to health. This is cheaper than many drugs, but since they're not prescribed, the patient has to pay. Once people feel the difference, most are more than happy to. Also, as a person gets healthier they need less additional supplements.

Each element of Zoe's food cure is well proven by proper scientific evidence – for instance, the benefits of digestive enzymes, probiotics and glutamine, and IgG food allergy as causative factor in IBS. A study conducted by researchers from York University in the UK, and published in the prestigious science journal *Gut*, which is widely read by gastro-intestinal experts, tested 150 IBS sufferers with the same test kit Zoe had used. The team then gave the participants' doctors real or fake results, and an 'allergy-free' diet sheet that was either real or fake, yet equally difficult. Neither the patient nor the doctor knew which diet they were on. So this was a double-blind trial.

Three months later, they compared the results. Those on their real allergy-free diet had significantly better results, reporting fewer allergic reactions and a reduction in the severity of symptoms like bloating, wind, abdominal pain and urgency.[38]

Zoe was angry that she'd suffered for six years and her doctor hadn't explored the nutrition link. But was her doctor to blame? Why isn't this kind of approach part of mainstream medicine? It's a combination of factors. Doctors don't have time to read all the medical journals. Even if they did, they might not put all the pieces together. This kind of 'network thinking', focusing on health and function rather than on symptom reduction isn't part of the medical curriculum, and certainly wasn't when most doctors trained. There are no reps flogging enzymes or glutamine, no sponsored conferences pushing non-patentable probiotics and, even if there were, most of the tests and supplements we've described can't be prescribed in most health-care systems.

It also takes time. This kind of medicine can't be dispensed in five minutes. It's a paradigm shift and one that we hope this book will help along. In Part 4 we explore ways in which you can help make this happen. One way is to go to your doctor when you've got better to share what worked first hand. In Zoe's case, she went back to her doctor who sat back in his chair and listened, but she wasn't convinced he was going to take this approach on board.

Leaving that aside, how healthy are you and what changes do you need to make to feel great and stay free of disease, without the need for drugs? How do you find out what your level of health is, and your balance across the six key pillars of health? The next chapter shows you how.

7.

Your 100% Health Check-up
Find out how healthy you are and how healthy you could be

JUST LIKE ZOE and Elaine, you too can find out how healthy you really are out of 100 per cent – and how to improve your health and prevent disease in the future. In much the same way that you get your car checked every couple of years, it's well worth assessing your own health before something breaks down – and you go from 'vertical' to 'horizontal' and are more at risk of having to take prescription drugs.

To get a picture of your basic health, answer the questionnaires below. This is like a snapshot of how healthy you are in relation to the six essential body functions – blood sugar and neurotransmitter balance, digestion, hormonal health, inflammatory response and immune response. Your 'health snap' allows you to understand which areas of your health need the most attention.

If you want to go for a more comprehensive health profile, more in-depth advice on how to make nutritional and lifestyle changes, and support while you're doing it, see Appendix 1, page 392, for details on the 100% Health Profile and related services.

Your basic health profile

For a basic check-up across the six key systems, answer these questions, scoring 1 for each answer to which you'd answer 'often' or 'frequently' or 'always'. Add up your score for each section.

Blood-sugar balance

☐ Are you rarely wide awake within 15 minutes of rising?

☐ Do you need tea, coffee, a cigarette or something sweet to get you going in the morning?

☐ Do you crave chocolate, sweet foods, bread, cereal or pasta?

☐ Do you add sugar to your drinks, have sugared drinks or add sugared sauces, such as ketchup, to your food?

☐ Do you often have energy slumps during the day or after meals?

☐ Do you crave something sweet or a stimulant after meals?

☐ Do you often have mood swings or difficulty concentrating?

☐ Do you get dizzy or irritable if you go six hours without food?

☐ Do you find you overreact to stress?

☐ Is your energy now less than it used to be?

☐ Do you feel too tired to exercise?

☐ Are you gaining weight, and finding it hard to lose, even though you're not noticeably eating more or exercising less?

☐ Do you have diabetes?

_____Total

Male hormonal balance (men only)

☐ Are you gaining weight?

☐ Do you often suffer from mood swings or depression?

☐ Have you at any time been bothered with problems affecting your reproductive organs (prostate or testes)?

☐ Do you have difficulty urinating?

☐ Do you suffer from reduced libido or loss of interest in sex?

☐ Do you suffer from impotence?

☐ Do you awake less frequently with a morning erection or have difficulty maintaining an erection?

☐ Do you suffer from fatigue or loss of energy?

☐ Have you had a drop in your motivation and drive?

☐ Do you feel that you are ageing prematurely?

☐ Have you had a vasectomy?

☐ Do you have an underactive or overactive thyroid?

_____Total

Female hormone balance (women only)

☐ Do you use the contraceptive pill or are you on HRT, or have you been on either for more than three years in the last seven years?

☐ Do you often suffer from cyclical mood swings or depression?

☐ Do you experience cyclical water retention?

☐ Do you especially crave foods premenstrually?

☐ Have you at any time been bothered with problems affecting your reproductive organs (ovaries, womb)?

☐ Do you have fertility problems, difficulty conceiving or a history of miscarriage?

☐ Do you suffer from breast tenderness?

☐ Do you experience cramps or other menstrual irregularities?

☐ Are your periods often irregular or heavy?

☐ Do you suffer from reduced libido, impotence or loss of interest in sex?

☐ Do you have menopausal symptoms such as sweats, hot flushes, weight gain, pain with intercourse, loss of libido and depression?

☐ Do you have an underactive or overactive thyroid?

_____Total

Mind and mood

☐ Is your memory deteriorating?

☐ Do you find it hard to concentrate and often get confused?

☐ Are you often depressed?

☐ Do you easily become anxious or wake up with a feeling of anxiety?

☐ Does stress leave you feeling exhausted?

☐ Do you often have mood swings and easily become angry or irritable?

☐ Are you lacking in motivation?

☐ Do you sometimes feel like you're going crazy or have distorted perceptions where things don't look or sound right or you feel distant or disconnected?

☐ Do you suffer from insomnia?

☐ Does your mind ever go blank?

☐ Do you often find you can remember things from the past but forget what you did yesterday?

☐ Do you wake up in the early hours of the morning?

☐ Are you prone to premenstrual tension?

☐ Is your mood noticeably worse in the winter?

_____Total

Digestion

☐ Do you fail to chew your food thoroughly?

☐ Do you suffer from bad breath?

☐ Do you get a burning sensation in your stomach or regularly use indigestion tablets?

☐ Do you often have an uncomfortable feeling of fullness in your stomach?

☐ Do you find it difficult digesting fatty foods?

☐ Do you often get diarrhoea?

☐ Do you often suffer from constipation?

☐ Do you often get a bloated stomach?

☐ Do you often feel nauseous?

☐ Do you often belch or pass wind?

☐ Do you fail to have a bowel movement at least once a day?

☐ Do you feel worse, or excessively sleepy, after meals?

_____Total

Detoxification

☐ Do you suffer from headaches or migraine?

☐ Do you have watery or itchy eyes or swollen, red or sticky eyelids, bags or dark circles under your eyes?

☐ Do you have itchy ears, earache, ear infections, drainage from the ear or ringing in the ears?

☐ Do you suffer from excessive mucus, a stuffy nose or sinus problems?

☐ Do you suffer from acne, skin rashes or hives?

☐ Do you sweat a lot and have a strong body odour, including from your feet?

☐ Do you have joint or muscle aches or pains?

☐ Do you have a sluggish metabolism and find it hard to lose weight, or are you underweight and find it hard to gain weight?

☐ Do you suffer from nausea or vomiting?

☐ Do you have a bitter taste in your mouth or a furry tongue?

☐ Do you easily get a hangover and feel considerably worse the next day even after a small amount of alcohol?

_____Total

Allergy and inflammation

☐ Do you suffer from allergies?

- [ ] Do you suffer from IBS?
- [ ] Can you gain weight in hours?
- [ ] Do you sometimes get really sleepy and tired after eating?
- [ ] Do you suffer from hayfever?
- [ ] Do you suffer from rashes, itches, eczema or dermatitis?
- [ ] Do you suffer from asthma or shortness of breath?
- [ ] Do you suffer from headaches?
- [ ] Do you suffer from joint aches or arthritis?
- [ ] Do you suffer from colitis, diverticulitis or Crohn's disease?
- [ ] Do you suffer from other aches or pains?
- [ ] Do you get better on holidays abroad, when your diet is completely different?
- [ ] Do you use painkillers most weeks?

_____Total

Immunity

- [ ] Do you get more than three colds a year?
- [ ] Do you get a stomach bug each year?
- [ ] Do you find it hard to shift an infection (cold or otherwise)?
- [ ] Are you prone to thrush or cystitis?
- [ ] Do you take at least one course of antibiotics each year?
- [ ] Has more than one member of your immediate family had cancer?
- [ ] Had you been diagnosed with cancer, or any precancerous condition?
- [ ] Do the glands in your neck, armpits or groin feel tender?
- [ ] Do you suffer from allergy problems?
- [ ] Do you have an auto-immune disease?

☐ Do you have an inflammatory disease such as eczema, asthma or arthritis?

_____Total

Hair, skin and nails

☐ Do you have dry or greasy hair?

☐ Do you have acne?

☐ Do you have eczema or dermatitis?

☐ Do you have red pimples on your skin?

☐ Do you have white spots on your fingernails?

☐ Do your nails peel, crack or break easily?

☐ Do you have stretch marks?

☐ Do you bruise easily?

☐ Is your hair thinning or are you losing your hair?

☐ Do you often get mouth ulcers?

☐ Does your skin take a long time to heal?

_____Total

Health indicators

(You will find information on these tests in Part 3)

☐ Is your homocysteine level above 7?

☐ Do you have a raised cholesterol level (above 5.5mmol/l)?

☐ Are you overweight (BMI above 25)?

☐ Do you have high blood pressurc (above 140/90)?

☐ Is your pulse more than 70 beats a minute?

☐ Do you exercise less than one hour a week?

What's your health score?

Blood-sugar balance   _____

Hormonal balance   _____

Mind and mood   _____

Digestion   _____

Detoxification   _____

Allergy and inflammation   _____

Immunity   _____

Hair, skin and nails   _____

Health indicators   _____

Your total health score __ ____ subtract from 100 = _____ per cent

If you have answered yes to:

- **Less than 4 in any section:** you are unlikely to have a problem with this key function.

- **4 to 7 in any section:** you are beginning to show signs of sub-optimal function in that system.

- **7 or more in any section:** that key function needs a boost.

The ideal is to not answer 'yes' to any of these questions, which would give you a score of 100 per cent health. Your total health score is your number of 'yes' answers, subtracted from 100. If you score:

80–100	You are in optimum health
60–79	You are in moderate health
40–59	You are in poor health
0–39	You are in very poor health

Tuning up your health

Now you have some sense of where you are on the scale of health, and where there's room for improvement, what do you do about improving your health and reducing your risk of becoming 'horizontally ill' in the future?

If you have a specific problem – for example, diabetes or depression, high blood pressure or asthma – turn to the chapters in Part 3 where we compare nutritional approaches to the current most commonly prescribed drugs, so you can decide which avenue you wish to pursue. At the end of each chapter there's an action plan for you to follow.

If you don't have any specific health problems but do wish to up your health rating by tuning up your digestion or your blood-sugar balance, for example, you'll find an action plan below that details changes to make to your diet and your lifestyle, and the most effective supplements to take for each key factor. Focus on the two key factors that are most out of balance and commit to these changes for three months. Reassess using this questionnaire after three months and adjust your supplement regime accordingly. The healthier you become, the less you'll need, although everyone can benefit from basic supplementation:

- A high-strength multivitamin and mineral (ideally one twice a day)

- Extra vitamin C (500mg to 1,000mg twice a day)

- Omega-3s (600mg of EPA and 400mg of DHA) and omega-6s (200mg of GLA) a day.

The details and science behind these recommendations are explained in Part 3.

Action points for balancing your blood sugar

Diet and lifestyle

- Supplement the 'energy' nutrients (vitamin C and the Bs, plus chromium, which help turn food into energy)

- Exercise every day

- Follow a low-glycemic load (GL) diet (see Chapter 8) and eat low-GL foods – maximum 40 GLs to lose weight and 60 GLs a day to maintain it

- Graze rather than gorge, eating three meals and two snacks a day

- Eat carbs with an equal amount of protein

- Avoid sugar

- Avoid caffeine (tea, coffee, caffeinated drinks), choosing non-caffeine drinks

- Don't smoke

- Minimise alcohol.

Supplements	AM	PM
High-strength multi	1	1
Vitamin C 1,000mg	1	
Chromium 200mcg	1	
Adrenal support formula*	2	

* If you're tired or coming off stimulants, try supplementing 1g of tyrosine or 'adaptogenic' herbs such as rhodiola, ginseng, Siberian ginseng (eleutheroccus) or reishi mushroom. These appear to regulate adrenal hormones.

Also read Chapter 8 which gives you more guidance on balancing your blood sugar, especially if you have diabetes.

Action points for balancing your hormones

Diet and lifestyle

- Balance your blood sugar (as above) – reduce stress

- Eat organic

- Filter all drinking water or drink natural mineral water

- Reduce your intake of animal fats and milk

- Ensure optimal intake of essential fats from seeds, fish and supplements

- Eat organic/wild salmon, trout, sardines, mackerel, herring or kippers three times a week. (If you like tuna steak, eat it only twice a month maximum due to its higher mercury content. Tinned tuna has little omega-3 in it because of the way it is processed)

- Ensure a regular intake of phytoestrogens from soya, beans and lentils.

- Don't go on the pill

- Avoid HRT with oestrogen or progestin

- Ask a nutritionist to check your salivary hormone levels. If progesterone is low, consider progesterone cream.

Supplements	AM	PM
High-strength multi	1	1
Vitamin C 1,000mg	1	1
Omega-3s and omega-6s	1	1
Agnus castus*/dong quai† (women)	1	1
or saw palmetto‡/pygeum (men)	1	1

* 90mg per day of standardised extract with one per cent agnusides

† 600mg per day of standardised extract with one per cent lingustilides

‡ 240mg per day

Also read Chapter 9, which will give you more guidance on balancing your hormones, especially if you have PMS or menopausal problems.

Action points for your mind and mood

Diet and lifestyle

- Balance your blood sugar (as above)

- Avoid colourings and additives

- Eat seeds and fish for essential fats

- Eat fish and organic/omega-3 eggs for the phospholipids

- Ensure adequate protein for amino acids, the precursors for neuro-transmitters

- Drink water and diluted juice, not caffeinated drinks

- Minimise caffeine, nicotine and alcohol.

Supplements	AM	PM
High-strength multi	1	1
Vitamin C 1,000mg	1	
Omega-3s and omega-6s	1	1
'Brain food' formula with phospholipids*	1	1
5-HTP 100mg	1–2	1–2

* Phospholipids include phosphatidyl choline, serine and DMAE. These are all found in the brain

Also read Chapters 10 and 11, which give you more guidance on balancing your mood and improving your memory, especially if you suffer from depression and memory problems.

Action points for digestion

Diet and lifestyle

- Test for and avoid your food allergies

- Minimise wheat and other gluten grains

- Limit alcohol

- Limit fried foods, especially deep-fried foods

- Eat something raw with every meal

- Eat some fermented foods, such as yogurt

- Choose whole, not refined, foods.

Supplements	AM	PM
High-strength multi	1	1
Vitamin C 1,000mg	1	
Omega-3s and omega-6s	1	1
Digestive enzymes	1 with each main meal	
A probiotic supplement or powder*	1	
L-glutamine powder (5g)	1 tsp in water last thing at night	

* Look for supplements that provide both *Lactobacillus acidophilus* and *Bifido bacteria* and millions of viable organisms per serving or capsule

Action points for detoxification

Diet and lifestyle

- Begin your detox at the weekend for nine days (two weekends and the week in between)

- Do yoga, t'ai chi or Psychocalisthenics (see Resources, page 405) every day

- Drink two litres of natural mineral water a day

- Have a large glass of fruit or vegetable juice – carrot/apple juice with water with grated ginger, or fresh watermelon juice – every other day

- Eat fruit, and especially berries, in abundance

- Eat vegetables such as tenderstem broccoli, asparagus, kale, spinach and artichokes

- Eat in moderation grains such as brown rice, corn, millet and quinoa, and oily fish such as salmon, mackerel, sardines and herring (limit tuna steak to twice a month maximum because of its higher mercury content)

- Use cold-pressed oils only

- Have a handful a day of raw nuts or seeds a day

- Avoid all wheat, meat and dairy produce.

Supplements	AM	PM
High-strength multi	1	1
Vitamin C 1,000mg	1	
Omega-3s and 6s	1	1
Antioxidant formula*	1	1
MSM 1,000mg	1	

* Antioxidants are team players. A good antioxidant formula should provide a combination of key players, namely vitamin E, C, co-enzyme Q10, lipoic acid, beta-carotene, and glutathione or N-acetyl-cysteine

Action points for allergy and inflammation

Diet and lifestyle

- Reduce environmental toxins (eat organic)

- Identify and avoid allergens

- Balance blood sugar

- Reduce oxidants and increase antioxidant-rich foods

- Eat garlic, ginger and turmeric

- Increase fish and flax seeds (sources of omega-3s)

- Reduce meat and milk (sources of arachidonic acid).

Supplements	AM	PM
High-strength multi	1	1
Vitamin C 1,000mg	1	1
Omega-3s and omega-6s	1	1
MSM/glutamine/quercetin for allergies	1	1
Or MSM/glucosamine for joint problems	1	1

Also read Chapter 13, which gives you more guidance on how to reduce inflammation, especially if you have an inflammatory health problem such as arthritis. If you suffer from eczema or asthma, read Chapter 14 too.

Action points for your immune system

Diet and lifestyle

- Don't smoke

- No more than one unit of alcohol a day, and preferably not every day

- Get enough sleep – between six and a half and eight hours a night is ideal

- Exercise regularly, preferably in natural daylight

- Eat a carrot every day

- Eat something blue/red every day

- Eat lots of fresh fruit and vegetables

- Don't eat foods you are allergic to

- Have half your diet raw and avoid fried foods

- Supplement 2–4g of vitamin C a day.

Supplements	AM	PM
High-strength multi	1	1
Vitamin C 1,000mg	1–2	1–2
Omega-3s and omega-6s	1	1
Antioxidant formula	1	1
Echinacea/black elderberry	1	1

Action points for skin, hair and nails

Diet and lifestyle

- Follow an 'optimum nutrition' diet

- Drink two litres of water/non-caffeine teas a day

- Get enough omega-3 and omega-6 fats and severely limit fried food

- Avoiding sugar and foods with a high glycemic load

- Identify and avoid food allergens

- Apply vitamin A and C to the skin, plus sunscreen, daily.

Supplements	AM	PM
High-strength multi	1	1
Vitamin C 1,000mg	1	1
Omega-3s and omega-6s	1	1
Antioxidant formula	1	1

Also read Chapter 14, which gives you more guidance on reducing inflammation in the skin, especially if you suffer from eczema or dermatitis.

Weighing it all up

In this part of the book we've seen how the body is, in essence, an ecosystem. Anything we put into it or do with it will affect the whole for better – or worse. Prescription drugs, designed to target one aspect of this complex system, end up affecting more of it than they should because of the body's myriad interconnections. Like ripples in a pool from a thrown stone, these unwanted side effects can disrupt the equilibrium of the whole and set up vicious circles, where drugs generate new symptoms of ill health that then need to be treated with new drugs.

But as we've been saying all along, you don't have to go that way. Optimum nutrition, exercise and keeping stress at bay can ensure you stay healthy and drug-free, with your six key body functions operating smoothly, as we've explored in this chapter.

What if one or more of those six key functions has already gone awry, though? You may be facing anything from type 2 diabetes to the menopause, depression or memory loss. In Part 3, we look at all these conditions in detail and at how nutrition, exercise and simple lifestyle changes weigh up against the pharmaceutical heavyweights.

Part 3

Drugs vs Food as Medicine

8.

Arresting Diabetes
Diabetes drugs vs balancing your blood sugar

EVERY FIVE MINUTES, someone in the UK is diagnosed with diabetes. There are currently at least two million diabetic Britons, and by decade's end there could be a million more. In Australia, 275 people develop diabetes every day, and most developed countries are seeing a massive rise in this insidious disease.[1] Meanwhile, in South Africa, 40 per cent of the female population is classified as obese or overweight, making the prediction that every second or third woman in the country will be diabetic by 2025 all too possible.[2]

In short, we're in the middle of a diabetes epidemic – type 2 diabetes, that is. This used to be known as 'mature onset' because it usually develops after the age of 40, and in fact if you are over 40, you have a one in ten risk of developing the condition. (Type 1 diabetes is the rarer form, often developing in childhood and treated with daily insulin injections. We focus on type 2 in this book.)

If trends hold, the incidence of type 2 diabetes in the over-forties will be one in six for most countries where the Western diet prevails. Your risk is even higher if you are Asian and have a family history of diabetes, cardiovascular disease and high cholesterol.

Even more disturbing than all this is the possibility that as many as half the over-forties in the West have 'dysglycemia' – the technical term for the blood-sugar imbalance that is the forerunner of type 2 diabetes. So the odds are not in your favour.

The prevalence of diabetes has led to a raft of drug treatments. But there are simple, extremely effective ways of controlling this condition that don't involve drugs and focus instead on balancing blood sugar. We'll look at both later. For now, let's examine the condition in more detail.

The bitter truth – type 2 rising

Basically, diabetes is what happens when you have too much sugar in your blood. This is risky because glucose – blood sugar, which fuels our brain and body – is highly toxic in large amounts, damaging arteries, brain cells, kidneys and the eyes. Glucose also feeds infections, chronic inflammation and promotes the formation of blood clots; some 80 per cent of people with diabetes die from cardiovascular disease. Every year, a thousand people with diabetes start kidney dialysis, while others go blind. Half of all diabetics have one or more of these complications. So the human cost is very high.

Unsurprisingly, diabetes is also a drain on health services in the West. In the UK alone, diabetes costs the National Health Service more than £5 billion a year – over £10 million a day. In Australia, it's one of the top five causes of death.

As we've seen, the chances are that you already have some degree of blood-sugar imbalance. This is the prerequisite to developing diabetes. Check yourself out on the questionnaire below.

How is your blood sugar balance?

☐ Are you rarely wide awake within 15 minutes of rising?

☐ Do you need tea, coffee, a cigarette or something sweet to get you going in the morning?

☐ Do you crave chocolate, sweet foods, bread, cereal or pasta?

☐ Do you often have energy slumps during the day or after meals?

☐ Do you crave something sweet or a stimulant after meals?

☐ Do you often have mood swings or difficulty concentrating?

☐ Do you get dizzy or irritable if you go six hours without food?

☐ Do you find you overreact to stress?

☐ Is your energy now less than it used to be?

☐ Do you feel too tired to exercise?

☐ Are you gaining weight, and finding it hard to lose, even though you're not noticeably eating more or exercising less?

☐ Are you losing weight, and find it hard to gain?

☐ Do you get very thirsty and pee a lot – especially at night?

☐ Do you get blurred vision?

☐ Do you get genital itching or frequent thrush?

If you answered yes to:

Less than 4: your blood-sugar balance is reasonably good. The ideal is to have no 'yes' answers.

4 to 9: you have the indications of a potential blood-sugar problem and need to take our advice in this chapter seriously. Recheck your score in one month. If your number of yeses hasn't gone down, see a nutritional therapist.

10 or more: you have a major blood-sugar problem. The last four questions, particularly, are potential indicators of undiagnosed diabetes. We recommend you go to your doctor or practice nurse and get your blood-sugar level checked.

See page 136 below for a discussion of diabetes tests you might encounter at your doctor's.

Normally the amount of glucose in your blood is kept within a healthy range by a set of hormones. Insulin is the one involved in lowering blood sugar, whereas three other hormones – glucagon, cortisol and adrenalin – help counterbalance the effect of insulin and raise blood sugar if it is falling rapidly or when it is low.

After a meal, the carbohydrates that you have eaten are broken down into the simplest sugar, glucose, which is absorbed from the gut into your bloodstream. Then specific cells in the pancreas, called beta cells, begin to pump out insulin, whose job it is to clear the glucose away, stashing it either in the muscles where it provides instant energy, or in fat cells, where it's stored. As part of this system, glucose is also stored and released by the liver.

If this system goes wrong and your blood-sugar levels start skyrocketing, it's for one of two reasons: either you are not making enough insulin, or the insulin you produce isn't doing its job. Both of these are most commonly the result of a combination of genetic predisposition, a lack of physical activity, chronic stress and overloading your bloodstream with glucose, over and over again, until your cells either become 'resistant' to insulin or just can't produce enough any more.

Glucose overload will happen if you're eating lots of refined carbohydrates – say, cornflakes, white bread, white pasta, cakes and biscuits. Eating a big bowl of refined cereal or a large portion of refined pasta, for instance, will cause sudden peaks of blood glucose, triggering the release of extra insulin to deal with it. As this is 'fast-release' carbohydrate, you'll then experience a sudden slump. Eating refined carbohydrates at every meal puts you on a blood-sugar rollercoaster.

Eventually, you can develop type 2 diabetes. This accounts for eight out of every ten cases. This form of diabetes is a diet and lifestyle disease that simply doesn't happen in countries where a traditional, wholefood diet and a lot of physical activity still prevail. After 30 or 40 years of a typical Western diet with little exercise, the excessive demands for insulin take their toll and eventually the pancreas just can't produce enough any more. So about a third of type 2 diabetics end up needing insulin injections in order to sustain this unhealthy diet and lifestyle.

Insulin resistance and obesity

But there is also a change in the way the body responds to insulin. As a person edges towards diabetes, their cells become less sensitive to its effects. Normally insulin sends a message to cells like those in your muscles and fat deposits, telling them to open up and start storing glucose. But after years of levels that are higher than the system was designed for, the storage cells start to ignore the message insulin is sending out. Known as 'insulin resistance', this state is made worse by the damage that raised glucose levels have been inflicting on your arteries.

There's another factor at work here, also related to our lifestyle, and that's obesity. There's a strong link between overweight and type 2 diabetes (around 80 per cent of people with diabetes are also over-weight), and as everyone knows, obesity levels in the West are soaring. Until recently it wasn't clear why, but current thinking is that fatty acids and proteins released from fat stores[3] – especially the fat around your middle, known as 'visceral fat' – actively interfere with the messages that normally allow glucose to be stored.

Although it might seem strange to think of it this way, insulin resistance in muscles and fat stores may have originated as a valuable adaptation to maintain glucose supplies in times of starvation and other forms of stress, giving the brain enough to keep going.[4] So you can think of this common combination of health problems, often called 'syndrome X' – fat round the middle (the so-called 'apple shape'), insulin resistance, blood sugar problems and cardiovascular disease (itself a combination of high cholesterol and blood pressure) – as your body's best effort to adapt to an unhealthy diet and lifestyle that's become the norm in the twenty-first century.

Testing, testing

If you've done the questionnaire on page 133 or feel you fit the criteria for syndrome X, you may want to ask your doctor to run a diabetes test on you. The standard way of testing is to check how efficiently your body can clear glucose out of the bloodstream. So after you haven't eaten for a while – such as overnight – a blood test is taken. Then you have a drink containing a measured amount of glucose, and over the next two hours several more blood samples are taken to see how fast you are getting rid of it. By the end of the two-hour period, the level of glucose in your blood should normally be below 7.8 mmol/l (equivalent to 120mg/dl in the US). If it is between 7.8 and 11 mmol/l you've got dysglycemia, which means your system is not handling glucose as well as it should. Over 11mmol/l(200mg/dl) and you've probably got diabetes.

Another blood test measures how sugar-coated your red blood cells have become from too much blood glucose. It's called glycosylated haemoglobin, abbreviated to HbA1c. This should not be above eight per cent and ideally should be closer to four per cent.

Caught before it has done too much damage, type 2 diabetes should be a fairly straightforward disorder to treat. As we've seen, the main causes are a particular sort of diet and a lack of exercise, and the remedy is simply to eat a diet and follow a lifestyle that stabilises your blood sugar levels and restores insulin sensitivity. But this approach takes some time and effort to be effective, so most people with diabetes are prescribed drugs. Let's examine how effective these are.

Diabetes drugs

Diabetes drugs are big business. In Britain sales are now worth close to £1 billion a year and rising. They work by affecting different parts of the body's glucose balancing act – either by making cells more responsive to insulin or by boosting insulin production. If you've got diabetes, chances are you'll be on one or more of these drugs.

There are three main types of diabetes drugs on the market.

Biguanides

Metformin is the main one in this class. It's been around for about 30 years and is still the most widely used. Metformin works to lower your levels of blood sugar by increasing insulin sensitivity in the muscles so they take up more glucose. It also increases sensitivity in the liver, which means that organ doesn't release so much glucose. It doesn't cause weight gain –

which other treatments do – and may even result in some weight loss. It's the best of the bunch, but is even more effective if you are following the diabetes-friendly diet and lifestyle outlined later in this chapter.

SIDE EFFECTS When you start using metformin, it frequently causes gastrointestinal symptoms such as mild nausea, cramps and vomiting, and soft or loose stools, although a new, slow-release formulation minimises the likelihood of these side effects.

It has a black-box warning (the most serious sort) in the US because of a very small risk of a potentially fatal condition known as 'lactic acidosis'. That said, it's probably one of the better diabetic drugs.

Few doctors are aware that metformin knocks out vitamin B12 and may cause vitamin B12 deficiency in about a third of those who take it.[5] This in its turn is likely to allow homocysteine levels to rise (see page 301), which in turn increases the risk of heart attack. You can counter this by increasing your intake, perhaps by taking a supplement specifically designed to lower your homocysteine level, containing vitamin B6, B12 and folic acid (see page 304). Because metformin is processed in the kidneys, it shouldn't be used if you have serious kidney problems.

Sulfonylureas

Brands include Amaryl, Euglucon and Diamicron. These drugs stimulate the beta cells in the pancreas to produce more insulin. Most type 2 diabetics produce too much insulin already – the problem is that the insulin that's produced just does not function properly. It makes little sense to stimulate the pancreas to produce even more in order to accommodate the very same poor dietary choices that lead to the development of diabetes in the first place. When you get your diet right, these drugs often become unnecessary.

SIDE EFFECTS The most common side effect with sulfonylureas is an excess of insulin, causing too much glucose to the taken out of blood. This can lead to a potentially serious drop in glucose supplies to the brain, known as a 'hypo', which can lead to feeling dizzy, or fainting, as blood-sugar levels go too low. Watch out if you've suddenly improved your diet, as this side effect may become more common as your need for the drug decreases. For instance, within six weeks of eating our recommended 'low-glycemic load diet' (see page 143), one patient's blood-sugar level normalised and she started experiencing hypos when she took her Amaryl. Her doctor then stopped the drug.

Sulfonylureas can also cause gastrointestinal problems including nausea, vomiting and diarrhoea, or constipation and weight gain. The weight gain can be significant, triggered by rising insulin levels in people who typically have dangerously high levels to begin with. There is also evidence that they flog the pancreas into early failure, so control of sugar, although quick, is brief. Not surprisingly, we feel sulphonylureas are bad news.

Glitazones

Brands of this drug family include Actos (Pioglitazone) and Avandamet® (Rosiglitazone). Also known as thiazolilinediones, these are relatively new drugs that work by making cells more sensitive to the effects of insulin.

SIDE EFFECTS The first of these drugs to arrive on the market (Rezulin) was banned in the US in 2000 due to deaths from liver failure. In 2002 it was found that later versions can also damage the liver.[6] Glitazones may, according to a study published in 2003, also cause heart failure and a buildup of fluid in the lungs (pulmonary oedema).[7]

There is evidence that these drugs can cause weight gain.[8] This is, in part, the result of increased body water and more subcutaneous fat (that is, fat under the skin throughout the body), although visceral fat (fat in the abdomen and between the abdominal organs) is reduced, which is positive.

Newer drugs

The latest variant on glitazones both increases insulin sensitivity and increases levels of the 'good' cholesterol HDL. One of these, Pargluva (Muraglitazar) was recently approved by the US Food and Drug Administration. However, a controlled trial published at the same time, in 2005, found it more than doubled the incidence of deaths, heart attacks or strokes, even though this trial had excluded people with cardiovascular problems.[9]

Muraglitazar can also promote significant weight gain. Our advice is to tread carefully with these new drugs. Their long-term effects are largely unknown.

Yet more drugs?

It's very clear that the individual drugs used to control insulin and blood sugar levels come with a fairly hefty range of side effects, perhaps with the exception of metformin. People with diabetes also usually have two related problems – high blood pressure and overweight or obesity, which may have increased even more as a side effect of the insulin-boosting drugs they've taken. If this applies to you, your doctor might have recommended you take a drug to lose weight.

The main two are orlistat (Xenical) and sibutramine (Meridia/Reductil), but their effectiveness is not impressive and they come with side effects that can be lethal.

A recent review of 22 studies involving Xenical and Reductil (18 of which were carried out by the drug companies involved – see Chapter 3 for how that can skew the results) concluded that they 'may help type 2 diabetes patients to lose small amounts of weight' but that 'long term health benefits are unclear'.[10]

That is putting it politely. The actual average weight loss was 13lb (about 6kg) – after taking these drugs for four years – with patients who weighed nearly 250lb (113kg).[11] The side effects are such that the American consumer activist group Public Citizen has petitioned the Food and Drug Administration (FDA) to take both of them off the market. This is same group that petitioned the FDA to remove Vioxx three years before it was finally withdrawn.

Xenical may reduce your risk of diabetes but, because it reduces fat absorption in the gut, it can interfere with your absorption of fat-soluble vitamins and cause loose stools and anal leakage. More seriously, it has been linked with causing precancerous changes to the lining of the intestines.[12]

Reductil has been found to reduce glucose levels, but because it works by raising serotonin levels it can also cause raised blood pressure (serotonin constricts blood vessels). In his testimony to Congress in the wake of the Vioxx scandal, Dr David Graham, associate safety director of the FDA, named five drugs that he believed should also be withdrawn on safety grounds – one of them was Reductil.[13] According to the journal *Science*, 'Between February 1998 and September 2001, 150 patients taking Reductil worldwide were hospitalized and 29 died, 19 from cardio-vascular problems.'[14]

For hypertension, the American Diabetic Association recommends treatment with drugs that lower blood pressure. A 2003 study following 1,860 Swedish men, however, found that those with raised glucose levels had a higher risk of heart attack but that those who had been treated with the blood pressure-lowering drugs beta-blockers and diuretics had an added risk of heart attack.[15]

Recent research also shows that diabetics on the popular insulin-increasing sulfonylurea drugs are also further raising the risk of death from cardiovascular disease. A five-year study of 5,500 diabetics, published in 2006 in the *Canadian Medical Association Journal*, found that the higher the drug dose and the more consistently the patients took the drugs, the greater the risk of cardiovascular death.[16] So being on both blood pressure-lowering drugs and sulfonylureas is particularly bad news for some people.

Going down the drug route leads you into a maze of competing side effects, and yet more drugs to control them. Even if the drugs achieve the short-term goals of controlling your blood-sugar levels, there's evidence – which we'll come to below – that you can do it more effectively in the longer term with diet and exercise.

Natural alternatives

So just how effective is a healthy diet plus exercise in preventing or treating diabetes in the longer term? We should note that trials on lifestyle are much harder to do than trials on pills, but a good attempt was made by researchers at George Washington University in Washington DC, who published their findings in 2005.

The team selected volunteers who had signs of dysglycemia (glucose intolerance) and were therefore at high risk of developing diabetes, then split them into three groups. One received placebos, the next 850mg of metformin twice a day, and the third began to make lifestyle changes designed to lower weight by seven per cent, including two and a half hours of exercise a week (20 minutes a day). At the end of three years, among those who made the lifestyle changes, 41 per cent were no longer glucose intolerant. Among those who took metformin, 17 per cent were no longer glucose intolerant, compared to the placebo. So the lifestyle change was more than twice as effective.[17]

What's more, despite the prevailing medical view, the dietary approach is likely to be more cost-effective. Based on the data from a massive diabetes prevention programme launched in the US in 2002, Dr William Herman, professor of internal medicine at the University of Michigan School of Medicine, built a computer simulation to estimate the cost-effectiveness of changing one's lifestyle versus taking diabetes drugs.[18]

'There's been a debate about how to implement lifestyle intervention. Many say it can't be done. It's too expensive,' says Herman. However, his study – published in 2006 – showed that taking metformin might delay the onset of diabetes by three years, while diet and exercise change delays it by 11 years. His team estimated that the drug would cost $29,000 per year of healthy life saved, while the diet and exercise regime would cost $8,800. 'The bottom line,' says Herman, 'is that lifestyle intervention is more cost-effective than a pill.'

Another landmark study, which also found diet and exercise twice as effective as metformin in preventing at-risk patients from developing diabetes, estimated that the non-drug approach was also very cost-effective.[19] In this study, published in 2002, one case of diabetes was prevented in every seven people treated for three years.

A trial published in 2005 and involving obese and overweight people with diabetes or insulin resistance showed a 50 per cent reversal of insulin resistance and diabetes after only three weeks when placed on a high-fibre, low-fat diet, combined with 45 to 60 minutes of exercise on a treadmill each day.[20] The 31 volunteers in this residential trial at the Pritikin Longevity Center in California took on a diet that didn't even restrict the amount of food, but just gave better choices of unrefined carbohydrates, wholefoods and low-fat foods. In only three weeks the volunteers, aged 46 to 76, had lower glucose levels, better insulin resistance and a lower body-mass index. Not bad for three weeks!

The perfect diet for diabetes prevention

This kind of trial makes it glaringly obvious that the solution to diabetes is not going to be drugs – they just slow down the inevitable. The solution is changing the way of eating, and living, that led to diabetes in the first place. Then we need to find out what the best anti-diabetes diet is – along with the best way to motivate people to change.

The low-GL route

Luckily, we already know what the best diet to help people recover from type 2 diabetes is. It's the low-glycemic load (GL) diet, which we've already mentioned a few times in this book. Currently this is a very popular and effective way of losing weight, but on top of that, it is the absolute state-of-the-art diet for controlling blood sugar, preventing diabetes, and also for regaining energy.

This is how it works. The carbohydrates contained in foods are turned into glucose at different speeds. For example, the carbohydrates in strawberries are 'slow-releasing', which means they raise your blood-sugar level fairly gradually. But eat a date, and your blood-glucose level will begin climbing within minutes – they are very fast-releasing. The rate at which a food releases its sugar is known as its glycemic index (GI). The fastest-releasing food is pure glucose, which is given a score of 100 on the index, while apples, which raise blood sugar at less than half the rate of pure glucose, score 38.

The GI is a useful way of rating foods if you want to stabilise your blood glucose because it allows you to choose slow-releasing carbohydrates. But it has one big limitation. It doesn't tell you how much carbohydrate there is in a particular food. Watermelon, for example, has very little carbohydrate in it, as it's mostly water; but the carbs in it are fast-releasing, so it does have a very high GI. Sweet potatoes, on the other hand, have a low-GI carbohydrate, but lots of it. Basing your choice on GI alone, you'd probably opt for sweet potatoes and avoid watermelons, but in fact, the large amount of sugar in a portion of sweet potato would push your blood glucose up much more than a large slice of watermelon would.

This is where glycemic load comes in. A food's GL takes into account not just the type of carbohydrate in it – slow or fast-releasing – but also how much there is of that carbohydrate in the food. You work it out by multiplying a food's GI by the amount of carbohydrate in it. One date, for example, is five GLs, as is a large punnet of strawberries. Two bowls of oat flakes is five GLs – as is half a bowl of cornflakes!

To control your blood sugar, you need to eat no more than 65 GLs a day (45 if you want to lose weight), spread out throughout the day at roughly 10 to 15 GLs per meal plus 5 to 10 GLs for a snack (you should have two in-between snacks a day), with 5 GLs to spare for drinks or desserts. So if you were diabetic and wanted to stabilise your blood sugar, you'd eat a bowl of oat flakes or porridge with berries for breakfast. Your blood sugar level would stay even, you wouldn't need to produce so much insulin and, in time, you would actual regain insulin sensitivity and stabilise your blood sugar. Gradually, if you stuck with it, the need for diabetic drugs would become increasingly unnecessary.

The Holford Low-GL Diet explains how you put a low-GL diet together in detail, but for now the tables below give you an idea of which foods are high and which low GL, what to avoid, and how a day's healthy menu might look.

10 GL serving of common foods

Low-GL foods	High-GL foods
2 large punnets of strawberries	2 dates
6 oatcakes	1 slice of white bread
4 bowls of oat flakes	1 bowl of cornflakes
A large bowl of peanuts	A packet of crisps
1 pint (550ml) of tomato juice	Half glass of Lucozade
6 tablespoons of xylitol (a natural low-GL sugar)	2 teaspoons of honey
10 handfuls of green beans	10 French fries

'GOOD' LOW-GL DAY'S DIET		'BAD' HIGH-GL DAY'S DIET	
Breakfast	GL	*Breakfast*	GL
A bowl of porridge	2	A bowl of cornflakes	21
Half a grated apple	3	A banana	12
A small tub of yogurt	2	Milk	2
and some milk	2		
Total	9	Total	35
Snack		*Snack*	
A punnet of strawberries	5	Mars bar	26
Lunch		*Lunch*	
Substantial tuna salad,		Tuna salad baguette	15
plus 3 oatcakes	10		
Snack		*Snack*	
A pear		Bag of crisps	11
and a handful of peanuts	4		
Dinner		*Dinner*	
Tomato soup, salmon		Pizza with Parmesan and	
Sweetcorn, green beans	12	tomato sauce and some salad	23
'GOOD' DAY'S TOTAL GL	**40**	**'BAD' DAY'S TOTAL GL**	**110**

The protein connection

Going for slow-release carbohydrates is only part of the story, however. Another way to lower the GL of your diet is to eat more protein, fibre and healthy fats, as well as cutting out refined, sugary carb-rich foods such as biscuits. The controversial low-carbohydrate/high-protein Atkins Diet, for instance, has recently been shown to lead to both weight loss and improved glucose control in two small studies.

One, published in 2005, put ten obese diabetic patients on the Atkins Diet for two weeks. They spontaneously reduced their calorific intake by 1,000 calories a day[21] as well as improved their insulin sensitivity. And a 2004 study at the Metabolic Research Laboratory of the VA Medical Center in Minneapolis, Minnesota, put eight patients on a diet with 20 per cent carbs, 30 per cent protein and 50 per cent fat, which reduced glucose levels 'dramatically'.[22] While high-protein diets, especially those based on meat, milk and cheese, may create other problems such as a heightened risk of kidney problems, osteoporosis, breast and prostate cancer, it seems that eating protein with low-GL carbohydrates does help stabilise blood-sugar levels. Examples would be chicken kebabs with a piece of brown pitta bread; chickpeas with a small portion of brown basmati rice; or fish with wholewheat pasta.

So choosing the best low-GL carbs and combining those with quality proteins is the cornerstone of diabetes treatment and prevention, and is also now recommended by most diabetes associations. But the potential for certain foods to lower glucose and improve insulin sensitivity and release will continue to shape the perfect anti-diabetes diet (see 'The best new anti-diabetic foods and nutrients' box below).

THE BEST NEW ANTI-DIABETIC FOODS AND NUTRIENTS

A spoonful of cinnamon

It's now been found that just half a teaspoon of cinnamon a day significantly reduces blood-sugar levels in diabetics, and could also benefit millions of non-diabetics who have blood-sugar problems but are unaware of it.

The discovery was initially made by accident. Dr Richard Anderson at the US Department of Agriculture's Human Nutrition Research Center in Beltsville, Maryland, was looking at the effect of common foods on blood sugar. He was surprised to discover that apple pie (spiced with cinnamon) was actually not bad for blood sugar.

The active ingredient in cinnamon turned out to be a water-soluble polyphenol compound called MHCP. In the lab, MHCP mimics insulin, activates its receptor, and works synergistically with insulin in cells – improving glucose metabolism twentyfold. In short, it helps insulin do its job of getting excess sugar out of the bloodstream and into the cells.

To see if it would work in people, volunteers with type 2 diabetes were given 1, 3 or 6g of cinnamon powder per day, in capsules after meals. As the paper, published in 2003, shows, all responded to the cinnamon within weeks, with blood-sugar levels 20 per cent lower on average than those of a control group.[23] Some of the volunteers taking cinnamon even achieved normal blood-sugar levels. Tellingly, blood sugar started creeping up again after the diabetics stopped taking cinnamon.

Cinnamon has other significant benefits. In the diabetic volunteers, it lowered blood levels of fats (triglycerides) and 'bad' LDL cholesterol, both also partly controlled by insulin. In the lab experiments, it neutralised damaging free radicals.

Luckily, cinnamon is a versatile spice. You'll need about half a teaspoon a day, added perhaps to oatmeal, fruit salads, marinades, stews or curries.

Get your oats – and xylitol

Oats, or specifically oat bran, contain a powerful anti-diabetes nutrient. It's called beta-glucan. Diabetic patients given oatmeal or oat-bran rich foods experienced much lower rises in blood sugar compared to those who were given white rice or bread. In fact, it's been known for nearly a decade that having ten per cent of your diet as beta-glucans can halve the blood-sugar peak of a meal.[24-25]

This level of effect is far greater than you'll get from taking metformin (see page 137), at a fraction of the price and with none of the side effects. Practically, that means eating half oat flakes, half oat bran, cold or hot as porridge, with a low-GL fruit such as berries, pears or apples, and snacking on oat cakes (rough oat cakes have the most beta-glucans). With over 1,000 studies on beta-glucans, the evidence really is overwhelming. (Oats have a relatively low GL, too.)

Other big contenders for anti-diabetic foods include buckwheat, green tea, cherries and plums and other fruits high in a very low-GL sugar called xylitol.[26] Xylitol has a ninth of the GL of sugar or honey; so while you can't scoff it indiscriminately, switching to it and using it sparingly will certainly cut your total GLs significantly if you like to indulge a sweet tooth.

Chromium – the forgotten mineral

While drugs like metformin increase sensitivity to insulin, there's a mineral that does the same thing – but with no significant downsides. It's called chromium, and insulin can't work properly without it.

Trivalent chromium was discovered to be an essential mineral back in the 1960s. This form of chromium, the kind found in foods, is completely different from the kind you find in old car bumpers. (This is called hexavalent chromium and can be quite toxic.) In the 1970s, chromium was proven to be essential for insulin to do its job properly, but the mechanism hadn't been discovered.[27] Now we know how it manages the job.

Chromium does two things. Firstly, insulin has to dock on to cells to open them up for the next delivery of glucose. Chromium is part of the docking port, or receptor, for the insulin. It also helps stop insulin from being changed in a way that stops it working. Both of these improve your sensitivity to insulin.

Today we also know that many of us are deficient in this mineral, which is absolutely essential for good health.[28] In other words, your doctor should really check that you are not chromium deficient, since this alone can cause blood-sugar problems and insulin resistance.

But how do you know if you're chromium deficient? Without testing, this isn't easy to ascertain.

Tell-tale signs are low energy, especially in the morning, feeling groggy, craving sweet foods and depression. The more sugar or refined food you eat the more likely you are to be deficient, not only because processed foods are low in chromium, but also because they rob the body of chromium. Every time your blood sugar goes up, whether due to sugar, stress or a stimulant such as coffee or a cigarette, you lose chromium. The older you are and more stressed you are, the lower your levels. And if you're diabetic, it is very likely indeed that you're deficient. (See page 150 for the evidence on chromium as a treatment for diabetes.)

So what's the evidence?

Now let's look at the evidence for all these claims, from low-GL diets to chromium supplementation as a way of regulating blood-sugar levels.

The lowdown on low GL

'There is no question that low-GL is pushing back the boundaries in terms of safe, rapid and permanent weight-loss diets and for diabetes. The evidence has been mounting for some time,' says Dr David Haslam, medical doctor and clinical director of the UK National Obesity Forum. Study after study has shown that low-GL diets not only cause rapid weight loss but also improve insulin resistance and fasting glucose (which is the concentration of glucose remaining in your blood after you have not eaten for eight to 12 hours).[29–30] In animal studies, it's well known that a low-GL diet rapidly improves blood-sugar control and pancreatic function.[31]

All of this translates into a massive reduction in risk of developing diabetes, as well as the ability to stop and even reverse the condition, especially for those in the early stages of type 2 diabetes.

Back in the early 1990s, researchers at the Harvard School of Public Health in the US monitored the health of over 100,000 middle-aged men and women for six years and found that those who ate a high-GL diet were one and a half times more likely to develop diabetes than those who ate a low-GL diet.[32–33] In a study published in 2003, another group of researchers at Harvard put obese adolescents on either an unlimited low-GL diet or a low-calorie, low-fat diet. In addition to losing more weight, those on the low-GL diet experienced less insulin resistance, while those on the conventional low-fat, low-calorie diet worsened theirs.[34]

There's really no question that a low-GL diet rapidly improves blood sugar and the symptoms of diabetes. More than that, its side effects are side benefits: increased energy, better sleep, better mood and less craving for carbohydrates. This is exactly what we found in our own research, a survey of 72 people who had followed the Holford Low-GL Diet, followed by a study of 20 people we placed on this diet. The weight loss was 1.7lb (0.8kg) a week in the survey and 10.25lb (4.6kg) in eight weeks (1.3lb, or about 0.6kg, a week) in the study, which was published in 2006. Most people's blood-sugar levels normalised and most reported more energy.[35]

A DOZEN ANTI-DIABETIC FOODS

- Apples
- Berries
- Buckwheat
- Cherries
- Chickpeas
- Cinnamon
- Green tea
- Lentils
- Oat bran and flakes
- Oat cakes
- Pears
- Plums

Can chromium take the place of drugs?

We know chromium restores blood-sugar balance and hence prevents or improves the symptoms of diabetes. But is it an alternative to drugs like metformin? There have been over 20 trials on chromium, not all of which have shown positive results. Generally, those that gave patients below 250mcg a day were less effective. Also, those using less bioavailable (that is, easily useable by the body) forms of chromium such as chromium chloride didn't work as well as those giving chromium picolinate, which is a highly bioavailable form.[36]

There aren't enough decent trials that have given sufficient chromium in the right form, but those that have are very encouraging. For example, a Chinese study published in 1999 gave 833 patients with type 2 diabetes 500mcg of chromium picolinate for 10 months. As you can see from the figure opposite, there was a major improvement in both the participant's fasting blood-sugar levels and blood-sugar levels after meals, and it also reduced the incidence of diabetes symptoms, including fatigue, thirst and frequent urination.[37]

Another study published in 1999 showed that the combination of chromium and the B vitamin biotin appears particularly effective, since biotin is essential for the release of insulin.[38] In the 30-day study, 12

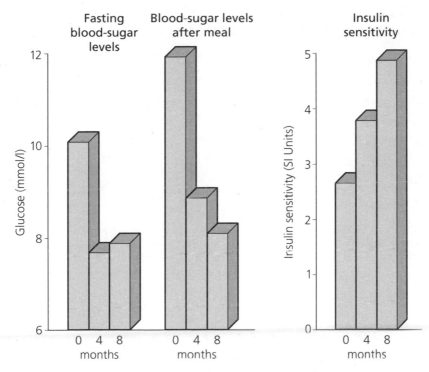

Fasting blood-sugar levels

Blood-sugar levels after meal

Insulin sensitivity

Glucose (mmol/l)

Insulin sensitivity (SI Units)

0 4 8 months

0 4 8 months

0 4 8 months

Length of time taking chromium supplements

The effects of chromium on blood sugar and insulin resistance

type 2 diabetics took a daily dose of 600mcg of chromium picolinate and 2mg of biotin, while another 12 took a placebo. All the subjects had previously taken anti-diabetic drugs, but still had difficulty managing sugar levels.

Those taking the chromium and biotin supplement had a 26mg/dl (1.43mmol/l) drop in fasting blood glucose with more than 70 per cent of the supplement group experiencing significant drops. LDL (bad) cholesterol levels also decreased substantially.[39] Compare that with what happened to patients taking metformin in a key 2002 study comparing metformin with diet.[40] During the first six months of taking metformin, the subjects' average fasting blood glucose dropped by only about 3mg/dl (0.17mmol/l) .

There's also good evidence that chromium can help prevent diabetes in people at risk. In a study published in 1999, a group of 29 people who were both overweight and had a family history of diabetes were given 1,000mcg of chromium a day for eight months or a placebo. Their insulin sensitivity improved dramatically on chromium, but not on the placebo, as the trial progressed.[41]

The US Food and Drug Administration is sufficiently convinced by the evidence so far, and have allowed one US supplement company to state that 'chromium picolinate may reduce the risk of insulin resistance, and therefore possibly may reduce the risk of type 2 diabetes'. However, any such claim in Europe or Australia, where laws on nutritional supplements are exceptionally tight, would lead to chromium being banned and classified as a medicine! (See Chapter 17.)

What are chromium's side effects? Fortunately, it is remarkably safe. According to a report published by the World Health Organization, based on a trial with rats, you'd need to take 20,000,000mcg of chromium – that's 100,000 regular chromium supplements a day – to reach toxic levels.[42] Suffice it to say that up to 1,000mcg is perfectly safe, even in pregnancy. Long-term studies of up to five years, published in 2004, have shown this to be the case.[43]

Finding the motivation

Tony is a typical example of someone who has benefited from a low-GL diet plus chromium. A year ago he was diagnosed with borderline diabetes following a minor stroke. He was put on medication to lower his high blood pressure, but not for his diabetes. Instead, he was told to monitor it twice a day and eat a low-sugar diet. His blood sugar, which should be below 7mmol/l, would fluctuate between 6.3 and 12.8mmol/l despite his attempts to eat healthily. He was also gaining weight.

Then he switched to a low-GL diet plus chromium. After eight weeks, his blood-sugar levels normalised and consistently fell below the ideal of 5.5mmol/l. As he says,

'I have a lot more energy, I feel fitter. I'm sleeping better, but fewer hours, and feeling less tired. I've also lost 28lb [13kg] in weight and I have also seen an improvement in my cholesterol, homocysteine and blood-sugar levels, and as a consequence I have been fully discharged by my hospital consultant. I'm managing to keep it off without too much difficulty. My blood pressure is now normal and my next goal is to reduce my medication for that.'

Linda experienced something very similar. Within six weeks on a low-GL diet plus chromium, she had not only stabilised her blood-sugar levels, lost her craving for sweet foods and 16lb (almost 8kg) to boot, she had to reduce her medication because she was getting hypos – low blood sugar. She had been taking Amaryl, a sulfonylurea drug, plus metformin (see pages 138 and 137 respectively). Once her blood sugar had normalised, she was able to stop her Amaryl. Six months later, eating low GL has become part of her life, she's lost 35lb (16kg), her blood sugar has remained stable and she no longer gets sugar lows. Her doctor has kept her on metformin.

It's best to approach changing your diet much as you would redecorating your house. You need to do the preparation, such as shopping for your new foods. Expect a week or two of disruption, then look forward to the results. For Tony and Linda, this way of eating has become the norm.

Food or drugs? The verdict

For diabetes and its precursors dysglycemia and insulin resistance, there is no doubt that making the right diet and lifestyle changes is essential. Eating a low-GL diet, taking supplements, staying away from sugar and taking regular exercise can both prevent and significantly reverse insulin resistance and diabetes, at least in the early stages, far more so than currently available medication. For those with more advanced diabetes these changes are highly likely to reduce the need for medication and, in the case of insulin-dependent diabetes, for insulin too.

Unlike the side effects from the drugs we discussed at the start of the chapter, the only ones you'll get from a low-GL anti-diabetes diet are more energy; a lowered risk for cardiovascular disease, cancer and arthritis; better mood and concentration; and weight control – to name only a few. In other words, no downsides and no risks.

What works

- Eat a low-GL diet (roughly 45 to 65 GLs a day)

- Combine protein foods with carbohydrate foods, which stabilise blood-sugar levels even further

- Avoid all sugar, except xylitol

- Sprinkle half a teaspoon of cinnamon on your food daily

- Eat oats with oat bran for breakfast and snack on rough oat cakes

- Exercise every day – for at least 30 minutes

- Take a supplement of a high-strength multivitamin and mineral, plus 2g of vitamin C and 200mcg of chromium (400 or 600mcg if you have diabetes, taken in the morning or at lunch – chromium can over-energise so it's best not taken in the evening)

- Dig deeper by reading books (see Recommended Reading, page 398), attending a workshop, seeing a nutritional therapist or joining a club or evening classes that can help you get and stay on track. (See Resources, page 392.)

Working with your doctor

Despite the undeniable evidence that changing your diet and lifestyle works better than just popping pills, you may need to persuade your doctor that this is the way you want to go. One of the best ways of doing this is to cite the evidence.

For instance, the attitude among too many doctors is that no patient can be bothered to make the necessary shifts. A major review of the causes of diabetes in the leading journal *Science*, for instance, described a dozen genes and proteins involved in the disorder and how they could all be targeted with new drugs. 'Other drugs are urgently needed to treat the diabetes epidemic,' it concluded, 'because people are unlikely to cut back on food intake and start exercising any time soon.'[44]

To add to the malaise, the most recent guidelines from NICE (the National Institute for Health and Clinical Excellence), which your doctor is likely to rely on for guidance, are distinctly lukewarm about non-drug treatments.[45] The main type of diet it considers is the low-fat/high-carbohydrate diet, which these days looks an odd way to handle a blood-glucose problem. The research it quotes found only 'modest improvements' and that they were 'short lived'. Educating people about their condition and teaching them to change their behaviour was 'partially effective' although none of these efforts at education was any better than the rest. But the issue here may be more about failing to motivate people to make the right kind of changes. For some ideas on how to change your relationship with your doctor see Chapter 21.

If you're lucky, your doctor will be delighted straightaway at your wish to pursue a low-GL diet and exercise. Others will need a bit of convincing, but you shouldn't give up. Just keep what we've discussed in mind. For instance, despite the evidence, most doctors are not that informed about chromium – so you can point out the studies that will do the job.

It's particularly important to work with your doctor if you're on drugs for your diabetes. If you are on sulfonylurea drugs, these should be the first to go as your blood sugar stabilises, but be aware that your blood-sugar level and use of these drugs will need careful monitoring as you improve your nutrition. Your doctor will be invaluable for helping you keep within safe blood-sugar limits.

9.

Balancing Hormones in the Menopause
The HRT scandal vs natural control

FOR MANY WOMEN approaching middle age, the most worrying aspect of the menopause is not the increased risk of illness – osteoporosis, breast cancer or heart disease. It's having to cope with the debilitating symptoms that will affect nearly half of them: hot flushes, fatigue, headaches, irritability, insomnia, depression and a decreased sex drive.

For years, doctors faced with women stressed out by feeling snappish, depressed or hounded by their own hot flushes handed out hormone replacement therapy, or HRT, as a kind of panacea. Many of these doctors promised that HRT would not only fend off disease and banish the symptoms, but even maintain sexual allure – although this wishful medical thinking had never been tested in proper clinical trials. In fact, by the 1970s HRT had become linked to a raised risk of endometrial cancer, and by the 1980s to breast cancer and blood clots.

Prescriptions plummeted, but HRT is still very much with us, and patients now have to juggle the risks: if you haven't got cancer in the family but are worried about osteoporosis, or suffering menopausal symptoms, is popping the pill worth the risk? Officially, doctors in the UK are now told that the risks outweigh the benefits, and not to prescribe it for osteoporosis prevention. But it is still commonly prescribed for this reason in other parts of the world.

Oestrogen and progesterone: a balancing act

What is it that makes the menopause so potentially dramatic in effect? It happens when a woman's production of the hormones oestrogen and progesterone begins to decline because they are no longer needed to prepare the womb lining for pregnancy. As oestrogen levels fall, the menstrual flow becomes lighter and often irregular, until eventually it stops altogether. Even before the menopause, often when a woman is in her forties, many cycles occur in which an egg is not released. These are known as anovulatory cycles. Whenever this happens, levels of progesterone, produced from the sac that's left once the egg has been released, decline rapidly.

Progesterone is oestrogen's alter ego and you need to keep the two in the right balance. Too much oestrogen relative to progesterone – the so-called 'oestrogen dominance' – results in too many growth signals to cells of the breast and womb, raising the risk of cancer. Consequently, many women in their forties, although low in oestrogen, are in a state of oestrogen dominance because their progesterone levels are even lower.

Symptoms of oestrogen dominance can include water retention, breast tenderness, mood swings, weight gain around the hips and thighs, depression, loss of libido and cravings for sweets. The symptoms of progesterone deficiency overlap these, and also include insomnia, irregular periods, lower body temperature and menstrual cramp.

Many of these symptoms also show up during menopause along with the usual hot flushes, vaginal dryness, joint pains, headaches and depression. So if your hormones are in real disarray, you can end up with a distressing burden of symptoms. There is much you can do about this, but women are rarely told by their doctors how they can help themselves to cope with the menopause naturally. The best way to start is to find out from the list below how well balanced your hormones are at the moment.

How is your hormone balance?

☐ Have you ever used or do you use the contraceptive pill?

☐ Have you had a hysterectomy or have you been sterilised?

☐ Do you experience cyclical water retention?

☐ Do you have excess hair on your body or thinning hair on your scalp?

☐ Have you gained weight on your thighs and hips?

☐ Have you at any time been bothered with problems affecting your reproductive organs (ovaries or womb)?

☐ Do you have fertility problems, difficulty conceiving or a history of miscarriage?

☐ Are your periods often irregular or heavy?

☐ Do you suffer from lumpy breasts?

☐ Do you suffer from a reduced libido or loss of interest in sex?

☐ Do you often suffer from cyclical mood swings or depression?

☐ Do you suffer from insomnia?

☐ Do you experience cramps or other menstrual irregularities?

☐ Do you suffer from anxiety, panic attacks or nervousness?

☐ Do you suffer from hot flushes or vaginal dryness?

If you answered yes to:

4 or less: you have a few symptoms of hormonal imbalance. This chapter will give you clues on how to further reduce any symptoms you do have.

5 to 10: you have a mild to moderate symptoms of hormonal imbalance. It's worth your while getting your hormone levels checked and working with a nutritional therapist to balance your hormones naturally (see page 392).

More than 10: you definitely have hormone imbalances. Besides following the advice in this chapter, we recommend you see a nutritionally oriented doctor.

HRT – hormonal hell?

Raising the risk of womb cancer

The first generation of HRT gave women massive amounts of oestrogen, usually in the form of 'conjugated equine oestrogens'. The equine stands for 'horse', since the oestrogens are derived from horse urine. While their chemical structure is close to human oestrogens, they are not identical. Premarin, one of the top selling brands, contains two – equilin and equilenin – that don't even occur in the human body.[46]

The real problem, however, is the dose. Women vary a lot in the amount of oestrogen they produce. Some women are naturally low oestrogen producers, making 50 to 200mcg a day. Others make up 700mcg a day. HRT provides an oestrogen dose of between 600 and 1,250mcg a day. For most women, this is just too high. (See the 'Inside story: oestrogens' box below for more information.)

Early trials of HRT, which contained only oestrogen, showed a vastly increased risk of endometrial or womb cancer because one of the jobs of oestrogen is to stimulate cell growth there, preparing the womb for a potential pregnancy. The increase ranged from 200 to 1,500 per cent, depending how long you had been taking it; and your risk would still be significantly raised several years after you stopped taking it.[47] So a synthetic progesterone-like hormone called progestin was added to the mix starting in the 1960s. The idea was that, by counteracting unopposed oestrogen, the womb lining would be protected from excess cell growth.

INSIDE STORY: OESTROGENS

Oestrogen is not one hormone but a family of three, namely oestradiol, oestrone and oestriol.

Oestradiol is the strongest, most often used in HRT preparations and most associated with side effects, including increased risk of breast and uterine cancer.

There is one HRT preparation, Hormonin, which contains all three — oestradiol, oestrone and oestriol. Physiologically this is more balanced, as it provides what the body produces. For post-menopausal women with low oestrogen and progesterone level this, taken together with progesterone cream in equivalent amounts to those a woman produces, is a more logical way to restore hormone balance.

Oestriol only is available as a cream and in tablets as Ovestin. The cream is excellent for vaginal dryness, while the tablets often help women with hot flushes, with a fraction of the associated risk of oestradiol. It is best given together with natural progesterone cream (see page 167).

Phyto-oestrogens are plant-based oestrogens that are very weak in comparison and appear to protect against oestrogen overload by occupying the same hormone receptor sites as oestrogen. These are found in beans, lentils, nuts and seeds and especially soya.

Xeno-oestrogens are environmental chemicals that mimic oestrogen and often attach to the same hormone receptor sites as oestrogen, triggering a growth message and potentially promoting cancer. These include alkylphenols, nonylphenols, octylphenols and bisphenol A, found in plastics and some detergents, PCBs and dioxins (which are industrial pollutants), and DDT, DDE, Lindane, Toxaphene, dieldrin, endosulphan, methoxychlor and heptachlor (used as pesticides and herbicides). One of the best ways to limit your exposure is to eat organic food.

Adding progestins to HRT did reduce the risk of endometrial cancer, although it didn't stop it.[48] However, the new progestins had to have a slightly different chemical structure to natural progesterone, so they could be patented. This turned out to be a serious problem because only the exact natural progesterone molecule can trigger a precise set of instructions that maintain pregnancy, bone density, normal menstruation and other 'acts' of the hormonal dance that occurs in every woman. Natural progesterone also has, even at levels considerably higher than those produced by the human body, remarkably little toxicity.

Yet almost without exception, every contraceptive pill or HRT prescription, be it a pill, patch or injection, contains synthetic progestins (also called progestagens) – altered molecules that are similar to but different from genuine progesterone. They are like keys that open the lock, but don't fit exactly – consequently generating a wobble in the body's biochemistry. They might be more profitable, but that profit comes at a high price in the form of an increase in the risk of breast cancer.

Raising the risk of breast cancer

Breast cancer is a major concern for any woman. The average risk of developing breast cancer during one's life is one in ten and its incidence is going up, not down, unlike that for other cancers. Survival, fortunately, is improving.

The first major warning sign of a link between breast cancer and HRT came in 1989. A study by Dr L. Bergkvist and colleagues involving 23,000 Scandinavian women showed that if a woman is on HRT for longer than five years, she doubles her risk of breast cancer.[49] But it also revealed that adding progestins to cut down the womb-cancer risk raised the risk of breast cancer. This was confirmed in a large-scale study, published in the *New England Journal of Medicine* in 1995, which showed that post-menopausal women in their sixties who had been on HRT for five or more years increased their risk of developing breast cancer by 71 per cent.[50]

The longer you were on HRT, the greater the risk. Overall, there was a 32 per cent increased risk among women using oestrogen HRT, and a 41 per cent risk for those using oestrogen combined with synthetic progestin, compared to women who had never used hormones. Another study in 1995, carried out by the Emory University School of Public Health, followed 240,000 women for eight years and found that the risk of ovarian cancer was 72 per cent higher in women given oestrogen.[51]

Evidence continued to accumulate year on year, but the real clincher came with the 'million women' trial in 2003. This trial, published in *The Lancet*, followed a million women aged 50 to 64, half of whom had used HRT.[52] It was found that those who had used oestrogen and progestin HRT doubled their risk of breast cancer.

The conclusion of the paper written by Professor Valerie Beral from the UK Cancer Research Epidemiology Unit at Oxford, who was in charge of this study, was: 'Use of HRT by women aged 50 to 64 years in the UK over the past decade has resulted in an estimated 20,000 extra breast cancers, 15,000 associated with oestrogen-progestagen; the extra deaths cannot yet be reliably estimated.'

THE DARK HISTORY OF HRT: 1940–1980

In the **1940s**, Wyeth Pharmaceuticals produced what they described as a 'natural' oestrogen replacement called Premarin, extracted from (*pre*)gnant (*ma*)res' u(*rine*).

In the **1950s**, oestrogen replacement therapy was being prescribed to women as an aid to easy and successful pregnancy and to help with 'women's problems' on the flimsiest of medical evidence. Millions of women, particularly in North America, were prescribed DES, one of the first synthesised oestrogens. Although it was originally given as a contraceptive, it was eventually given as a 'miracle cure' for any female reproductive problem, even prophylactically to prevent miscarriage.

In the **1960s**, sensing a billion-dollar market, pharmaceutical companies developed the argument that the menopause was a medical condition. HRT could, they suggested, relieve the adverse effects of menopause and return women to their younger sexual selves by resolving oestrogen imbalances, which occur naturally in women at menopause and also occur in women following surgical removal of their ovaries.

In the **1970s** it became apparent that the use by menopausal women of HRT increased their chance of endometrial cancer. One study found that women using the treatment for seven years or more had a 14-fold increase in the incidence of this cancer.[53] The drug companies' answer to this 'problem' was to add progestin to oestrogen in replacement therapy in the hope that this would suppress the action of the oestrogen. There was also a drive by some doctors and some pharmaceutical companies to get women to have their uteruses removed so that they could continue to take 'safe' oestrogen.[54] In 1977, Drs McDonald, Annegers and O'Fallon reported the growing incidence of endometrial cancer in relation to exogenous oestrogen. Their paper cited long-term therapy with estrogens for menopausal symptoms as the usual history in such cases.[55]

In the **1980s**, there was a flow of studies linking hormone replacement therapy to a variety of conditions, the evidence for which became undeniable in the 1990s.[56] Doctors also began to find a rare vaginal cancer in young women whose mothers had taken DES – a synthetic form of oestrogen. After a series of costly court cases, DES was taken off the market. Later research showed not only that the mothers who had taken DES had a slightly increased risk of breast cancer,[57] but that thousands of 'DES sons' and 'DES daughters' had cancers and malformations of the genitals.

Also in the 1980s, a series of studies showed that synthetic human hormones, introduced into women's bodies as contraceptives or as hormone replacement therapies, even as anti-cancer drugs, had the capability to produce cancer, thrombosis and cardiovascular problems. The fact that HRT could cause cancer had been known by manufacturers since the 1950s in any case. A British study published in the *British Journal of Obstetrics and Gynaecology* in 1987, which followed 4,544 women for an average of five and a half years, showed that breast cancer risk was one and a half times greater in HRT users, while the risk of endometrial cancer nearly trebled.[58] In 1989 a study in the *New England Journal of Medicine* showed that taking HRT for longer than five years doubles risk of breast cancer.[59]

The following background is taken from Martin Walker's book *HRT – Licensed to Kill and Maim: The Unheard Voices of Women Damaged by Hormone Replacement Therapy* (see page 400 for further details).

Here's what happened in the **1990s**:

1995 HRT for five plus years increases breast cancer risk by 71 per cent. *New England Journal of Medicine.*

1995 Ovarian cancer risk is 72 per cent higher on oestrogen HRT. *American Journal of Epidemiology.*

1997 Oxford University review of all research up to 1997 concludes 'HRT raises the risk of breast cancer by 25 per cent'.

2002 Combined oestrogen and progestin HRT for five years increases risk of invasive breast cancer by 26 per cent, strokes by 41 per cent and heart disease by 22 per cent. *Journal of the American Medical Association.*

2003 Combined oestrogen and progestin HRT for five years doubles the risk of breast cancer. *The Lancet.*

2004 Combined oestrogen and progestin HRT doubles the risk of developing blood clots (venous thrombosis). *Journal of the American Medical Association.*[60]

Still limping on

It was the death knell for HRT. Sales plummeted by almost a third from more than £30 million a year as the government advised doctors to review the medication on a case-by-case basis – and sales have continued to drop as more and more press reports confirm associated risks.

Despite initial press coverage suggesting that HRT might reduce cardiovascular disease, for instance, the evidence now clearly shows that it doubles the risk of thrombosis, moderately increases the risk of strokes, and slightly increases the risk of cardiovascular disease,[61] although not all studies have shown this. (For an account of how the drug companies 'educated' doctors in the face of mounting evidence of a link between HRT and heart attacks, see Chapter 3, page 61.)

You'd think all this negative science would finish off HRT. But to this day, a rearguard action is still being fought to mitigate the damage of this highly profitable medicine that has clearly killed thousands of women prematurely. In his excellent book *HRT – Licensed to Kill and Maim: The Unheard Voices of Women Damaged by HRT*, the investigative writer Martin Walker states:

> One thing that could be seen with certainty following the publications of these critical studies [quoted in the box on pp 163–4] was that, in the main, pharmaceutical loyal doctors used science to defend themselves only when it suited them. When science threatened the financial base of the pharmaceutical industry they suddenly cease to believe and put everything down to personal choice.

Over the period that the critical studies were published, all the research scientists, Department of Health officials, FDA staff, drug companies' representatives and general practitioners played the 'risk game'. They washed their hands of responsibility and suggested that it was patients who determined what happened, who 'make up their own minds', once they had been told all the facts by their physician.

Some medical experts did make plain statements about the catastrophe which science had begun to structure. In Germany, Professor Bruno Muller-Oerlinghausen, chairman of the German Commission on the Safety of Medicine, compared HRT to thalidomide, saying that it had been a 'national and international tragedy.' By March 2004, even WHO officials were making clear statements, distancing themselves from the treatment. On March 5th at a conference in Sydney, Australia, the co-ordinator of the World Health Organization said that hormone replacement therapy was 'not good for women'. Alexandre Kalache said that science sometimes makes big mistakes and it had done so with HRT. Professor Jay Olshansky, a public health professor at the University of Illinois, said 'scientists now suggest that in most cases HRT should not be used. It's harmful for some and of no use to others.'

Even when the full truth is out about the number of premature deaths caused by different forms of HRT, there are still questions to be answered. These questions go to the very heart of the relationship between pharmaceutical companies and doctors, the prescription of pharmaceutical medicines in a socialised health-care system and even the very nature of science and its links with medicine.

Does it work at all?

For a moment, let's put aside the considerable risks for cancer and circulatory disease laid on women who take HRT. And let's ignore the horrendous side effects that some women on HRT experience, which can include heavy or irregular bleeding if taken before the cessation of periods, water retention, weight gain, PMS-type symptoms and nausea.

Aside from these, just how effective is HRT as a treatment for menopausal symptoms, which is the main reason women choose to use it?

Hot flushes and night sweats are often cited by women as the worst of the menopausal symptoms. As a meta-analysis published in 2004 shows, there have been 24 good-quality trials of HRT for symptom relief, involving over 3,000 women,[62] and they show that it comes up trumps. HRT reduces hot flushes or night sweats by 74 per cent compared to placebos, although quite a few on HRT in these trials dropped out because of side effects. Placebos themselves were also quite effective, reducing reports of hot flushes or night sweats by 50 per cent, showing how important placebo-controlled trials are in this area.

When we look at the evidence for the effectiveness of HRT in preventing osteoporosis, however, it's a much less impressive record. In the Women's Health Initiative, a large trial involving over 16,000 women in the US on HRT for five years, researchers reported in 2002 that there was a small decreased risk of hip fracture.[63] One study involving 670 women, of whom nearly a third were taking HRT, found that bone mass was only preserved in those who had been on it for seven years or more.[64] But even when you take it for that long, bone mineral density rapidly declines once you stop taking it.

Younger women who use short-term HRT will probably gain little or no protection against fracture beyond the age of 70, according to a study from 1993.[65] At 75, the women's bone mineral density was found to be only just over 3 per cent higher than that of women that had never taken HRT. So, unless you are prepared to take HRT for life, it is unlikely to protect you against osteoporosis – and the longer you take it, the greater your risk of developing breast and womb cancer. (See 'Beyond calcium – bone-friendly minerals', page 170, for ways of building bone density nutritionally.)

If you don't have menopausal symptoms, don't go there. That's the conclusion of a 2004 review assessing the benefits versus the harms of HRT in the *British Medical Journal*. It concludes: 'HRT for primary prevention of chronic diseases in women without menopausal symptoms is unjustified. Women free of menopausal symptoms showed a net harm from HRT use.'[66] If you are concerned about osteoporosis, research is showing that changes in diet and exercise are a lot more effective, and certainly safer, than HRT. (See 'The dark history of HRT: 1940–1980' on page 162 for the full story.)

The natural alternatives

Fortunately, you can balance your hormones naturally. The main way is through lifestyle changes and specific foods, nutrients and herbs, which can lessen the severity of menopausal symptoms, and improve bone health safely and effectively. We'll look at those in a moment. But if you'd still like to go down the hormonal route, there is natural progesterone – a safe and effective alternative to HRT.

Natural progesterone – a safer way with hormones

If you still want to use a hormonal approach, 'natural' progesterone looks like a far better bet. A skin cream that must be prescribed by your doctor, natural progesterone is identical to the progesterone molecule your body produces. In France there is a prescribed progesterone pill called Uterogestan. Although this body-identical progesterone can be synthesised in a laboratory from diosgenein, which is found in wild yams, it is quite different from wild yam extract, which does not contain progesterone and is not effective – as was found in 2001 – against hot flushes.[67]

Progesterone is given in amounts equivalent to that normally produced by a woman who is ovulating (between 20 and 40mg a day) and, unlike oestrogen or synthetic progestins, it has no known cancer risk – in fact, as the late Dr John Lee discovered over a decade ago, quite the opposite.[68]

Since the body can make oestrogen hormones from progesterone, as well as the adrenal hormones and testosterone, which is important for sex drive, a natural progesterone patch is more likely to prevent oestrogen dominance while maintaining your libido. It's also good for the other menopausal symptoms. In one double-blind trial from 1999, some 83 per cent of women on progesterone found that it significantly relieved or completely arrested menopausal symptoms, compared to 19 per cent on the placebo.[69] As effective as HRT without the risks, it also has the pleasant side effect of improving skin condition and reducing wrinkles, according to a study published in 2005.[70] If given with oestradiol (see 'Inside story: oestrogens', page 159), it works better at relieving symptoms compared to oestradiol plus progestins and is better for you.[71]

Dr Lee's website (www.johnleemd.com), gives the full story on the use of natural progesterone, as do his excellent books, *What Your Doctor May Not Tell You About Menopause* and *What Your Doctor May Not Tell You About Breast Cancer* (both, Warner Books).

Eat your isoflavones

Four trials published in 2003 have shown that the oestrogen-like, plant-derived substances known as isoflavones, found in high concentrations in soy and red clover, approximately halve the incidence and severity of hot flushes.[72] While other studies have not found this effect (at least at a level of statistical significance), they have shown that the higher the isoflavone levels in the urine of the women studied, the lower the incidence of hot flushes.[73] This suggests that a high intake of isoflavones from diet or supplements is likely to help reduce hot flushes in some women, but not all, and not to the same extent as HRT.

However, unlike conventional HRT, isoflavones have also been shown to protect against cancer. For example, we know that Asians who consume a diet rich in phyto-oestrogens have much lower rates of breast, prostate and colon cancer than we do in the UK, elsewhere in Europe or the US. A 2003 review of the evidence by the Committee on Toxicology (COT), part of the UK's Food Standards Agency, also indicated that phyto-oestrogens may protect against breast cancer. According to the draft report of the COT Working Group on Phyto-ocstrogens, 'Most epidemiological studies . . . have reported an inverse association between soy consumption and breast cancer.'[74] In other words, the majority of research into the effects of one of the richest sources of phyto-oestrogens, soya beans or their products such as tofu, shows they reduce the incidence of breast cancer.

Nor are men left out of this equation. An American study from 1998 involving more than 12,000 men showed that frequent consumption (more than once a day) of soya milk was associated with a 70 per cent reduction in prostate cancer risk.[75]

Our advice is to eat some tofu, beans or chickpeas every day. You probably need the equivalent of 50g a day for an effect. An ideal intake is equivalent to a 340ml serving of soya milk or a 113g serving of tofu.

Isoflavone supplements, either soya or red clover, are an alternative, although we favour food as the best source. The effective amount is the equivalent of 80mg of isoflavones a day, as instructed on the supplements. Isoflavones take time to work, so try these for a couple of months.

Blood-sugar balance and vitamins

Research at the University of Texas at Austin, published in 2003, has proven what nutritionists have known all along. If you have dysglycemia – which means your blood-sugar level goes up and down like a yo-yo – you are much more likely to experience fatigue, irritability, depression and hot flushes. Specifically, the research found that when you have a blood-sugar low this can trigger a hot flush.[76] By keeping your blood-sugar level even through 'grazing' rather than gorging, and by choosing low-GL foods, you can considerably reduce the number of hot flushes you have. The advice here is no different to that for preventing diabetes – eat a low-GL diet and also consider supplementing chromium. For more details see page 143 in Chapter 8.

According to a 2003 study, other nutrients that may help during the menopause are vitamin C,[77] vitamin E and essential fats (both omega-3 and omega-6). Choose a vitamin C supplement that contains berry extracts rich in bioflavonoids, as there's some evidence that these help, too. Vitamin E has been reported to help alleviate vaginal dryness.

B vitamins may also play an important role in preventing symptoms, including osteoporosis. Two surveys from 2004 found a doubling to quadrupling in the incidence of fractures in people with high blood levels of the amino acid homocysteine.[78–79] As B vitamins lower levels of homocysteine, supplementing B6, B12 and folic acid, plus TMG, could be a good idea (see Chapter 15).

BEYOND CALCIUM – BONE-FRIENDLY MINERALS

The story sounds good. Your bones are made of calcium, so the more calcium you have, the stronger your bones. However, research has shown mixed results from supplementing calcium. Similarly, some trials have found an increased – not decreased – risk of fractures in people with a high milk intake.

Vitamin D is also needed for your body to utilise calcium, and a meta-analysis of five trials involving patients with corticosteroid-induced bone mass loss showed that this combination of nutrients was effective.[80] However, not all trials have tallied with this finding. A recent one involving more than 3,000 women at risk for osteoporosis found no protective effect from giving 1,000mg of calcium plus 800iu of vitamin D (as cholecalciferol).[81]

Another, published in the *New England Journal of Medicine* in 2006, found a mild improvement in bone mass density, but no significant reduction of risk for hip fracture from 1,000mg of calcium and 400iu of vitamin D.[82] Personally, we still recommend that you supplement calcium (500mg) and vitamin D (400iu). But we'd do so by taking a bone-friendly formula that also provides magnesium (250mg), silica (30mg) and boron (1mg) – all of which are needed for good bone health.

Going for helpful herbs

The most promising of the herbs used to treat the symptoms of menopause is black cohosh, which can help reduce hot flushes, sweating, insomnia and anxiety. Three double-blind trials have been published.[83] One showed no effect, the other was beneficial and the third showed reduced sweating but no reduction in the number of hot flushes. Also encouraging is new research that seems to indicate black cohosh neither increases cancer risk nor is anti-oestrogenic.[84] It also helps relieve depression by raising serotonin levels. Even so, we'd recommend that you take black cohosh three months on, one month off, and avoid it if you are taking liver-toxic drugs or have a damaged liver. Take 50mg twice a day.

The other 'hot' herb for hot flushes is dong quai, whose scientific name is *Angelica sinensis*. In one placebo-controlled study from 2003, 55 postmenopausal women who were given dong quai and chamomile instead of HRT had an 80 per cent reduction in hot flushes. These results became apparent after one month.[85] An earlier study didn't find this effect, however.[86] If you want to try dong quai, which doesn't appear to have oestrogenic or cancer-promoting properties, we recommend 600mg a day for relief from hot flushes.

St John's wort, a herb renowned for its anti-depressant effects, has been demonstrated to relieve other menopausal symptoms, including headaches, palpitations, lack of concentration and decreased libido. In fact, a German study found that 80 per cent of women felt their symptoms had gone or substantially improved at the end of 12 weeks.[87] The combination of black cohosh and St John's wort (300mg a day) can be particularly effective for women who are experiencing menopause-related depression, irritability and fatigue.[88]

SIDE EFFECTS There are no known serious adverse effects from black cohosh. Dong quai may thin the blood and is therefore contraindicated for women on the drug warfarin. St John's wort, at this dosage, has no reported serious adverse effects, but be aware that it is best to consult your doctor if you are on an anti-depressant (and read Chapter 10 to explore safer and more effective options).

HERBS FOR PREMENOPAUSAL HORMONAL HEALTH

Another popular herb, Chasteberry, or *Vitex agnus-castus*, while less helpful for menopausal symptoms, is proving very helpful for menstrual irregularities, PMS, and especially for the symptoms of breast tenderness. It has been used for at least 2,000 years by the Egyptians, Greeks and Romans. Chasteberry's therapeutic powers, proven in a series of double-blind trials in 2005, are attributed to its indirect effects on decreasing oestrogen levels while increasing progesterone and prolactin.[89] Raised prolactin is known to lower oestrogen levels. In most trials, 4mg a day of a standardised extract (containing six per cent agnusides – one of the active ingredients) was used.

Exercise – and take a deep breath

Both regular exercise and learning how to breathe deeply have proven benefits for menopausal symptoms. According to a 2003 study conducted at Lund University in Sweden, if you stay active, you can reduce the impact of menopausal symptoms. Researchers interviewed nearly 4,500 women 58 to 68 years old about their sociodemographic, lifestyle and current health conditions. They found that women who did more vigorous physical exercise were less likely to suffer from hot flushes.[90] Exercise also has profound effects on keeping your bones strong and protecting you from osteoporosis (see the 'Get moving on the menopause' box below).

GET MOVING ON THE MENOPAUSE

The two main forms of exercise that boost the health of your bones and increase bone mass are weight-bearing exercise and resistance exercise. Note that the recommendations here are for both younger people and women in the menopause, as prevention is vital.

A weight-bearing exercise is one where bones and muscles work against the force of gravity. This is any exercise in which your feet and legs carry your weight. Examples are walking, jogging, dancing and climbing stairs.

Resistance exercise involves moving your body weight or objects to create resistance. This type of exercise uses the body areas individually, which also strengthens the bone in that particular area.

For women before the menopause
You can either do all the following suggestions or a combination of them based on your level of fitness:

- Jumping or skipping on the spot (50 jumps daily)

- Jogging or walking for 30 minutes (five to seven days per week)

- Resistance weight training (two to three days per week)

- High impact circuit or aerobic style class (one to two times per week).

For postmenopausal women (and men over 50)

You can either do all of the following suggestions or a combination of them based on your level of fitness:

- Weight training (one set of eight to 12 repetitions using maximum effort. If 12 can be reached on a regular basis then the weight is slightly too light)

- Jogging/walking for ten to 20 minutes (five to seven days per week)

- Stair climbing (ten flights of ten steps per day)

- Exercise classes such as yoga or aqua aerobics (one to two per week).

With thanks to Joe Sharpe for compiling this information

BREATHING FROM THE BELLY

The basic principle of all breathing exercises is to use your diaphragm, rather than the top of your chest as we tend to do when we are anxious or stressed. If you're unsure where the diaphragm is, it's the dome-shaped muscle at the bottom of the lungs. Three trials have shown that this type of breathing can reduce the frequency of hot flushes by about 50 per cent.[91]

Breathing in this way works best at the start of a hot flush. Breathing from the diaphragm is part of many health systems such as yoga and the martial arts. (See Appendix 2, page 394, for more precise instructions on this kind of breathing.)

While you can try any of these recommendations individually, a combination of all these herbs, nutrients, diet and lifestyle suggestions will yield the best results.

Food or drugs? The verdict

Conventional HRT does relieve hot flushes in many women, although only as long as you take it, but are the long-term risks of HRT worth it? Many women think not. Natural progesterone, although under-researched, seems to help many women without the associated risks. Backed up with simple diet and lifestyle changes, as well as herbal and dietary supplements, the chances are you'll achieve an equivalent result, but sleep easy for the lack of risk of any problems in the future.

What works

- Eat beans, especially soya products such as tofu or soya milk, or chickpeas, every day. You probably need the equivalent of 50g a day for an effect. An ideal intake is equivalent to a 340g serving of soya milk or a 113g serving of tofu. Alternatively, have an isoflavone supplements, either soya or red clover, providing the equivalent of 80mg of isoflavones a day.

- Balance your blood sugar by eating a low-GL diet (see Chapter 8, page 143) and possibly supplementing chromium 200mcg in the morning.

- Take a high-strength multivitamin, with an additional vitamin C supplement (1 to 2g) that also contains berry extracts, and an essential fat capsule with both omega-3 and omega-6.

- Check your homocysteine level. If it's high, supplement additional B12, folic acid, B6 and B12 (see Chapter 15) accordingly.

- Consider using natural progesterone cream, prescribable by your doctor (see below).

- Try these herbs: black cohosh (50mg a day) or dong quai (600mg a day) with 300mg St John's wort a day if you're prone to depression, or *Vitex agnus-castus* (4mg a day of a standardised extract).

- Get fit with frequent weight-bearing exercise to minimise your risk of osteoporosis (see 'Get moving on the menopause', page 172).

- Learn 'belly breathing' (see Appendix 2, page 394, or join a yoga class).

Working with your doctor

Your doctor may not be aware of the science behind natural progesterone, and they may not know they can prescribe it. The Natural Progesterone

Information Society (NPIS) produce an information pack for doctors (see Resources, page 404), so it is best to go armed with this information. If the combination of natural progesterone and the nutritional and herbal recommendations above don't solve your symptoms, then there may be some value in a more balanced oestrogen-based preparation such as Hormonin, provided it is taken with progesterone cream to avoid oestrogen dominance. For vaginal dryness, Ovestin cream can also be helpful.

If your doctor is not up on, or interested in, these more natural approaches, the NPIS can refer you to a doctor who is.

10.

Beating Depression
'Let them eat Prozac' vs natural anti-depressants

We all know the hallmarks of depression – low mood, lack of motivation and feelings of hopelessness. Most people experience these as a fleeting reaction to life's trials and tribulations. The ONUK survey carried out by the Institute for Optimum Nutrition and involving 37,000 people in Britain found that as many as one in three people say they sometimes or frequently feel depressed and suffer from low moods.[92] Perhaps you are one of them.

A small proportion of people may slide into deeper depression, and cry uncontrollably, lose their appetite or have suicidal thoughts. People under this kind of pressure are more likely to go to their doctor to seek help, where they may be diagnosed with 'clinical' depression.

Whatever the degree, people in the industrialised world seem to be much more depressed than they used to be. Although it is entirely possible that depression is more readily diagnosed these days, the incidence has increased tenfold since the 1950s and, according to research by London University and Warwick University, has doubled in young people over the past 12 years.[93] Depression affects more than 95,000 children and teenagers in Australia each year, along with 800,000 adults.[94]

Overall in the UK, approximately 15 per cent of people are labelled clinically depressed, and half of them will consult their doctor.[95] In fact, an estimated one in three doctor consultations concern patients with mental health concerns such as depression.

One of the worst outcomes of depression is suicide, claiming 3,000 lives a year; it is now the second most common cause of death in young people aged 15 to 24. All in all, depression is a vast and growing health problem that costs Britain's National Health Service an estimated £2 billion a year.[96] The scale of the problem is such that pharmaceutical anti-depressants are out there in abundance, but as you'll see, this is hardly the whole story regarding ways to tackle this debilitating condition.

Unlike a physical condition such as diabetes that can be diagnosed by blood tests, depression is diagnosed by psychological tests, the most common being the Hamilton Rating Scale of Depression. This lists questions about mood, guilt feelings, suicidal thoughts, insomnia, agitation, anxiety, physical problems, sex drive, and so on. Depending on your total score, you will be diagnosed with either 'mild,' 'moderate,' or 'severe' depression. To compare the effectiveness of drug and food-based approaches we'll be using changes in the Hamilton Rating Scale, or HRS for short, to provide a concrete measure of improvement. You can too as you try out the approaches we'll be recommending.

Here's a simplified questionnaire to check your mood.

How depressed are you?

Check yourself out on this simplified Mood Check.

☐ Do you feel downhearted, blue and sad?

☐ Do you feel worse in the morning?

☐ Do you have crying spells, or feel like it?

☐ Do you have trouble falling asleep, or sleeping through the night?

☐ Is your appetite poor?

☐ Are you losing weight without trying?

☐ Do you feel unattractive and unlovable?

☐ Do you prefer to be alone?

☐ Do you feel fearful?

☐ Are you often tired and irritable?

☐ Is it an effort to do the things you used to do?

☐ Are you restless and unable to keep still?

☐ Do you feel hopeless about the future?

☐ Do you find it difficult to make decisions?

☐ Do you feel less enjoyment from activities that once gave you pleasure?

Score 1 for each 'yes' answer. If you answered yes to:

Less than 5: you are normal. You appear to be positive, optimistic and able to roll with the punches. This chapter will give you clues on how to handle those occasions when things aren't going so well for you.

5 to 10: you have a mild to moderate case of the blues. Read on to see how this can happen, and then, to the solutions. You might also consider seeking outside help.

More than 10: you are moderately to markedly depressed. Besides following the advice in this chapter, we recommend you seek professional help.

If you find you're depressed and go to your doctor, there's a good chance you'll be prescribed one of the anti-depressant drugs. Approximately half of those who seek help from their doctor are prescribed anti-depressants, while a quarter are referred for counselling. Psychological factors, including stress and not having someone to talk through your problems with, play a big part, as does nutrition, yet the emphasis on treatment usually veers towards pharmaceutical drugs. Before we examine what works for dealing with depression, let's look at just how effective they are.

Prozac and other anti-depressants

In 2004, some 3.5 million people in Britain received prescriptions for anti-depressants, costing the NHS about £300 million. But that pales into insignificance compared with the annual anti-depressant consumption in the US, where over 60 million prescriptions for these drugs are written each year at a cost of $10 billion.

One of the reasons so many people continue to take them, however, is that they can't get off them. Whether you call it 'cessation effects', 'withdrawal effects' or addiction, it's a major problem. More on this in a minute.

Most anti-depressants fall into one of three categories: monoamine oxidase inhibitors (MAOIs), tricyclic anti-depressants (TCAs) and selective serotonin reuptake inhibitors (SSRIs). There's also a fourth generation of anti-depressants starting to replace the SSRIs as their patents run out. These are known as serotonin and noradrenalin re-uptake inhibitors, or SNRIs.

The model used by the drug companies to explain how anti-depressant drugs work is that depression is essentially a deficiency disease, the result of low levels of the brain's own 'feel-good' neuro-transmitters – serotonin for mood and noradrenalin for motivation. Neurotransmitters are the chemical signals that allow messages to pass between brain cells; too little of one or other, so the story goes, and you feel gloomier and less enthusiastic. The action of these drugs is to increase the amount of one or more of these neurotransmitters. This is almost certainly not all that is going on biologically in depression. It's very likely, for example, that inflammation is involved as well.[97] But let's stick with this story for now.

MAOI anti-depressants

Monoamine oxidase inhibitors, including drugs such as Parnate, were the first generation of anti-depressants. They block the monoamine oxidase enzyme (hence MAO inhibitor) that normally clears away the neurotransmitter dopamine, which is linked with feelings of pleasure. This class of drugs includes phenelzine (Nardil) and trifluoperazine (Parstelin).

SIDE EFFECTS They can cause dangerously high blood pressure if taken with substances containing yeast, alcohol and caffeine.

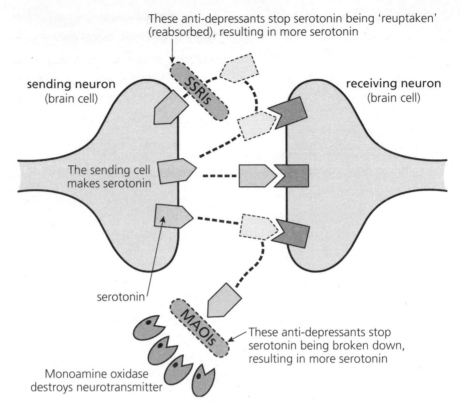

How anti-depressants work

Tricyclic anti-depressants

Tricyclics were the forerunners of today's SSRIs. They work in a similar way to MAOIs but they increase the availability of serotonin and noradrenalin. Commonly prescribed brands are amitriptyline (Elavil), desipramine (Norpramin), imipramine (Tofranil), and trimipramine (Surmentil).

SIDE EFFECTS These have the undesirable effect of depressing acetylcholine — a neurotransmitter involved, among many other things, in memory and muscle control. This in turn can cause such side effects as dry mouth, blurred vision and drowsiness.

SSRI anti-depressants

Most people are familiar with selective serotonin reuptake inhibitors or SSRIs, as they've been heralded in books and debated hugely in the media. SSRIs have largely replaced tricyclic anti-depressants, although as a review of the research in 2005 showed, most studies show little difference in effectiveness.[98] SSRIs are more 'selective', in the sense that they only target the enzyme that clears away serotonin, the key mood neurotransmitter. Their major advantage was supposed to be fewer side effects and it is less easy to overdose on them than on tricyclics. The most commonly prescribed are fluoxetine (Prozac), paroxetine (Seroxat/Paxil) and sertraline (Lustral/Zoloft).

SIDE EFFECTS SSRIs can increase the risk of suicide (for details of the long concern over suicide links, see Chapter 2). SSRIs can also cause patients to feel 'fuzzy' and may promote sexual problems. On top of this, recent research at Duke University is suggesting that SSRIs might dramatically increase the risk of death in those with cardiovascular disease.[99]

SNRI anti-depressants

Serotonin and noradrenalin reuptake inhibitors or SNRIs, such as Effexor and Cymbalta, are being prescribed more frequently and are said to be more effective at promoting motivation. Apathy, lack of drive and motivation is a hallmark of depression, thought to be due to a lack of noradrenalin. Although targeting the same neurotransmitters as tricyclics, SNRIs are said to be more precise.

SIDE EFFECTS Nausea, headaches, insomnia, sleepiness, dry mouth, dizziness, constipation, weakness, sweating, nervousness and, as with SNRIs, serious sexual dysfunction.

So what's the evidence?

Effectiveness

Just how effective are these drugs? The short answer is: not very. A recent report on all treatments for depression from the UK's National Institute for Health and Clinical Excellence (NICE) says: 'There is little clinically important difference between anti-depressants and placebo for mild depression.'[100] For mild depression, NICE does not recommend anti-depressants, favouring instead exercise, 'guided self-help' (effectively, keeping a journal) and counselling. Unfortunately, nutrition has not yet made it on to their agenda.

For moderate to severe depression, three major reviews show a significant but hardly spectacular improvement comparing anti-depressants to placebo.[101] One from 2005, for example, found that 58 per cent of people taking an anti-depressant improved, compared to 45 per cent of those on placebos.[102] So, not much difference.

Another found that the difference in HRS scores between those taking SSRIs and placebos was only 1.7 points – a result that could have been obtained by answering just two out of the 17 questions differently (for example, that you're sleeping better and have gained weight).

A major review in 2000 of all the published studies finds that these 'state of the art' SSRI anti-depressants lower HRS scores by a 10 to 20 per cent.[103] This might not mean much to you now, but when we look at the evidence for certain key nutrients, you'll find that these drugs are less than half as effective at dealing with depression. And the most recent review of anti-depressants, from 2005, suggests that even this unimpressive difference may have more to do with the way double-blind placebo controlled trials are conducted by the drug companies than proof that these drugs are even slightly effective.[104]

The criticism goes like this. In a classic drug trial you compare two groups – one getting the drug and one the placebo. You assume that any improvement in the placebo group is because they think they are getting a drug, but that any improvements in the drug group are believed to be due only to the drug. But suppose the patients in the drug group correctly guess they are getting a drug because they start getting side effects – dry mouth and so on? When that happens, and there is good evidence that it often does, the placebo effect kicks in to boost the drug's effect because the volunteers think they're getting the real thing.

When researchers have used 'active' placebos that produce similar side effects to those triggered by the drugs, the differences between the two were even smaller.[105]

Another factor that makes anti-depressants less effective in reality, as compared to during drug trials, is compliance – that is, taking the drugs as prescribed. While compliance is close to 100 per cent in drug trials, in real life many people, perhaps as many as one in four, don't take them as prescribed by their doctor. That could make the anti-depressants a quarter as effective in practice.

Some studies show that neither anti-depressants nor alternative remedies such as St John's wort are very effective on their own for severe depression. For example, a 2002 study of 900 patients with severe depression gave a third an SSRI anti-depressant (sertraline), a third St John's wort, and a third a placebo. None worked.[106]

As you'll see in a minute, nutritional approaches, as well as exercise and counselling, have already been proven to be much more effective – without the side effects.

How bad are anti-depressants' side effects?

Anti-depressants may work, although not spectacularly, but it's the side effects that are truly depressing. You had a taste of them in the discussion of anti-depressants above, so you can see they're not pleasant and in some cases constitute a huge risk.

Up to a quarter of the people taking anti-depressants experience side effects – the milder of which include nausea, vomiting, malaise, dizziness, and headaches or migraines. Prozac, the original market leader and prescribed to more than 38 million people worldwide, has 45 listed side effects. And more: there is the increased risk of suicide, as we have seen, and there can also be severe withdrawal problems with SSRIs. They are far from being the magic bullet many believed they were in the 1990s.

The most comprehensive review, a study of 702 trials involving 87,650 patients published in the *British Medical Journal* in 2005,[107] shows a doubling to tripling of suicides in patients on SSRIs versus placebos. As these are trials of depressed patients, you would expect the opposite, so this really is a serious indictment of these drugs. The study came in the wake of a decade of denial – by both the pharmaceutical industry and the British government's drug watchdog the MHRA – that there was any cause for concern (see also Chapter 2, page 36). Now, however, the official recommendation is not to prescribe most of these anti-depressants to children and teenagers.

Does that mean doctors should switch back to earlier 'tricyclic' anti-depressants? According to the *British Medical Journal* review, there was no difference in the incidence of suicides between tricyclic anti-depressants and SSRIs. And suicide is not the only major risk of these drugs.

According to a study from the *British Journal of Cancer*, published in 2002, the heavy use of at least six different tricyclics was shown to double your risk of breast cancer.[108] The ones that caused an increased risk were amoxapine, clomipramine, desipramine, doxepin, imipramine and trimipramine. A similar study from 2000, published in the *American Journal of Epidemiology*, found that women who used tricyclics for more than two years could double their risk of breast cancer.[109]

What about the new generation of SNRI anti-depressants such as Effexor and Cymbalta, which are said to be superior because they affect both serotonin, for mood, and noradrenalin, for motivation? Here again the news is far from good.

Dr David Healy, the psychiatrist in the North Wales Department of Psychological Medicine in Bangor who blew the lid on the link between suicides and SSRIs, says this about SNRIs: 'We can have absolutely no confidence at all that SNRIs will be any better. At this stage Effexor appears, from adverse event reports worldwide, to have just the same rates of people becoming suicidal as the SSRIs.' In a 'healthy volunteer' trial (when a drug is given to people with no illness to check for reactions) of duloxetine (Cymbalta), one volunteer committed suicide. However, just as with the SSRI saga, it will probably take some years before enough evidence accumulates, and probably even longer before the authorities will take action.

If 'guilty' is the verdict from the court of science, what about the court of law? There have now been 90 legal actions against the manufacturers of SSRIs in the US, one ending with the plaintiffs being awarded $6.4 million dollars.[110] 'I estimate that about one person a day in the UK alone has committed suicide as a direct result of taking SSRIs since they were introduced,' says Healy, who has been petitioning the MHRA for years to issue a warning to doctors and users about these potential adverse reactions. In the US they could have resulted in up to 10,000 suicides and 100,000 attempts.[111]

Are they addictive?

The MHRA now tells pharmaceutical companies to change the wording on their list of cautions from 'cessation effects' to 'withdrawal effects'. Of all the side effects, the addictive quality of most anti-depressants may be the most worrying, and a major reason why so many people are taking these potentially dangerous and rather ineffective medicines. There is now considerable evidence that some 50 per cent of those who try to quit get alarming withdrawal effects. One study testing withdrawal showed that as many as 85 per cent of the volunteers – people with no previous hint of depression – suffered agitation, abnormal dreams, insomnia and other adverse effects on withdrawal.[112] In studies on duloxetine, the new kid on the block, 44 per cent of people report adverse symptoms on discontinuation, compared to 22 per cent on placebo.[113] A Canadian study also found about a quarter of people had withdrawal symptoms on stopping SSRIs.[114]

Christianne is a case in point. At the age of 18, she was prescribed Prozac and then Seroxat for her depression and panic attacks. Here's what happened when she started taking the drug, and then when she tried to stop.

Since being on Seroxat I've started self-harming, cutting myself, and I also have a disturbed sleep pattern. When I do sleep, I have very vivid weird dreams and violent nightmares and sweat excessively. I have feelings of inadequacy and suicidal thoughts on a daily basis and I hate myself for it. I often wanted to overdose on my sleeping tablets so I wouldn't have to wake up in the morning and sometimes took two instead of one before I went to bed. I feel more withdrawn than before, I have difficulty getting up in the mornings and have violent mood swings, which is quite out of character for me. I suffer from extreme headaches and spells of light-headedness which makes me sometimes lose my balance. I also become confused quickly and have spells of feeling 'spaced-out' and an awful span of concentration. I get upset and emotional very quickly, sometimes for the silliest of reasons. Sometimes I have no appetite at all.

I feel worse now than I ever did before. I mentioned these feelings to my doctor at the mental heath clinic and she told me that these feelings weren't side effects from the drug, but totally psychological and down to the development of my condition, which I do not believe to be the case. When I asked her what she was going to do about the way I was feeling, she said she would refer me to a psychologist. Six months later, I am still waiting for an appointment to come through. She also suggested upping the dosage to 40mg, which I refused.

My last spell of self-harm led to an argument between my long-term boyfriend and me. It was after this that I decided to come off my tablets completely as my thought was that I couldn't feel much worse than I do now. However, no more than a day or two after, I began suffering severe withdrawal symptoms. These included an extreme feeling of weakness, excessive and painful diarrhoea, and stomach cramps, intense nausea and shakes and I felt as though I needed to cry. I felt so ill that I began taking the tablets again that evening and I am still taking them today.

I am still on these tablets and want to come off them. I wonder if I will ever feel 'normal' again. These tablets have ruined my life. I believe that it is these tablets that make me feel and behave the way I do. I feel enormously angry with the doctors and medical associations for dismissing these symptoms out of hand.

That was three years ago. Since then Christianne has attended the Brain Bio Centre in London, where she was treated with the nutritional approach suggested below. It has been so effective that she no longer needs anti-depressants and no longer suffers from depression or panic attacks.

Like Christianne, many people have huge difficulty in getting off these drugs. For more details on withdrawal problems, see http://www.socialaudit.org.uk.

Natural alternatives

A truly scientific approach

There is a curious contradiction at the heart of the drug-based approach to depression. The treatment is based on correcting a biochemical imbalance in the brain. So you might think a scientific approach would be to check whether depressed patients actually had an imbalance and if so, exactly which neurotransmitters were low so they could be given a boost. But that is not what happens. Instead, the diagnosis of depression is based solely on a checklist of psychological symptoms, which doesn't tell you anything about what is going on with brain or indeed body chemistry.

In fact, it has taken a nutritionally minded doctor to take this obvious scientific step. Professor Tapan Audhya from New York University Medical Center in the US first showed that the level of serotonin found in platelets, which are tiny disc-like bodies in the blood, correlates with the level of these neurotransmitters in the brain.[115] Next he investigated whether people with depression do actually have abnormal levels of platelet serotonin by measuring platelet levels in 52 normal and 74 depressed volunteers. The difference was striking. In 73 per cent of depressed patients, serotonin levels were barely a fifth of those in the normal subjects.[116]

Knowing that this neurotransmitter is made directly from amino acids found in food, Audhya then gave his patients 5-hydroxytryptophan (5-HTP), the amino acid that's a direct precursor to serotonin, from which it is made. This corrected the deficiency and resulted in major and rapid relief from depression.[117]

When it comes to treating depression or any other chronic condition, nutrition is a real alternative as it is based on finding out what is actually going on in the patient's system and then sorting out any specific imbalances. That makes a lot more sense, and is far more scientific, than giving millions of people precisely the same chemical regardless of what is actually wrong with them.

At the Brain Bio Centre, filling in the Hamilton Rating Scale questionnaire is just the beginning. You will also be asked about your diet and other health symptoms and then given blood and urine tests to discover how well you are functioning in four key areas that can affect depression:

- Serotonin levels – do they need boosting?

- Your homocysteine level – is it too high?

- Essential fats – are your levels high enough?

- Blood-sugar balance – is yours within the healthy range?

Each of these can, if necessary, be improved with one or other of the top five natural anti-depressants, which include B vitamins, omega-3 fats and amino acids.

Unlike drugs for related problems such as anxiety, depression and insomnia, which often interact with each other in damaging ways, the various elements of a nutritional approach all complement one another. As we saw in Chapter 5, to begin to cure any chronic disorder you need to be sure that the various biochemical elements involved are balanced in an optimum way. So what has to happen to lift depression?

First, you'll need the building blocks for the relevant neurotransmitters (see diagram below). These are tryptophan or 5-hydroxytryptophan (5-HTP), both amino acids found in protein foods. But they are no good without the catalysts that turn them into neurotransmitters, which are B vitamins, magnesium, zinc and something called trimethylglycine (or TMG for short). These nutrients will also keep levels of an amino

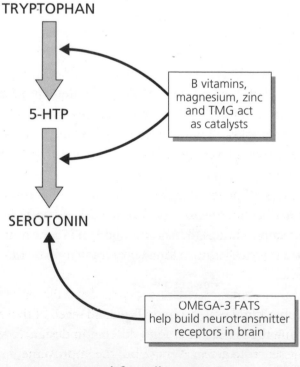

Mood-friendly nutrients

acid known as homocysteine low in the blood, which is important for holding depression at bay.

Omega-3 fats, especially one called EPA, are vital. Not only do they act as catalysts, but they are also needed to build the receptors – the docking ports in brain cells that serotonin and the other neurotransmitters attach themselves to. Finally, the whole system needs a constant and stable supply of energy, which is why blood-sugar levels need to be maintained within healthy limits. Other elements of the new medicine package for depression could include exercise and increased exposure to natural light, both of which raise serotonin, along with psychotherapy.

But what is the evidence that each one of these elements not only works on its own but is more effective than anti-depressants? Just one of them may do the trick for you or you may benefit from several in combination. However, once you see how they all work together, it becomes clear just how limited the standard drug style clinical trials are for testing this sort of medicine.

So what's the evidence?

5-HTP

We've now seen how serotonin is made in the body and brain from 5-HTP. In its turn, 5-HTP is made from another amino acid, tryptophan. Both can be found in food: many protein-rich foods such as meat, fish, beans and eggs contain tryptophan, while the richest source of 5-HTP is the African griffonia bean. Not getting enough tryptophan is likely to make you depressed: people fed food deficient in tryptophan became rapidly depressed within hours.[118] Both have been shown to have an anti-depressant effect in clinical trials, although 5-HTP is more effective. There have been 27 studies, involving 990 people to date, most of which proved positive.[119]

So how do they compare with anti-depressants? Eleven of the 5-HTP trials were double-blind placebo controlled, and seven of those measured depression using the HRS. The studies differed in design, so you cannot just add up the scores to get an average, but the improvement rated 13, 30, 34, 39, 40, 56 and 61 per cent. It doesn't take a scientist to realise these results are a lot better than the average 15 per cent improvement reported for anti-depressants.

In play-off studies between 5-HTP and SSRI anti-depressants, 5-HTP comes out slightly better. One double-blind trial headed by Dr W. P. Poldinger at the Basel University of Psychiatry gave 34 depressed volunteers either the SSRI fluvoxamine (Luvox) or 300mg of 5-HTP. At the end of the six weeks, both groups of patients had had a significant improvement in their depression. However, those taking 5-HTP had a slightly greater improvement, compared to those on the SSRI, in each of the four criteria assessed – depression, anxiety, insomnia, and physical symptoms – as well as their own self-assessment.[120]

Since in some sensitive people, anti-depressant drugs could theoretically induce an overload of serotonin called 'serotonin syndrome' – characterised by feeling overheated, high blood pressure, twitching, cramping, dizziness and disorientation – some concern has been expressed about the possibility of increasing the odds of serotonin syndrome with the combination of 5-HTP and an SSRI drug. However, a recent review on the safety of 5-HTP concludes that 'serotonin syndrome has not been reported in humans in association with 5-HTP, either as monotherapy [on its own] or in combination with other medications.'[121]

Are there any side effects with 5-HTP? Some people experience mild gastrointestinal disturbance on 5-HTP, which usually stops within a few days. Since there are serotonin receptors in the gut, which don't normally expect to get the real thing so easily, they can overreact if the amount is too high, resulting in transient nausea. If this happens, just lower the amount you take and take it with a fruit snack.

B vitamins and the homocysteine link

People with either low blood levels of the B vitamin folic acid, or high blood levels of the amino acid homocysteine, are both more likely to be depressed and less likely to get a positive result from anti-depressant drugs.

A study published in 2003 found that having a high level of homocysteine doubles the odds of a woman developing depression, for instance.[122] Ensuring homocysteine stays low means that your brain will methylate well, keeping its chemistry ticking over and in balance. So one way of staving off depression is to keep your homocysteine levels in check (see pages 197 and 301 for how this works). The ideal level is below six, and the average level is 10–11. The risk of depression doubles with levels above 15.

Normalising homocysteine levels is mainly down to getting enough vitamins B2, B6, B12, zinc, TMG – and folic acid. In fact, the higher your blood homocysteine level, the more likely folic acid will work for you. In a study from 2000, comparing the effects of giving an SSRI with either a placebo or with folic acid, 61 per cent of patients improved on the placebo combination but 93 per cent improved with the addition of folic acid.[123]

But how does folic acid, a cheap vitamin with no side effects, compare to anti-depressants? Three trials published in 2003 and involving 247 people addressed this question.[124] Two, with 151 participants, assessed the use of folic acid in addition to other treatment, and found that adding folic acid reduced HRS scores on average by a further 2.65 points. That's not as good as the results with 5-HTP but as good, if not better, than anti-depressants. These studies also show that more patients treated with folic acid experienced a 50 per cent greater reduction in their HRS after ten weeks, compared to those on anti-depressants.

As for side effects, there are none, except a lower risk for heart disease, strokes, Alzheimer's and improved energy and concentration. However, if you are vegan – which can potentially leave you B12 deficient – taking folic acid on its own can mask symptoms of fatigue, but the underlying nerve damage caused by B12 deficiency anaemia, the symptoms of which are tingling and numbness of the extremities, can persist. So don't take folic acid without also supplementing vitamin B12. (Pregnant women should also ensure they take a recommended multivitamin if they are supplementing folic acid.)

Omega-3s

The richest dietary source of omega-3 essential fats is fish, specifically carnivorous coldwater fish such as salmon, mackerel and herring. As a 1998 *Lancet* article reveals, surveys have shown that the more fish the population of a country eats, the lower their incidence of depression.[125] The omega-3 fat EPA seems to be the most potent natural anti-depressant.

There have been six double-blind placebo-controlled trials to date, five of which show significant improvement in levels of depression.[126–127] The first, by Dr Andrew Stoll from Harvard Medical School, published in the *Archives of General Psychiatry*, gave 40 depressed patients either omega-3 supplements or a placebo, and found a highly significant improvement in those given the omega-3s.[128]

The next, published in the *American Journal of Psychiatry*, tested the effects of giving 20 people suffering from severe depression and who were already on anti-depressants, but still depressed, a highly concentrated form of omega-3 fat called ethyl-EPA versus a placebo. By the third week, the depressed patients on the EPA were showing major improvement in their mood, while those on placebo were not.[129] A 2006 trial by Dr Sophia Frangou from the Institute of Psychiatry in London gave a concentrated form of EPA, versus a placebo, to 26 depressed people with bipolar disorder (otherwise known as manic depression) and again found a significant improvement.[130]

In these trials, which used the HRS, the average improvement in depression in those taking omega-3s over the placebo hovered around the 50 per cent mark. Again, it doesn't take a rocket scientist to realise that these results are a quantum leap ahead of anti-depressant drugs – and *without* the side effects. This is because omega-3s help to build your brain's neuronal connections as well as the receptor sites for neurotransmitters, so the more omega-3s in your blood, the more serotonin you are likely to make and the more responsive you become to its effects.

Top fish for brain-boosting fats

Amount of EPA in 100g (3oz)

Mackerel	1,400mg
Herring/kipper	1,000mg
Sardines	1,000mg
Tuna	900mg
Anchovy	900mg
Salmon	800mg
Trout	500mg

What about side effects? Participants in some earlier studies, who were consuming 14 fish oil capsules a day, experienced mild gastro-intestinal discomfort – mainly loose bowels. However, nowadays you can buy more concentrated EPA-rich fish oils, so you get more omega-3 with less oil. Supplementing fish oils also reduces the risk of heart disease, alleviates arthritic pain and may improve memory and concentration.

Balancing your blood sugar

If you went to your doctor complaining of depression, you'd hardly expect them to say, 'Eat less sugar.' But they should, because there is a direct link between mood and blood-sugar balance. As we've already seen, all carbohydrate foods are broken down into glucose and your brain runs on glucose. The more uneven your blood-sugar supply, the more uneven your mood.

Eating lots of sugar is going to give you sudden peaks and troughs in the amount of glucose in your blood. You will experience this as fatigue, irritability, dizziness, insomnia, excessive sweating (especially at night), poor concentration and forgetfulness, severe thirst, depression, crying spells, digestive disturbances and blurred vision. (For more details on blood-sugar problems, see Chapter 8.) Since the brain depends on an even supply of glucose, it is no surprise to find that sugar has been implicated in aggressive behaviour,[131–136] anxiety,[137 138] depression,[139] and fatigue.[140]

Lots of refined sugar and refined carbohydrates (white bread, pasta, rice and most processed foods) are also linked with depression because these foods not only supply very little in the way of nutrients, but also use up the mood-enhancing B vitamins. And the body needs B vitamins to turn each teaspoon of sugar into energy. Sugar also diverts the supply of another nutrient we highlighted in our discussion of diabetes in Chapter 8 – chromium. This mineral is vital for keeping your blood-sugar level stable because insulin, which clears glucose from the blood, can't work properly without it. In fact, it turns out that just supplying proper levels of chromium to certain depressed patients can make a big difference.

CHROMIUM AND 'ATYPICAL' DEPRESSION

'Atypical' depression is so-called because it differs markedly from so-called 'classic' depression, where sufferers have little appetite, don't eat enough, lose weight and can't sleep. Let's look at some of the symptoms of atypical depression; if you answer yes to five or more of these questions, you might be suffering from it.

• Do you crave sweets or other carbohydrates?

• Do you tend to gain weight?

• Are you tired for no obvious reason?

• Do your arms or legs feel heavy?

• Do you tend to feel sleepy or groggy much of the time?

• Are your feelings easily hurt by the rejection of others?

• Did your depression begin before the age of 30?

Atypical depression is estimated to affect anywhere from 25 to 42 per cent of the depressed population, and an even higher percentage among depressed women, so it's actually extremely common (and misnamed).

A chance discovery by Dr Malcolm McLeod, clinical professor of psychiatry at the University of North Carolina in the US, suggested that people who suffer from it might benefit from chromium supplementation.[141] In a small double-blind study published in 2003, McLeod gave ten patients suffering from atypical depression chromium supplements of 600mcg a day, and five others a placebo, for eight weeks.[142]

The results were dramatic. Seven out of the ten taking the supplements showed a big improvement, as opposed to none on the placebo. Their HRS dropped by an unheard-of 83 per cent: that is, from 29 – major depression – to five, which is classed as not depressed. A larger trial at Cornell University in the US, involving 113 participants, confirmed the finding in 2005. After eight weeks, 65 per cent of the people taking chromium had had a major improvement, compared to 33 per cent on placebos.[143]

SIDE EFFECTS None, except more energy, better weight control and less risk of diabetes. Chromium has no toxicity, even at amounts 100 times those used in the trials above.

Light, exercise, air and friends

Exercise is a key part of the new medicine model's non-drug approach. It also turns out to be as effective as taking anti-depressants. A number of studies in which people exercised for 30 to 60 minutes three to five times a week found a drop of around five points in their HRS – more than double what you'd expect from anti-depressants alone.[144] In an Australian study published in 2005, involving 60 adults over the age of 60, half took up high-intensity exercise three days a week, while the other half did low-intensity exercise. Of those doing high-intensity exercise, 61 per cent halved their HRS, while only 29 per cent of those doing low-intensity exercise halved their score.[145]

And if you exercise in bright light, you get a double dose of natural 'anti-depressant', as a number of studies using full-spectrum lighting (versus normal room lighting) have shown. Unlike normal 'yellow' lighting, sunlight is white and contains a stronger and fuller spectrum of light. Although more expensive, full-spectrum light bulbs are a worthwhile addition, especially if you are prone to the winter blues – known as SAD or seasonal-affective disorder. (See Resources, page 405, for suppliers of full-spectrum lighting.)

In one study published in 2004, a third of depressed volunteers who exercised in full-spectrum lighting experienced a major improvement in their depression (a 50 per cent or more decrease in their HRS).[146] Other studies from 2005 have also found a definitive improvement, even among those not specifically prone to SAD.[147] The effect could be due to the direct effect of light on raising serotonin.[148]

One other gadget, or lifestyle change, you might want to consider to beat the blues is an ioniser. These give off negative ions, which are naturally generated by turbulent water – think waterfalls and the seaside – and are thought to be good for you, while positive ions, produced especially by electronic equipment such as computer screens, air-conditioning and TV sets, are not. In one controlled trial, depressed patients exposed to both full-spectrum lighting plus a high-intensity ioniser reported major improvements in their depression.[149] By leaving an ioniser on overnight you might substantially improve mood (see Resources, page 405, for the best ionisers).

Counselling and psychotherapy

Probably the biggest non-nutritional factor in recovering from depression is having someone to talk to about life's inevitable problems and stresses. Much depression is linked to, or triggered by, stressful life events such as a death, the loss of a job, or the break-up of a relationship. Or you may have felt that your life was out of kilter and lacking in essential elements – a circle of supportive friends or relatives or good standing at work, for example – for some time, and feel that you're tipping over from the blues into a real depression.

Feeling bad about yourself and lacking someone supportive to listen to you can be a major cause of depression however good your diet might be.[150] A problem shared is a problem halved. While good nutrition might give you more mental and emotional energy to solve your problems, it doesn't take away the underlying issues that fuel depression. For this reason, we recommend counselling and psychotherapy as well as nutritional approaches.

Food or drugs? The verdict

The evidence suggests that the nutritional approach it not only more effective. It's also practically free of serious negative side effects. So why not do it? Well, you could argue that there's not enough research to conclusively prove all the benefits we've discussed here. You might be thinking that many of the trials are small, although well designed. That's true to an extent, and it's also unlikely to change: there's little profit to be made from non-patentable nutrients such as omega-3, folic acid or 5-HTP.

Psychiatrist Dr Erick Turne from the Mood Disorders Center in Portland, Oregon, who uses 5-HTP in his practice, says: 'Unfortunately, because 5-HTP is a dietary supplement and not a prescription pharmaceutical, there is comparatively little financial incentive for extensive clinical research.' Also, since no benefits for nutrients can be put on their packaging, and there's no army of reps or marketing budget, most people simply don't know about these highly effective, and considerably safer, nutritional options.

But then there's the other, now-familiar problem: most doctors are also unacquainted with food-based medicine. 'A doctor receives virtually no training in nutritional approaches to depression. It's an obvious oversight, given the wealth of evidence,' says André Tylee, professor of primary care mental health at the Institute of Psychiatry. But that is no reason why you shouldn't try it yourself with the help of a nutritional therapist.

What works

- Set up the building blocks. Most of the studies we've cited used 300mg of 5-HTP, but we recommend ideally testing to see whether you are low in serotonin with a platelet serotonin test (see Resources, page 406) and starting with 100mg, or 50mg, twice a day. Be aware that 5-HTP is best absorbed either on an empty stomach or with a carbohydrate snack such as a piece of fruit or an oat cake. Otherwise, make sure you eat enough protein from beans, lentils, nuts, seeds, fish, eggs and meat, which are all high in tryptophan. If your motivation is low, you could also supplement 1,000mg of tyrosine.

- Put the catalysts in place. Test your homocysteine level, which can be done using a home-test kit (see Resources, page 406). Your doctor can also test you, although few do. If your level is above 9mmol/l, take a combined 'homocysteine' supplement of B2, B6, B12, folic acid, zinc, and TMG, providing at least 400mcg of folic acid, 250mcg of B12 and 20mg of B6. If your homocysteine score is above 15mmol/l, double this amount. Also eat whole foods rich in the B vitamins – whole grains, beans, nuts, seeds, fruits and vegetables. Folic acid is particularly abundant in green vegetables, beans, lentils, nuts and seeds, while B12 is only found in animal foods – meat, fish, eggs and dairy produce.

- Take omega-3s. You need about 1,000mg of EPA a day for a mood-boosting effect. That means supplementing a concentrated omega-3 fish oil capsule providing 500mg twice a day, and eating a serving of either sardines, mackerel, herring, or wild or organic salmon, three times a week. Tuna steaks are also a good source but should be eaten only once a fortnight because of possible mercury contamination, whereas tinned tuna has very little omega-3s because of the way it's processed. Very little, perhaps 5 per cent, of the omega-3 fats found in flax or pumpkin seeds convert into EPA, so while these are good to eat they don't have the same anti-depressant effect.

- Keep your fuel supply stable. Eating a diet that will stabilise your blood-sugar (see page 143), and supplementing 600mcg of chromium, will help tremendously in keeping your moods stable. Chromium supplements generally come in 200mcg pills. Take two with breakfast and one with lunch. After a month, cut down to one with breakfast and one with lunch. Don't take chromium in the evening, as it can have a stimulating effect.

- Exercise for at least 15 minutes most days. Psychocalisthenics (see Resources, page 405) is especially good for balancing your mood.

- Consider psychotherapy (see Resources, page 403, for help with referrals).

Working with your doctor

Much of what we recommend you can either do for yourself or by seeking the guidance and support of a nutritional therapist. However, the process of weaning yourself off anti-depressants is something you must do with the support and guidance of your doctor.

We recommend that 5-HTP not be taken in significant amounts, above 50mg, if you are on an anti-depressant – 5-HTP helps the body make serotonin while SSRI anti-depressants stop it being broken down. If your doctor is willing to wean you off anti-depressants it helps, at the same time, to wean you on to 5-HTP, gradually building the daily amount up to a maximum of 300mg, but no more than 100mg before you are completely off the anti-depressant. In our experience, this minimises and shortens the withdrawal effects that many people experience when coming off anti-depressants.

All the other mood-boosting factors we've discussed – from omega-3s to exercise – can safely be added while you're on medication and will probably help you reduce your need, them come off anti-depressants with fewer withdrawal effects.

11.

Preventing Memory Loss and Alzheimer's
Memory drugs vs natural mind boosters

IF YOU ARE over 35, it's time to think about Alzheimer's. As strange as this may sound, we now know that it takes approximately 40 years to develop Alzheimer's and there are no obvious signs, except perhaps a minor deterioration in memory and concentration, for at least the first 20 years of the disease process. Many people think of this as 'getting old', but you can age without excessive memory loss, as we'll see in this chapter.

For many people over the age of 60, it becomes harder to concentrate. Their short-term memory isn't as good as it used to be, and problems become harder to solve. When these symptoms become more severe, usually around age 80, a person may be diagnosed with dementia. Every year in Europe, a million people are diagnosed with memory decline, and 400,000 of them go on to be diagnosed with dementia. In Australia, half a million people live with this harrowing condition.[151]

Devastating diagnosis

There are many causes of dementia – for example, poor blood supply to the brain – and all these will be investigated and ruled out. If no other causes are identified and the deterioration continues, a person may be diagnosed with probable Alzheimer's. About three out of four people diagnosed with dementia end up with this diagnosis.

The human cost is, of course, massive, both for sufferers and their families. And so is the cost to health services. In the UK, treating Alzheimer's costs an estimated £14 billion a year, paid for partly by the National Health Service and partly by the families involved. That's 20 per cent of the NHS budget!

But Alzheimer's is not simply degeneration that happens as you get old. All the evidence now points to a specific disease process that occurs in some people, but not all, which causes brain cells in an area called the 'median temporal lobe' – involved in both memory and emotion – to begin to die off. The evidence also suggests that it's a long time coming, with the degeneration beginning perhaps 30 years before the first symptoms develop. That's why prevention makes far more sense than treatment – especially since there is currently no way to significantly reverse the condition, although there may be ways to stop it from getting worse. Check yourself out on the questionnaire below.

How is your memory and concentration?

☐ Is your memory deteriorating?

☐ Do you find it hard to concentrate and often get confused?

☐ Do you sometimes meet someone you know quite well but can't remember their name?

☐ Do you often find you can remember things from the past but forget what you did yesterday?

☐ Do you ever forget what day of the week it is?

☐ Do you ever go looking for something and forget what you are looking for?

☐ Do your friends and family think you're getting more forgetful now than you used to be?

☐ Do you find it hard to add up numbers without writing them down?

☐ Do you often experience mental tiredness?

☐ Do you find it hard to concentrate for more than an hour?

☐ Do you often misplace your keys?

☐ Do you frequently repeat yourself?

☐ Do you sometimes forget the point you're trying to make?

☐ Does it take you longer to learn things than it used to?

Score one for each 'yes' answer. If your score is:

Below 5: you don't have a major problem with your memory – but you'll find that supplementing natural mind and memory boosters will sharpen you up even more.

5 to 10: your memory definitely needs a boost – you are starting to suffer from some memory loss. Follow all the diet and supplement recommendations here.

More than 10: you are experiencing significant memory decline and need to do something about it. As well as following all the diet and supplement recommendations in this chapter, see a nutritionist.

Memory drugs – marginal benefits

As the brain cells of someone with Alzheimer's start dying off, levels of the memory neurotransmitter acetylcholine, which they produce, begin to decline. Most of the current medications work by replacing the lost acetylcholine, but they don't deal with the underlying causes of the damage. The drugs seem to be able to produce an improvement in about 20 per cent of people, but only as long as they have enough neurons to produce the acetylcholine, which can then be 'spared' by the drug. As the disease progresses and more neurons die off, the drugs soon stop working.

Acetylcholinesterase inhibitors

These drugs work by blocking an enzyme that normally clears acetyl-choline away – hence their name. The big brands include donepezil

(Aricept), rivastigmine (Exelon) and galantamine (Reminyl). They can temporarily improve or stabilise the symptoms of dementia by improving communication between neurons, but once you stop your prescription, you'll deteriorate rapidly and within six weeks you will be no better than someone who has never taken the drug.

Just how marginal the benefits are was revealed in a five-year trial of Aricept – the most widely prescribed brand – published in *The Lancet* in 2004.[152] Regardless of the dose given, it found no difference in 'worthwhile improvements' in a range of categories: rates of disease progression, the rate at which patients were placed in nursing homes, care-giver time, or how fast behaviour deteriorated. The one benefit is that during the first two years of the study, patients taking Aricept did do slightly better in tests measuring thinking and functional ability.

Here, 'slightly better' means an improvement in the scores on a questionnaire called the Mini Mental State Exam, or MMSE for short. It includes questions like, 'Count backwards from 50 in 5s,' 'What street are we in?' and 'You'll be asked to name pictures of objects, and then remember them.' The average score for someone aged 18 to 24 is 29 out of a possible 30, whereas a healthy 80-year-old could expect to score 25. The NHS used to recommend Aricept for people with a score of 12 or less. In the study quoted above, those on the drug had an MMSE score 0.8 points higher after two years than those on the placebo. So we are not talking about major improvement, and at the end of five years there was no difference at all.

Even this study's lead researcher, Richard Gray, admitted: 'Realistically, patients are unlikely to derive much benefit from this drug.' At best, one could say that up to half those taking this kind of drug derive a ten per cent improvement in memory for up to two years. They then decline rapidly to the same place they would have been without the drug.

SIDE EFFECTS For one in three people taking acetylcholinesterase inhibitors such as Aricept, the side effects can include nausea, vomiting, diarrhoea, stomach cramps, headaches, dizziness, fatigue, insomnia and loss of appetite.

NMDA-receptor agonists

Another drug, Memantine – an NMDA-receptor agonist – works by regulating the activity of a brain chemical called glutamate. Glutamate plays an essential role in learning and memory, but too much glutamate allows excess calcium into nerve cells, killing them off. This is where Memantine's regulatory role comes into its own. But a review of studies on Memantine, published in 2005, shows it produces minor benefit after six months in moderate-to-severe Alzheimer's, but not in milder cases.[153]

What's left out of this picture is that one of the causes of dangerously raised levels of glutamate is excess homocysteine in the bloodstream, which is a characteristic of Alzheimer's. As we'll see later, a safer alternative to preventing excess of this otherwise vital brain chemical is to lower homocysteine levels with B vitamins.

SIDE EFFECTS Possible side effects for Memantine include hallucinations, confusion, dizziness, headaches and tiredness.

That's the best current memory drugs have to offer: a short-lived improvement for a few, but no change in the underlying disease progression. For many there is no improvement and a range of what we can clearly see are undesirable side effects. That's why the UK's National Institute for Health and Clinical Excellence (NICE), which advises doctors on prescribing, concluded that drugs such as Aricept – even at the relatively low cost of £1.20 a day – are not worth it. They recommend that none of these drugs be used for mild to moderate Alzheimer's disease.[154]

Natural alternatives

The real solution to dementia and Alzheimer's lies in prevention – and there's plenty of evidence that that is entirely possible. For instance, some one in five people who end up with dementia are diagnosed with vascular dementia. The cause of this is almost identical to cardiovascular disease: blood vessels become increasingly blocked up, so the brain cells just don't get enough oxygen and nutrients. Chapter 15 goes into the nutritional solutions for this condition. But the majority of people with dementia go on to be diagnosed with Alzheimer's.

The real roots of Alzheimer's

There are two common myths about Alzheimer's that need debunking. The first is that it's caused by ageing, so there's nothing you can do about it. The second is that it's 'in your genes'.

There's no question that Alzheimer's is age-related. In other words, the older you are, the more likely you are to get it: while only two in 100 people aged 65 to 69 have dementia, one in four aged 90 or more are affected. For every five years you age, your chances of developing dementia double. But that doesn't mean that ageing *causes* it. Heart attacks are more likely to happen the older you are, but ageing doesn't cause them, either. In fact, in some countries and regions, such as rural China, there's remarkably little incidence of Alzheimer's among 90-year-olds, which tells us something. We'll come to that shortly.

As for genes, it is true that there are specific gene variations that increase your chance of developing Alzheimer's. But they are exceedingly rare and account for perhaps one in 100 cases. This kind of dementia starts early – usually when people are in their fifties – and runs in families.

The rest of the cases are caused by a combination of risk factors (see diagram overleaf), of which diet is probably the single most important. For example, if you have the ApoE4 gene variation, you are far more likely to develop the disease if you also have other risk factors: smoking, for instance, raises risk four times. If you don't have ApoE4 – and only ten per cent of the population do – smoking makes no difference. In fact, there is some evidence that nicotine has a protective effect (although this doesn't cancel out the considerable downsides of the habit!).

Conventionally, research into Alzheimer's has involved trying to understand the workings of a rogue protein, beta-amyloid. This is what forms the plaques and 'tangles' that are the signature of the disease and are found with the destroyed brain cells. The aim of this work has been to reduce the amount of beta-amyloid – but so far, it hasn't met with much success. However, there is evidence that a nutritional approach can

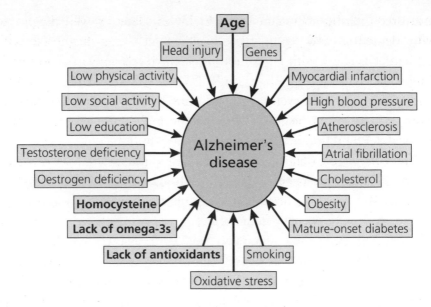

Risk factors for Alzheimer's disease

certainly reduce the risk of its developing in the first place, so let's examine the three hottest diet-related risk factors – high homocysteine, a lack of omega-3s and oxidant exposure – and what you can do to reverse them.

So what's the evidence?

Homocysteine and Alzheimer's prevention

At the moment, the single most important nutritional discovery is that your risk of developing Alzheimer's is strongly linked to the level of homocysteine in your blood. The lower your level throughout life, the smaller your chances of developing serious memory decline. Homocysteine is an amino acid, but it's also a neurotoxin capable of directly damaging the medial temporal lobe, which is the area of the brain that rapidly degenerates in Alzheimer's.[155] Homocysteine, as you will see, is easily lowered with inexpensive B vitamins such as folic acid.

A study in the *New England Journal of Medicine*, published in 2002, charted the health of 1,092 elderly people without dementia, and measured their homocysteine levels. Eight years later, 111 were diagnosed with dementia, and 83 of these participants were diagnosed with Alzheimer's. Those with blood homocysteine levels above 14 had nearly double the risk of getting Alzheimer's.[156] There's also evidence, in another study from 2002, that even before a decline in mental function starts to show up in so-called 'healthy' elderly people, high homocysteine predicts physical degeneration in certain parts of the brain.[157]

In Scotland, researchers have found that reduced mental performance in old age is strongly associated with high homocysteine and low levels of vitamins B12 and folic acid. Following up participants in the Scottish Mental Surveys of 1932 and 1947, which surveyed childhood intelligence, they found that the most mentally agile had the highest levels of B vitamins and lowest levels of homocysteine, whereas high homocysteine was linked with a seven to eight per cent decline in mental performance.[158]

A similar Californian study from 2006 asked 579 men and women aged 60 and over to keep track of their diet and the supplements they took. After nine years, 57 of them developed Alzheimer's. Those with the highest folic acid intake reduced their risk of developing Alzheimer's by 55 per cent.[159]

A research group led by Dr Teodoro Bottiglieri at the Baylor University Metabolic Disease Center in Dallas, Texas, suggests that low levels of folic acid may cause brain damage that triggers dementia and Alzheimer's. Their research has found that a third of those with both dementia and homocysteine levels above 14 units were deficient in folic acid.[160]

So there is a lot of research that points to a link between high homocysteine, low B vitamin intake and a raised risk of brain degeneration. But why? What is the link between B vitamins and damaged brain cells? This is what Bottiglieri has to say:

What is extraordinary is that B vitamins have been excluded from the Alzheimer picture for so long. The link between brain deterioration – memory loss, cognitive deficits, depression, and personality breakdown – and B vitamin deficiency is standard neurology textbook stuff. You get it with severe alcoholism, with some genetic disorders that prevent B vitamins functioning properly and with pernicious anaemia. The trouble is that there is a lot of money tied up in the amyloid protein story.

The reason for the B vitamin-Alzheimer's link is that the body needs B vitamins to handle homocysteine. Normally, they turn homocysteine into two very useful chemicals called glutathione, an antioxidant, and the amino acid SAMe. SAMe, in turn, is vital for the manufacture of one of the main neurotransmitters – acetylcholine. Alzheimer's patients have very low levels of SAMe and also of acetylcholine. So we can see how high homocysteine levels and low B vitamin levels – indicating less homocysteine is being converted to SAMe – would make for low levels of that vital neurotransmitter.

As we've seen already, the pharmaceutical approach is to raise acetylcholine levels directly. But the nutritional one is to go to the other end of that biochemical chain and supply the B vitamins needed to produce the amino acid that in turn produces not just acetylcholine, but also a range of other beneficial effects.

The theory makes sense, but does supplementing with vitamins prevent, or actually reverse memory loss? In truth, it's early days; but large amounts of the Bs do seem to be effective. There are trials going on right now giving B vitamins to people with age-related cognitive decline and Alzheimer's. A Dutch study involving 818 people aged between 50 and 75 was completed in 2005. Participants either got a vitamin containing 800mcg of folic acid a day – almost three times the RDA and the equivalent of the amount you'd get in 2.5lbs (1.1kg) of strawberries – or a placebo.[161] After three years, supplement users had scores on memory tests comparable to people 5.5 years younger. On tests of cognitive speed, the folic acid helped users perform as well as people 1.9 years younger.

Megadoses are also being used in a trial currently being run by Professor David Smith of the Optima Project at the University of Oxford. Smith is giving people with age-related memory decline 1,000mcg of folic acid, 20mg of B6 and 500mcg of B12, which is 250 times the RDA and a far cry from the amount you could get by eating 'a well-balanced diet'.

Such high amounts are being used for the simple reason that they work. 'The lowest dose of oral cyanocobalamin [B12] required to normalize mild vitamin B12 deficiency in older people is more than 200 times the recommended dietary allowance,' concludes a paper by scientists at the University of Wageningen in Holland, one of the world's top B12 research centres.[162]

Although more needs to be done to find out both how early supplementation has to begin in order to halt or even reverse memory loss, and what is the most effective combination of diet and supplements, it certainly makes sense to ensure an optimal intake of B6, B12 and folic acid. And along with this, it's a good idea to supplement the amino acid N-acetyl-cysteine (NAC), which is used to make the valuable brain antioxidant glutathione. A look at the case of Dr Tudor Powell will help make this real.

Tudor Powell, a retired teacher and doctor of philosophy, began to have problems with his memory when he reached the age of 71. 'Four years ago my short-term memory was getting worrying. I often lost things. Sometimes I'd go upstairs and didn't know why. My wife was becoming increasingly concerned about my driving.'

He went to see Dr Andrew McCaddon, a medical doctor in Wrexham, Wales, who specialises in the nutritional approach to Alzheimer's. He did what every doctor should immediately do for patients with worsening memory – gave Tudor a simple memory test and measured his homocysteine level.

Tudor's homocysteine level was 14.6 μmol/l, which is too high, although quite common among people in their seventies. On a standard memory test he scored 16 out of 39 (the higher the score the better). This score certainly indicated that Tudor had dementia. (An actual diagnosis of Alzheimer's is hard to make without a specialised, and very expensive, brain scan – which is why 'probable Alzheimer's' is so often diagnosed.)

McCaddon gave him high levels of supplements to take every day, including B12 (1,000mcg), folic acid (5,000mcg) and N-acetyl-cysteine (600mg). Within two weeks, Tudor started to notice a difference. 'I felt much better, my memory was sharper, I had more energy. I rejoined the local choir because I could remember the music.' After six months his homocysteine level had dropped to 8.3μmol/l, which is close to ideal for his age and equates to more than halving his Alzheimer's disease risk. His score on the memory test improved by 12.5 per cent.

Today, three years later, his memory has not declined any further – exactly the opposite of what normally happens. 'He's reading again. He interested in life once more,' says his wife. 'I feel like I've got my husband back. We've always had a pretty good diet. It's the nutritional supplements that have made the world of difference.'

Nutritional supplements aimed at lowering homocysteine not only produce a reduction in symptoms, but also potentially stop the progression of the disease. Although this has not yet been proven in double-blind controlled studies, case studies do show this type of improvement.

Reducing brain inflammation with omega-3s

In Chapter 10 we saw how omega-3 fats — most prevalent in carnivorous coldwater fish such as sardines, mackerel, salmon and herrings — have significantly helped people battling with depression and bipolar disorder. And according to a recent study by Dr Martha Morris and colleagues at Chicago's Rush Institute for Healthy Aging, eating fish once a week reduces your risk of developing Alzheimer's by 60 per cent.

The researchers followed 815 people aged 65 to 94 for seven years, and found that a dietary intake of fish was strongly linked to the risk of developing Alzheimer's. The strongest link was the amount of DHA, which along with EPA is a primary omega-3 found in oily coldwater fish. In essence, the finding was that the higher a person's level of DHA, the lower their risk of developing Alzheimer's. The lowest amount of DHA per day that offered some protection was 100mg. While the participants' intake of EPA did not seem significant in this study, possibly because the highest intake of EPA consumed was only 30mg a day.[163]

But why exactly does fish have this protective effect? One theory is that it helps to ease brain inflammation, which can damage brain cells (see Chapter 13 to read more about inflammation and the role of omega-3 fats). Omega-3 fats are also a vital component of brain cell membranes and help control the flow of calcium in and out of cells. This is important because too much calcium inside brain cells is known to contribute to the production of beta-amyloid protein, which is found in excessive levels in the brains of most people who develop Alzheimer's.

Boosting antioxidant levels

Along with inflammation in the brain, another characteristic of Alzheimer's is a rise in the level of free radicals or oxidants as a result of the spreading amyloid plaques and the death of brain cells. This adds to the problem because oxidants reduce the effectiveness of B vitamins in transforming homocysteine. Taking antioxidants such as beta-carotene and vitamins A, C, and E, all of which have been shown to be low in people with Alzheimer's, can help counteract such oxidative damage.

For instance, a study published in the *Journal of the American Medical Association* in 2002 found that the risk of developing Alzheimer's was 67 per cent lower in those with a high dietary intake of vitamin E, as compared to those with a low intake.[164] Vitamin E not only plays a key role in early prevention, but also in slowing down the progression of the disease. In another study from 1997, Alzheimer's patients received either 2,000iu of vitamin E, the drug Selegiline or a placebo.[165] Of the three, vitamin E was shown to reduce progression most significantly.

More studies are definitely needed but, to date, most of the evidence points to a protective role for vitamin E.

Keeping mind and body active

There is plenty of evidence that keeping both your mind and body active will help to prevent a decline in mental function.[166–171] For example, researchers at the Albert Einstein College of Medicine in New York tested the link between leisure activities and the risk of developing dementia or Alzheimer's in the elderly.

In the study, published in 2003, they followed 469 people over the age of 75, who had no signs of dementia when the study began, over five years. The team found that reading, playing cards and board games, doing crossword puzzles, playing musical instruments and dancing were all associated with a reduced risk of dementia, memory loss and Alzheimer's. Overall, the study participants who did these kinds of activities about four days a week were two-thirds less likely to get Alzheimer's compared with those doing them once a week or less.[172]

At the Rush Alzheimer's Disease Center in Chicago, researchers found the same things in a group of 801 Catholic nuns, priests and brothers who showed no signs of dementia over four and a half years. The team compared the amount of mentally stimulating activity each person engaged in and measured their rate of mental decline. The study, published in 2002, found that a boost in mental activity was associated with a reduced decline in overall mental function by 47 per cent, memory by 60 per cent, and perception by 30 per cent.[173]

But it's not just your brain that needs a workout. Physical exercise has a direct effect on mental powers, probably for a number of reasons. First, since your brain and body are made up of the same stuff, and we know that exercise keeps your body healthy, it stands to reason that exercise will keep your brain healthy too. Also, people at greater risk of cardiovascular disease are at greater risk of Alzheimer's. Secondly, part of the benefit of exercise is likely to be because exercise reduces stress (stress is a contributor to dementia and the risk of Alzheimer's because high levels of the stress hormone cortisol cause dendrites, the connections between neurons, to shrivel up). Thirdly, exercise increases blood flow to the brain, bringing more oxygen and nutrients.[174–175] And lastly, there is evidence that being overweight increases the risk of Alzheimer's, so part of the positive effect of exercise is likely to be that it helps you keep to a healthy weight.

Evidence for the importance of keeping fit was found in a five-year study of 5,000 Canadian men and women over the age of 65, published in 2001. Those who had high levels of physical activity, compared to those who rarely exercised, halved their risk of Alzheimer's disease.[176] Another study, from 1995, found that regular walking improved memory and reduced signs of dementia. About 1,000 steps, or a little over a mile a day, was the minimum distance required to achieve the positive effect.[177]

But the most convincing evidence for the value of exercise comes from a six-year study, published in 2006, of 1,740 elderly people. Those who exercised three or more times a week had a 30 to 40 per cent lower risk of developing dementia, compared with those who exercised fewer than three times per week.[178]

Exercise also prevents physical deterioration of the brain. Our brains become less dense and lose volume as we age and with that loss of density and volume comes mental decline. Researchers at the University of Illinois used MRI scans to examine the brains of 55 elderly people. When they compared their scans with their level of physical exercise they found that the people who exercised more and were more physically fit had the densest brains.[179] So the old saying 'Use it lose it' takes on greater significance in this context. Basically, if you don't use your body, you're at risk of losing your mind.

Exercise is not only protective against Alzheimer's, it can also lift your mood. In fact, it's more effective than anti-depressants for mild depression, as we've seen. Depression is a common problem among Alzheimer's patients. A 2003 study at the University of Washington in Seattle showed that exercise significantly improved the mood and physical health of depressed Alzheimer's patients and meant they were less likely to need to be moved into a care home.[180]

Food or drugs? The verdict

What all this adds up to is that Alzheimer's, which accounts for the vast majority of cases of dementia, is preventable. What is equally clear is that there is no drug that can do anything except, at most, briefly delay the debilitating symptoms. The nutritional approach, however, could play a role beyond the preventative, as valuable as that is. It may also reverse early signs of memory and mental impairment without any associated side effects. If this proves to be so in ongoing trials, the nutritional approach should certainly be the first port of call for anyone with memory problems.

What works

- Test your homocysteine level. If you have a relative whose mental gears are starting to slip, make sure they have a simple memory test, just to get a measure of the situation, plus a homocysteine test (see page 406), which is the best indicator of risk. If their (and in fact, your) homocysteine level is above nine units and there any signs or symptoms of memory problems, we recommend supplementing with a homocysteine-lowering formula. This should provide a daily vitamin B6 (20 to 100mg), B12 (100 to 500mcg), and folic acid (1,000 to 2,000mcg) or, better still, take an all-round homocysteine-lowering formula containing TMG and B2 as well. Also supplement N-acetyl-cysteine (500mg a day). Alternatively, choose a homocysteine formula incorporating a special form of B12, methyl B12, which works best for lowering homocysteine.

- Up your omega-3s. To help reduce brain inflammation, we recommend supplementing with omega-3 fish oils, as well as eating oily fish two to three times a week. The ideal amount for maximising memory and mental health is likely to be in the region of 300mg of EPA and 200mg of DHA daily, doubling this if you have age-related memory decline.

- Increase your antioxidants. To ensure you are getting the proper types and amounts of antioxidants, eat lots of fruit and vegetables with a variety of colours. Think blueberries, raspberries, apples, broccoli, red cabbage, sweet potatoes, carrots and so on – antioxidants such as the anthocyanidins found in red and purple fruit and vegetables are powerful and highly efficient at scavenging free radicals. On top of this, supplement 2,000 mg of vitamin C a day, taken in two divided doses, plus 400iu (300mg) of vitamin E, as part of an all-round anti-oxidant that contains N-acetyl-cysteine and/or reduced glutathione.

- Stay mentally and physically active. Keep learning new things and using your mind, and exercise at least three times a week. Even walking 15 minutes a day makes a difference.

Working with your doctor

Doctors like Andrew McCaddon (see page 209) routinely measure homocysteine in patients with memory decline, and there's no reason why your doctor cannot do the same. If your level is high, you should take a supplement with the B vitamins (shown on page 213), as well as zinc, TMG and NAC, and top up daily with plenty of B-rich fruit and green, leafy vegetables.

What if your doctor draws a blank or needs convincing? Show them the evidence: either lend them a copy of *The Alzheimer's Prevention Plan* by Patrick Holford and colleagues, or refer them to the work of Oxford's Optima Project or the Alzheimer's Research Trust.

If you, or a relative of yours, is prescribed Aricept, monitor changes in memory. If it makes no difference, there's little point in taking this drug.

12.

Relieving Anxiety and Insomnia
The sleeping pill scandal vs natural insomnia busters

SLEEP IS A wonderful thing, yet for quite a few of us it's an elusive pleasure. In the Institute for Optimum Nutrition's UK survey of 37,000 people, 53 per cent said they had difficulty sleeping or experienced restless sleep, while 63 per cent said they needed more sleep.[181] Somewhere between 2.2 and 5 million adults in the UK have a serious problem with insomnia, finding it hard to fall asleep, or wake in the night or the early morning and fail to get back to sleep.

You are more likely to suffer from it the older you are and it's more likely to affect women. Long-term insomnia may be linked to an illness like diabetes or a painful condition such as arthritis. If poor sleep continues for more than a week or so, it may start to affect your days because you feel so drowsy and woozy.

When you can't switch off

The problem usually begins before bedtime. You may feel unable to switch off from feelings of stress, tension and anxiety – the buzz words for the twenty-first century. According to the Institute for Optimum Nutrition's UK survey 63 per cent of people say they suffer from stress and more than half of all doctor visits are for stress-related conditions, including anxiety and insomnia. And that is a clue to the best way of treating it.

According to a review from 2004, published in *The Lancet*,[182] the various forms of counselling and psychological help are not only more effective than pills at tackling chronic insomnia – they are also, inevitably, far safer. But in the UK, for instance, good therapeutic help can be hard to find on the National Health Service. As a consequence, over 16 million prescriptions for what are called hypnotic (sleeping) and anxiolytic (anxiety-reducing) drugs were written out in 2004, at a cost of £37 million.

Do you suffer from insomnia/anxiety?

☐ Do you have difficulty getting to sleep?

☐ Do you wake in the night more than once?

☐ Are you a light sleeper?

☐ Do you wake up in the early hours of the morning feeling unrested?

☐ Would you describe yourself as anxious?

☐ Are you easily stressed?

☐ Do you have difficulty relaxing?

☐ Do you find yourself feeling irritable?

☐ Do you get angry easily?

☐ Do you find you are impatient with others?

☐ Are you prone to low moods?

☐ Are you easily upset or offended?

☐ Do you suffer from tense muscles?

Score 1 for each 'yes' answer. If you answered yes to:

Less than 4: you are not particularly anxious or stressed although the ideal is to have no 'yes' answers.

4 to 9: you have the indications of increased stress, anxiety or insomnia and need to take our advice in this chapter seriously. Recheck your score in one month. If your number of yes responses has not fallen, go and see a nutritional therapist.

10 or more: you have a major issue with anxiety and sleep. We recommend you pursue all the options here, including seeing a psychotherapist and a nutritional therapist. If you are taking anti-anxiety medication or sleeping pills, you will need to speak to your doctor about switching to some of these safer alternatives.

Before exploring the drugs and natural remedies on offer, it's important to understand what goes wrong in the brain to make a person more anxious and unable to sleep. Many insomniacs suffer from 'hyperarousal' – their body stays revved up towards evening, when most people are winding down. The root cause is often psychological (stress, anxiety or depression), linked to a body chemistry that's out of balance. It is a state likely to be associated with increased amounts of the hormone adrenalin.

Normally, in the evening as the light level decreases, we start to produce less adrenalin as it is turned off by the inhibitory neurotransmitter GABA (gamma aminobutyric acid). Alcohol, cannabis, benzodiazapine drugs such as Valium and most sleeping pills all target GABA. Stress and stimulants such as caffeine counteract GABA by promoting adrenalin, which is why they keep you awake. Caffeine also suppresses melatonin, a neurotransmitter that helps you to sleep. Melatonin is the cousin of serotonin, the happy neurotransmitter, and without enough of it it's hard to sleep through the night.

The sleeping pill scandal

Real downers – barbiturates

Remember the Rolling Stones' song, 'Mother's Little Helper'? Written in the late 1960s, it describes a woman relying on the 'shelter' of a yellow pill to get her through her day.

From the early 1900s until the mid-1950s, barbiturates such as pheno-barbital and Seconal were the mainstay for treating both anxiety and insomnia. Unfortunately, they were also associated with thousands of suicides; accidental deaths, both of children who took them and adults who overdosed on them; widespread dependency and abuse; and chemical incompatibility with other drugs and alcohol. By 1954, they were being replaced by the new, 'non-addictive' meprobamate (Miltown) as the calming agent of choice, which turned out to be as addictive as the old drugs.

The new breed – benzodiazepines

Then, in the 1960s, a new group of drugs were launched – the benzo-diazepines. These included diazepam (Valium), chlordiazepoxide (Librium), clonazapine (Klonopin) and then the shorter-acting alprazolam (Xanax), lorazepam (Ativan) and temazepam (Restoril). In the UK, 16 million prescriptions are still written annually for these so-called 'minor tranquillisers' to treat anxiety and insomnia. Their calming effect is due to their action on GABA: by increasing GABA activity, the benzodiazepines dull both awareness and overall brain activity. However, they also turned out to be nearly as addictive as the older ones, although not so easy to overdose on. What happened to Mary is an example of what these drugs can do.

> In her thirties, Mary found herself stuck in an unhappy marriage with a young child, and she began taking large doses of Valium to shut out the pain. One day, while filling yet another prescription for her, the pharmacist said, 'In case you don't know it, you're addicted. Speak to me when you're ready to stop.' This was Mary's wake-up call.
>
> In shocked response, she simply stopped the drug cold. She was too ashamed to face the pharmacist, who would have advised a slow withdrawal programme under medical supervision. Then, not knowing she was suffering from withdrawal symptoms, she simply, in her words, 'went crazy' for the next two months or so. It took that long for her brain to readjust itself.
>
> As with all addictive drugs, Valium had caused Mary's brain to 'down regulate' its production of the brain chemical involved, in this case GABA.

Without its calming influence Mary suddenly found herself in a state of extreme agitation, which is how withdrawal symptoms generally manifest. Eventually, normal production of GABA resumed as her brain readjusted itself.

'When I finally got my mind back, I decided to leave my husband. I never looked back. Nor did I ever dare take another tranquilliser,' declares Mary, now, at 48, a successful writer and a proud grandmother.

Mary was lucky with her pharmacist. Many other prescription-drug addicts, however, go for years having their prescription refilled in large, impersonal pharmacies, or rotate between several different stores so that nobody notices there is a problem. Harried physicians who have little time to really listen to patients find it easier to renew a prescription than to deal with someone's symptoms. And the prospect of detoxification is a tough one for both pharmacists and their addicted customers to deal with.

Although benzodiazepines suppress the symptoms of anxiety for a few hours, they do not treat underlying causes, and the anxiety returns as soon as the drug wears off. Moreover, there is a 'rebound effect', where you experience even worse symptoms than when you started because you have become dependent on the drug. Often, they will develop tolerance, meaning that even higher doses are needed for the same anti-anxiety effect. These factors – difficulty with withdrawal and tolerance – describe an addiction that can be as difficult to break as heroin. A combination of physical and emotional dependency develops. Ignoring the National Institute for Health and Clinical Excellence (NICE) warning that they 'should not be used beyond two to four weeks',[183] overburdened doctors may continue to renew a prescription for months or even years.

The dangers and addictive qualities of benzodiazepines are well known. Despite this, they are still widely prescribed, even though an editorial published in a 2004 issue of the *British Medical Journal* concluded that not only was there plenty of evidence that they cause 'major harm' but that there was 'little evidence of clinically meaningful benefit'.[184]

A recent trial found that people on these drugs for 18 months had 'negative effects on crisis reaction, intensified defence mechanisms and reduced cognitive, emotional and cognative [behavioural or active] functions and passive coping'.[185] A 2005 review of 37 trials examining whether benzodiazepines were effective for insomnia concluded that none were well enough designed to reach any conclusions.[186] Despite this, 6.5 million prescriptions were written out in 2004 for Diazepam and Nitrazepam alone.

SIDE EFFECTS Tolerance is a problem: after taking them for some time, a higher dose is required to get the same effect. People often experience forgetfulness, drowsiness, accident-proneness and/or social withdrawal. Other side effects include 'rebound' anxiety as a result of withdrawal and insomnia; hangover (grogginess the next morning, accidents caused not only right after ingestion, but the following day); and addiction (the person on the prescription must continue to take it just to stay 'even'). Benzodiazepines trigger serious withdrawal effects on quitting, including anxiety, insomnia, irritability, tremors, mental impairment, headaches – possibly even seizures and death. Combining these drugs with alcohol is especially dangerous.

The next generation – getting some Zs

All these terrible side effects were the major motivator for the development of a new class of drugs, the nonbenzodiazepines. These are a class of related but more targeted drugs, colloquially known as the 'Zs' – zolpidem (Ambien), zalephon (Sonata) and zopiclone (Zimovane). They were introduced in the 1990s amid claims that they were a safe and non-addictive alternative to earlier drugs.

However, a review in 2005 by NICE concluded that 'there was no consistent difference between the two types of drug for either effectiveness or safety.'[187] They too can cause tolerance and withdrawal. 'This medicine is generally only suitable for short-term use. If it is used for long periods or in high doses, tolerance to and dependence upon the medicine may develop, and withdrawal symptoms – rebound insomnia or anxiety, confusion, sweating, tremor, loss of appetite, irritability or convulsions – may occur if treatment is stopped suddenly,' advises one drug bulletin regarding zopiclone.[188] You are also not advised to take nonbenzodiazepines for more than a few weeks.

But these are the sleeping pills you are more likely to be offered on prescription these days: in 2004, there were close to 4 million prescriptions made for Zimovane in the UK alone. They will certainly help if you have a short-term problem with sleeping due to a crisis, but in the long term they are not what's needed. 'If you have chronic insomnia,' says Professor Jim Horne of Loughborough University's Sleep Research Centre, 'it's because you have an underlying problem and just getting an extra half an hour's sleep, which is about all the drugs give you, is not going to help tackle it.'

SIDE EFFECTS With nonbenzodiazepines, you can experience daytime drowsiness, which normally diminishes after the first few days of treatment, and a bitter taste in the mouth. Persistent morning drowsiness or impaired co-ordination are signs that your dose is too high. Zopiclone failed to get licensed in the US because of its association with cancer in animal studies. Combining these drugs with alcohol is especially dangerous. Zolpidem, the most commonly prescribed sleeping pill in the US, is associated with dizziness, difficulty with co-ordination and amnesia – people don't remember what has happened for several hours after taking the pill.

Yet more drugs?

Because of the problems with benzodiazepines, their use declined by over 50 per cent in the ten years since 1987, while at the same time the use of 'sedating anti-depressant' drugs went up by nearly 150 per cent. The most widely used of these is trazodone, whose side effects, along with nausea, dizziness and agitation, actually include insomnia! Yet again there was no evidence base for this move – it is another example of off-label prescribing (see Chapter 3, page 65). In 2004, the chairman of the Department of Psychiatry and Behavioral Medicine at Wake Forest University reported to the American National Institutes of Health that none of the sedating anti-depressants had actually been licensed to treat insomnia.

Meanwhile, yet another generation of sleeping pills is coming off the production line. First in the ring was eszopiclone (Lunesta), licensed in 2005 for long-term use after studies apparently showed no addiction and no need for increased dose after six months. It is a variation on zopiclone and is little different in effect. Trials found it increased the amount of time people slept before waking, but a common side-effect is drowsiness the next day.

Next is ramelteon (Rozerem) which, rather than targeting receptors on the GABA molecule as all the hypnotics do, affects two of the receptors on the sleep hormone melatonin. Because studies showed no signs of dependence, it is available over the counter. On its way is Indiplon, described as a 'unique non-narcotic, non-benzodiazepine agent', although like the other hypnotics it also targets one of the receptors on the GABA molecule. Remember, these are new drugs and nobody knows for sure what their long-term effects are likely to be.

Competition between the companies for a share of this market, which could rise to over $5 billion in a few years, has become so intense that commentators are talking of 'insomnia wars'. Spending on advertising is predicted to reach $145 million in the US alone. However, Professor Horne noted drily that 'claims of greater effectiveness and safety have been made for all new sleeping pills'.

WARNING: WITHDRAWAL RISKS

Be very aware that if you are addicted to any of these drugs, withdrawal needs to be taken seriously. It can be fatal if not done correctly and under medical supervision. See www.foodismedicine.co.uk/comingofftranquillisers for details about how to come off hypnotics and minimise withdrawal symptoms using safe, non-addictive herbal remedies. The organisation Counselling for Involuntary Tranquilliser Addiction (CITA) offers support, information and advice for those who are suffering from withdrawal and their families, and gives advice to health professionals to help people through withdrawal. If you live in the UK contact CITA at Cavendish House, Brighton Road, Waterloo, Liverpool L22 5NG, or call their National Telephone Helpline on 0151 932 0102, or visit www.liv.ac.uk/~csunit/community/careorgs/cita.htm.

Natural alternatives

Given the addictive nature of most anti-anxiety and insomnia drugs, their considerable side effects, and the fact that they don't address the underlying cause of the anxiety or insomnia in the first place, what are the natural, non-addictive alternatives?

These follow the same biochemical pathways in the body as the drugs – switching off the 'awake' neurotransmitter adrenalin, boosting GABA and restoring adequate levels of serotonin and melatonin – but without causing addiction. In addition to the nutritional solutions, there are many lifestyle solutions on offer. The first, and most obvious, is to deal with psychological issues and reactions that stress you out in the first place.

Psychotherapy

A small study published in a 2004 issue of the *Archives of Internal Medicine* found that just two hours of cognitive behavioural therapy (CBT) was able to cure insomnia by encouraging patients to acknowledge the stress that was preventing them from sleeping and then helping them develop ways of dealing with it.[189] One way CBT works is by helping the patient identify negative or unhelpful thoughts – 'I just can't sleep without my pills' – and then encouraging them to challenge them – 'I didn't have a problem until six months ago', 'I fell asleep with no trouble after that long walk.'

Such techniques are often combined with progressive muscle relaxation or a form of biofeedback to reduce the amount of active beta brain waves before going to bed. This involves hooking a patient up to a machine that displays their brain waves on a screen so they can see them slowing down as they do things like slowing their breathing. 'The challenge,' declared *The Lancet* review (referred to on page 216), 'is to move these therapies out of specialised sleep clinics and into everyday applications.'[190] Ask your doctor about getting psychological help or contact the Sleep Assessment Advisory Service (see Resources, page 405).

Sleep hygiene

A piece of essentially common-sense advice, rather quaintly known as 'sleep hygiene', forms part of most sleep regimes. Keep the bedroom quiet, dark and at a temperature that's good for you, wear comfortable clothing, don't have a big meal in the evening and avoid coffee and alcohol at least three hours before bed. Also exercise regularly but also not within three hours of bedtime. Be aware that certain prescription medications can cause insomnia, such as steroids, bronchodilators (used for asthma) and diuretics.

The idea is to create regular sleep-promoting habits. A similar but more systematic approach is known as 'stimulus control therapy' (SCT). This involves ensuring that the bed is only associated with sleeping. Patients are advised against having naps, and to go to bed when sleepy, to get up within 20 minutes if they haven't fallen asleep, to do something relaxing till they feel drowsy and to try again – but to get up again if it fails.

Although sleep hygiene is widely recommended, there have been very few studies of it as an individual treatment and what ones there have been have only found a 'limited improvement'. The evidence for the effectiveness of SCT is much stronger.

As a study from 2005 showed, doing regular exercise also helps you sleep better.[191] This may be because exercise helps 'burn off' excess adrenalin and generally helps stabilise blood-sugar levels.

Brain music

New York psychiatrist Dr Galina Mindlin, an assistant professor at Columbia University's College of Physicians and Surgeons, uses 'brain music' – rhythmic patterns of sounds derived from recordings of patients' own brain waves – to help them overcome insomnia, anxiety and depression. The recordings sound something like classical piano music and appear to have a calming effect similar to that generated by yoga or meditation. A small double-blind study from 1998, conducted at Toronto University in Canada, found that 80 per cent of those undergoing this treatment reported benefits.[192]

Another study found that specially composed music induced a shift in brain-wave patterns to alpha waves, associated with the deep relaxation before you go to sleep, and that this induced less anxiety in a study of patients going to the dentist.[193] This music, composed by John Levine especially to induce a relaxation response, has also been shown to calm down hyperactive children. Our favourite CD is called *Silence of Peace* (see Resources, page 405).

The right nutrition

Stay away from sugar and stimulants

Along with stress and stimulants like caffeine, there is one widely used substance that can also raise the activity of the two adrenal hormones, adrenalin and cortisol – sugar. When your blood sugar dips too low the adrenal hormones start rising. Raised cortisol levels at night have another drawback. it suppresses the growth hormone, essential for daily tissue repair, effectively speeding up the ageing process.

So a sensible starting place for a good night's sleep is to eat a low-GL diet, as explained in Chapter 8. A nutritionist can run a saliva test for you to determine whether your cortisol rhythm is out of sync, and give you specific supplements to bring your system back into balance.

Caffeine keeps you awake not only because it is a stimulant but also because it depresses the sleep hormone melatonin for up to ten hours. So avoid caffeinated drinks in the afternoon. Coffee drinkers take twice as long to go to sleep, and sleep on average one to two hours less than those given decaf, according to research from 2002 at Tel Aviv University in Israel.[194]

Alcohol, although classified as a relaxant precisely because it promotes GABA, which switches off adrenalin, actually promotes anxiety because of its after-effects. A couple of hours after drinking some alcohol, you get rebound low levels of GABA. To bring your brain chemistry back into balance, it's better to avoid alcohol as well, rather than depending on it to get you to sleep.

Get more GABA

If you suspect that switching off adrenalin is your problem, one obvious solution is to raise your level of GABA, the main inhibitory or calming neurotransmitter. Because GABA regulates the neurotransmitters noradrenalin, dopamine and serotonin, it can both shift a tense, worried state towards relaxation, and a blue mood to a brighter one. When your levels of GABA are low, you feel anxious, tense and depressed and have trouble sleeping.[195] When your levels increase, your breathing and heart rate slow down and your muscles relax.

GABA, unlike the other neurotransmitters we've been looking at here, is actually an amino acid. Logically, it's an obvious alternative to GABA-promoting drugs, but there's no money in it as a non-patentable nutrient and, as a consequence, not enough research has been done. In many parts of the world you can buy it over the counter or on the Internet, but in the UK it's recently been classified as a medicine so you can't buy it in health food stores (see Chapter 17 for how this catch-22 works). That's a shame because taking 500mg twice daily after meals is very calming.

Any side effects? Just don't exceed the dose of 500mg twice a day, because high amounts can cause nausea. Infrequently, this is also experienced with lower amounts.

How serotonin and melatonin help you sleep

So far we've been talking about ways of switching off stress and adrenalin. Of course, there are many other methods, from yoga to meditation, walking the dog and listening to soothing music. However, there's another factor at play here. During the daytime, adrenalin levels are higher and keep you stimulated. As you start to wind down, serotonin levels rise and adrenalin levels fall. As it gets darker another neurotransmitter, melatonin, kicks in. Melatonin is an almost identical molecule to serotonin, from which it is made, and both are made from the amino acid tryptophan. Melatonin's main role in the brain is to regulate the sleep/wake cycle.

Many people, especially women, become serotonin deficient.[196] A number of theories as to why have been proposed, some psychological, some social, but the truth is that women and men are biochemically very different. The research of Mirko Diksic and colleagues at McGill University in Montreal demonstrates this. They developed a technique using PET neuro-imaging to measure the rate at which we make serotonin in the brain.[197] What they found was that men's average

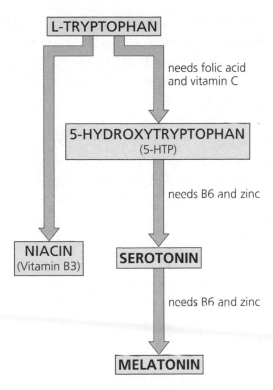

How the brain makes melatonin

synthesis rate of serotonin was 52 per cent higher than women's. This, and other research, has clearly shown that women are more prone to low serotonin.

In any case, without enough serotonin, you don't make enough melatonin. Without melatonin it is difficult to get to sleep and stay asleep. Waking far too early in the morning and not being able to get back to sleep is a classic symptom of a deficiency in these essential brain chemicals.

One way to improve matters is to provide more of the building blocks that are used to make serotonin and that means 5-HTP (5-hydroxy-tryptophan), which in turn is made up of various nutrients including folic acid, B6, vitamin C and zinc, plus tryptophan. So you've got a bio-chemical chain stretching straight from foods that are particularly high in tryptophan, like chicken, cheese, tuna, tofu, eggs, nuts, seeds and milk, up to melatonin. Other foods associated with inducing sleep are lettuce and oats. To support your brain's ability to turn tryptophan into serotonin and melatonin, it's best to supplement a high-potency multi-vitamin that contains at least 200mcg of folic acid, 20mg of vitamin B6 and 10mg of zinc, as well as 100mg of vitamin C.

Or you could supplement with these natural chemicals directly. Melatonin, which is a neurotransmitter, not a nutrient, is proven to help you get to sleep but needs to be used much more cautiously than a nutrient. In controlled trials it's about a third as effective as the drugs, but has a fraction of the side effects.[198] Even so, supplementing too much can have undesirable effects such as diarrhoea, constipation, nausea, dizziness, reduced libido, headaches, depression and nightmares. However, if you do sleep badly you may want to try between 3mg and 6mg before bedtime. In Britain melatonin is classified as a medicine and is only available on prescription. Discuss this option with your doctor. It is available in other countries, such as the US and South Africa, over the counter.

Another option is to take 5-HTP – which if you remember is the direct precursor of serotonin. If you are deficient, this will allow you to normalise your levels of both melatonin and serotonin.[199] 5-HTP is very highly concentrated in the seeds of the African griffonia plant, an extract of which is used for supplements. Supplementing 100 to 200mg of 5-HTP half an hour before you go to bed helps you get a good night's sleep.[200] It's also been shown to reduce sleep terrors in children when given at an amount equivalent to 1mg per pound of bodyweight before bed.[201] 5-HTP is best taken on an empty stomach, or with a small amount of carbohydrate such as an oatcake or a piece of fruit, one hour before sleep.

Tryptophan has also proven consistently effective in promoting sleep if taken in amounts ranging from 1 to 4g.[202] Smaller doses have not proven effective. You also need to take it at least 45 minutes before you want to go to sleep, again ideally with a small amount of carbohydrate such as an oat cake. The reason for this is that eating carbohydrate causes a release of insulin, and insulin carries tryptophan into the brain.

Sometimes supplementing tryptophan, 5-HTP or melatonin for a month can bring you back into balance, re-establishing proper sleep patterns. Doing this will make it much easier for you to wean yourself off more harmful sleeping pills. Once you're off the sleeping pills, continue with melatonin or 5-HTP for a month, then switch from melatonin to 5-HTP for a month or continue taking 5-HTP, then try stopping this. By this time your brain chemistry should be back in balance and you may find you sleep just fine. Pauline is a case in point. Prescribed Zimovane, she managed to come off it with a carefully balanced nutritional plan. As she says,

> 'After a very bad viral infection my doctor put me on Zimovane because I needed to sleep. I remained on it. I tried so many times to come off it and failed. Once I didn't have any for three days, couldn't sleep and drove into the back of a car! I decided I wanted to come off it and followed your advice. I took a supplement containing 5-HTP, B vitamins and magnesium, plus some valerian and, after a week, I was off Zimovane. To this day I still take these nutrients and I feel great. Goodbye Zimovane!'

And what about side effects? Tryptophan can make you drowsy if you take it in the daytime. And there's one important caution. If you are on SSRI anti-depressants, which block the recycling of serotonin, and you take large amounts of 5-HTP, this could theoretically make too much serotonin. An excess of serotonin can be as risky as too little (see Chapter 10, page 190). While this hasn't been reported, we don't recommend combining the two.

Minerals that calm

If you're not getting enough calcium and especially magnesium, that can trigger or exacerbate sleep difficulties. That's because these two minerals work together to calm the body and help relax nerves and muscles, thus reducing cramps and twitches. In fact, the sleeping pill Lunesta is believed to work by increasing the amount of calcium flowing into brain cells, which in turn dampens down activity.

If you are very stressed or consume too much sugar, your magnesium levels may be low. Including some magnesium in the evening, perhaps even in a supplement, may help. In one study, from 1998, it both helped insomnia and restless legs.[203] Your diet is more likely to be low in magnesium than in calcium – so make sure you are eating plenty of magnesium-rich foods such as seeds, nuts, green vegetables, wholegrains and seafood. Milk products, green vegetables, nuts, seafood and molasses are particularly good sources of calcium. Some people find it helpful to supplement 500mg of calcium and 300mg of magnesium at bedtime.

Herbal nightcaps

It's really best to resort to sleeping aids – whether natural or pharmaceutical – only as a last resort. There are many herbs and other natural substances that can help you sleep, although again, they should be used when other avenues have been exhausted and then only occasionally. You'll find a number of them, especially the herbs, sold as blends. Although they've stood the test of time, there's a need for more research on these sleep-promoting and anti-anxiety herbs.[204]

Valerian is sometimes referred to as 'nature's Valium'. As such, it can interact with alcohol and other sedative drugs and should therefore be taken in combination with them only under careful medical supervision. It seems to work in two ways: by promoting the body's release of GABA, and also by providing the amino acid glutamine, from which the brain can make GABA. Neither of these mechanisms make it addictive.[205]

One double-blind study in which participants took 600mg of valerian 30 minutes before bedtime for 28 days found it to be as effective as oxazepam, a drug used to treat anxiety.[206] Another found it to be highly effective in reducing insomnia compared with placebos.[207] While the evidence for valerian's effectiveness is definitely growing, with nine positive trials reported so far, some would say that the number and quality of these trials is not yet enough to get too excited about.[208]

Passion flower's mild sedative effect has been well substantiated in numerous animal and human studies. The herb encourages deep, restful, uninterrupted sleep, with no side effects. The dosage varies with the formula, but it's generally 100 to 200mg of a standardised extract.

St John's wort, or hypericum, has both serotonin and melatonin-enhancing effects, making it an excellent sleep regulator. However, it takes time to work and is better taken in the morning. It doesn't create daytime drowsiness. The dosage is 300mg to 900mg of a supplement standardised to 0.3 per cent hypericin.

Hops have been used for centuries as a mild sedative and sleeping aid. Its sedative action works directly on the central nervous system. Take around 200mg per day.

For more detailed advice on herbal remedies, contact the National Institute of Medical Herbalists at www.nimh.org.uk/index.html.

Food or drugs? The verdict

Taking drugs for sleeping problems and anxiety is very dangerous. While this route has a place in a short-term crisis when you're completely stressed out and need to sleep, most drugs on offer end up creating dependency if you take them for anything longer than a week. Combinations of nutrients, herbs and lifestyle changes are likely to be as effective, but without the downsides. These should be the first resort, not the last, if you are feeling stressed or anxious, or can't sleep.

What works

There are a number of routes you can take to vanquish anxiety and sleeplessness. Although it's safe to combine behavioural techniques such as sleep hygiene with, say, taking GABA, it's best to avoid taking a number of the substances below in combination. Read this chapter carefully to see what's safe. For example, take either melatonin or 5-HTP or tryptophan, possibly with some GABA or valerian, but not all of them together.

- Find the right kind of psychotherapy, especially cognitive behavioural therapy.

- Take 500mg of GABA an hour before bed. (Be aware that GABA is not available in the UK.) Don't combine with drugs that target GABA, such as most sleeping pills, unless under the guidance of a health professional.

- Take 3 to 6mg melatonin before bed; it's available on prescription in Britain, or take 100 to 200mg 5-HTP, or 2 to 4g of L-tryptophan, both one hour before bed with a light carbohydrate snack. Don't combine

5-HTP with anti-depressants unless under the guidance of a health professional.

- Practise sleep 'hygiene' (see page 224), and exercise regularly.

- Listen to alpha-wave-inducing music while in bed.

- Eat more green leafy vegetables, nuts and seeds to ensure you're getting enough magnesium, and consider supplementing 300mg of magnesium in the evening with or without calcium (500mg).

- Consider taking valerian, hops, passion flower, St John's wort or a 'sleep formula' combining several of them. Choose a standardised extract or tincture and follow the dosage instructions.

- Avoid sugar and caffeine and minimise your intake of alcohol. Don't combine alcohol with sleeping pills or anti-anxiety medication.

Working with your doctor

Many of the recommendations we have made above are easy for you to put into action. You may wish to work with a nutritional therapist who can devise a more personalised plan of action and support you through the process.

If you are currently taking sleeping pills, and have some level of dependence, it is extremely important to enrol your doctor's support to help you come off gradually. Most sleeping pills create 'down-regulation' to GABA – which means you become less responsive to your body's own GABA – the net consequence being rebound anxiety when you reduce the dose. The body can 'up-regulate', making you more sensitive to your own relaxing GABA, but this takes time: hence the need to reduce the dose gradually.

13.

Reducing Your Pain
Anti-inflammatories vs natural painkillers

THE SINGLE MOST common cause of pain is inflammation – the redness and swelling that are the immune system's way of responding to any kind of challenge, such as infection or an imbalance in the system. Most chronic diseases, including artery disease, cancer and Alzheimer's, involve inflammation. But it's those that actively cause pain, particularly arthritis, that are most often treated with drugs to bring down the inflammation.

Arthritis is a huge problem in the West. According to the UK's Arthritis Research Campaign, nearly nine million adults in Britain (that's 19 per cent of the adult population) have seen their doctors in the last year for arthritis or a related condition, and as many as 13 million Britons suffer from it.[209] Among the over-sixties, approximately three-quarters have osteoarthritis, which is the most common form. In Australia, 5.3 per cent of the total health spend for 2004 went on helping people with arthritis, who now make up 16.7 per cent of the population and are estimated to nudge 20 per cent by 2020.[210]

'Itis' means inflammation, whether it's inflammation of the joints (arthritis), inflammation of the colon (colitis), inflammation of the lungs (bronchitis), or inflammation of the sinuses (sinusitis). There are, however, some linguistic exceptions such as eczema, which is inflammation of the skin; asthma, which is inflammation of the air passages; and other conditions such as headaches that often respond to anti-inflammatory drugs.

Pain and painkillers – double-edged swords

There's a good and a bad side to inflammation and to the drugs used to treat it. When it first appears, it's a sign that your body is responding to a problem and trying to deal with it. It's the way we fight off infections, for instance. But if an area is still inflamed after the problem has been dealt with, that can get in the way of healing. When this happens, using anti-inflammatory drugs in the short term can improve healing – as long as the problem that triggered the inflammation in the first place has gone. If it hasn't, then taking anti-inflammatory drugs for any length of time just allows you to ignore the underlying causes. In the case of arthritis, this could be a food allergy, a lack of omega-3 fats or a physical misalignment.

But anti-inflammatory drugs don't just mask the problem, they are also dangerous. They come in several forms but by far the most commonly used are a type known as NSAIDs (nonsteroidal anti-inflammatory drugs), which include aspirin and ibuprofen. Prescriptions for NSAIDs cost the UK's National Health Service about £250 million a year.

It may seem extraordinary, but this class of drug is responsible for more deaths than any other. Of the 10,000 deaths in the UK every year from prescribed drugs, anti-inflammatory drugs account for 2,600. In the US, the figure is 16,500 deaths a year – more than from asthma, cervical cancer or malignant melanoma.

The other, more heavyweight drugs are the corticosteroids such as prednisone. They are based on the steroid cortisone (hence the phrase 'non-steroidal' to distinguish the aspirin-type drugs) and can be very dangerous over the long term. This is because they suppress the production of cortisol, the body's natural anti-inflammatory hormone, which is reserved for emergencies and acts as an immediate painkiller following serious accidents.

The long-term use of painkillers is also associated with 'chronic daily headache'. Painkillers should never be taken more than one day in four, or seven days a month. Despite this danger the average person takes in excess of 300 doses of these painkillers a year! That's six a week.

Before we look at what happens in your body when pain occurs, and the mechanism behind painkilling drugs and natural painkilling nutrients and herbs, let's gauge your pain level.

Unlike diabetes, which is principally measured by your blood-sugar level, the main indicator of pain and inflammation is simply how you feel. The effectiveness of treatments is rated by how much patients say their pain has gone down. Different types of questionnaires are used for different kinds of pain. (For example, the WOMAC check is used for hip and knee pain, while the Oswestry test is used for back pain.) Check yourself out on the questionnaire below.

How's your pain?

- [ ] Do you have aching or painful joints?
- [ ] Do you suffer from arthritis?
- [ ] Do you have painful or aching muscles?
- [ ] Do you suffer from muscle stiffness which limits your movement?
- [ ] Do you wake up with physical pain?
- [ ] Do you suffer from headaches?
- [ ] If so, how often? On average once a week (score 1), twice a week (score 2) or more (score 3)?
- [ ] Does your level of pain make you feel tired?
- [ ] Does it make you feel weak?
- [ ] Does it limit your ability to move around?
- [ ] Does it limit your ability to sit for more than 30 minutes?
- [ ] How intense is your pain, without medication? No pain (score 0); mild (score 1); discomforting (score 2); distressing (score 3); horrible (score 4); excruciating (score 5)

Score 1 point for each 'yes' answer (unless the question states otherwise). If you answered yes to:

Less than 5: your level of pain may be reduced by following the advice in this chapter. If not, we recommend you seek advice from a nutritional therapist or nutritionally oriented doctor.

5 to 10: you have a moderate level of pain and should definitely explore each of the options in this chapter as well as seeking advice from a nutritional therapist or nutritionally oriented doctor.

More than 10: you have a high level of pain and we advise you to consult a nutritional therapist or nutritionally oriented doctor.

INSIDE STORY: PAIN

The experience we call pain is triggered by certain chemicals called 'inflammatory mediators', which our bodies produce in response to some sort of damage. There are many of these, including interleukin, cytokines and leukotrienes. These in turn promote the accumulation of the substances that cause swelling and redness. Eventually, if pain and inflammation persist over the long term, body tissues will begin to break down. In the case of arthritis, for example, the joint becomes increasingly hard and stiffened – calcified – until you can't use it at all.

If you have joint problems you may have had your erythrocyte sedimentation rate (ESR) measured. A high ESR means your body is in a state of inflammation, as does a high level of C-reactive protein (CRP).

The problem with anti-inflammatories

By now it will probably come as no surprise that the drug approach to dealing with pain is to block one or more of the inflammatory chemicals. NSAIDS, for instance, work by stopping the formation of prostaglandins, which in turn are made from one of the omega-6 fats, arachidonic acid, which is abundant in meat and milk. The human body needs some of this fat, but too much can be harmful. Here's why.

Arachidonic acid makes two inflammatory chemicals known as type 2 prostaglandins and leukotrienes. The NSAIDs go to work on an

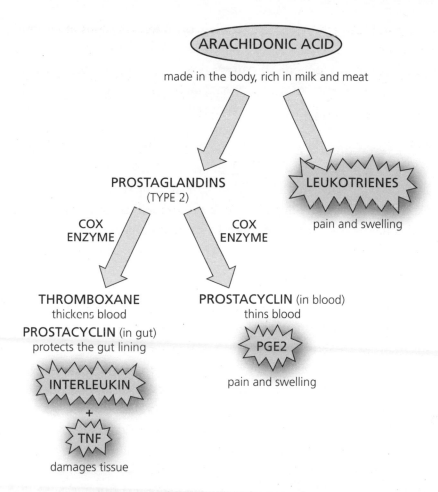

How your body's chemistry makes pain

enzyme involved in a crucial step in these chain reactions, which turns arachidonic acid into a type of prostaglandin called PGE2, which in turn causes pain. The enzyme's name is 'cyclo-oxygenase' or COX, which comes in two varieties. Blocking one or both of these COX enzymes is where all the action is, as far as NSAID drugs are concerned.

Why some NSAIDS cause heart problems

As we have seen in this book, blocking some element – such as an enzyme – that is part of a network as complex as the body almost never has just one effect, which is why drugs nearly always have damaging side effects. To see exactly why NSAIDS can be so harmful we need to delve a bit further into their biochemical pathways. The diagram below shows the effect of blocking each of the COX enzymes – COX-1 and COX-2.

We've encountered the COX enzymes in Chapter 1. You could think of COX-1 as the 'good' COX, because it helps to protect the gut and the kidneys and promotes normal blood clotting, while COX-2 is the 'bad' one because it leads to the painful prostaglandins. One of the first NSAIDs was aspirin, which targets both of these enzymes. Thus it's good for stopping pain and inflammation, but its also likely to put patients at risk by causing gastrointestinal bleeding when used over the long term, and also taxes the liver. Ibuprofen also targets both enzymes.

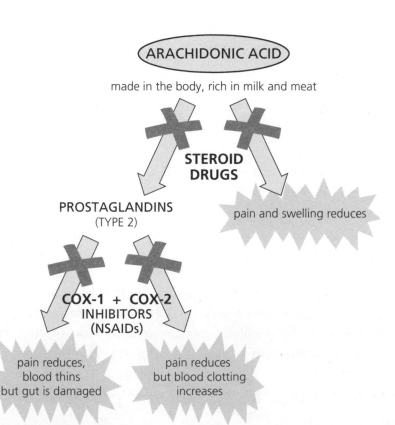

How COX-1 and COX-2 painkillers induce side effects

Because of the gastrointestinal problems, the thinking was that the ideal NSAID would be one that blocked only COX-2 and left COX-1 alone. And the launch of drugs such as Vioxx and Celebrex caused huge excitement because that's exactly what they did. But problems with these drugs also began emerging a few years after they appeared on the scene.

As you can see from the diagram on page 237, the COX-1 pathway, besides making mucus to protect the guts, also makes a fatlike substance called thromboxane A2. This promotes the narrowing of blood vessels and makes blood cells called platelets more 'sticky'. The COX-2 pathway, on the other hand, makes what might be thought of as the antidote – a substance called prostacyclin which helps prevent platelets from clumping together and helps dilate the blood vessels.

In a healthy system, the action of these two would be balanced. But by powerfully inhibiting the COX-2 pathway (and so blocking prostacyclin in the blood), the new generation of so-called 'coxib' drugs created a fresh problem, doubling or in some cases quadrupling a person's risk of a heart attack.[211] This effect of coxibs also caused another problem, increasing the level of damage to brain cells in the event of a stroke.[212] As discussed on page 33 in Chapter 2, as many as 140,000 Americans may have been damaged or killed by just one of them – Vioxx.

These 'new-generation', 'safer' painkillers were principally designed for patients who were at increased risk of gastrointestinal damage from NSAIDS. However, according to a study by researchers at the University of Chicago, '63% of the growth in COX-2 use occurred in patients with minimal risk of suffering gastrointestinal bleeding with NSAIDS.'[213] Robert Green is a case in point.

'I've had two heart attacks in the last four months,' says 57-year-old Robert Green who is now suing Merck. He had been taking Vioxx for four years, during which time his blood pressure rose and he began to have chest pains. 'I have no history of heart problems in my family,' he says. 'No one warned me about any dangers of heart attacks. I'm not taking anything for my arthritis now and getting out of bed in the morning can be murder.'

Since these drugs were no better at controlling pain, there was probably no benefit to switching them at all. In fact, the decision to prescribe them, say the Chicago team, had nothing to do with science or the evidence but was simply driven by 'heavy marketing and the tendency of physicians and patients to equate newer with better'. Until the withdrawal of Vioxx in September 2004, the COX-2 drugs had made up 25 per cent of all NSAID drugs prescribed in the UK, but accounted for 50 per cent of the costs.[214] These were highly profitable drugs.

However, it isn't just coxib drugs you need be concerned about. As a study published in 2005 shows, other NSAIDs, including ibuprofen, can also raise the risk of heart attacks, although not by as much as Vioxx.[215]

Back to aspirin?

Given the dangers of COX-2 inhibitor painkillers, should we be switching back to aspirin, which also blocks COX-1? Unfortunately, it looks like a case of out of the frying pan back into the fire. Out of every 1,000 people aged 55 to 59 who take a low-dose daily aspirin, about two will be prevented from getting a heart attack. But that comes at a high price.

SIDE EFFECTS The effect of preventing heart attacks is about evenly weighted with the risk of having serious gastrointestinal problems – two in 1,000 will suffer a major gastrointestinal bleed at age 60.[216]

Many other NSAIDs also cause gastrointestinal symptoms, including ulcers, which kill several thousand people in the UK every year.[217] (In the UK, there are 25 million annual NSAID prescriptions, 12,000 hospital admissions and 2,600 related deaths.) One small study published in 2005, using new scanning technology, has recently found that NSAIDS may damage more than the stomach. Seventy per cent of patients who had been on NSAIDS for just three months had visible damage to their small intestine.[218]

One other rarely mentioned side effect of aspirin and some other NSAIDs is that they can actually make the damage caused by arthritis worse. They stop the production of the collagen and other materials in the matrix that, with minerals and water, makes up the substance of bone; and in the process they speed up the destruction of cartilage in joints.[219] They can also worsen the key problem arthritis sufferers are wrestling with in another way: aspirin lowers blood levels of vitamin C, which is vital for the formation of collagen.

So in the short term, the use of aspirin may relieve symptoms, but in the long term it is more likely to cause further problems. When you do come off NSAIDS you should do it slowly; stopping abruptly often makes symptoms flare up.

Paracetamol and the liver

Paracetamol (called acetaminophen in the US), although classified as an NSAID, works in a different way from the others. There is little evidence that it suppresses the COX enzyme, or that its analgesic effect comes from reducing inflammation and swelling. Instead, as a study from 2000 shows, it seems to mainly reduce pain by boosting chemicals called opioids in the brain, making you less sensitive to the pain.[220]

An Australian study from 2004 showed that 66 per cent of patients found that paracetamol was better than ibuprofen, aspirin or the newer and much more expensive COX-2 inhibitors,[221] although most studies on arthritic patients has shown the opposite – that it is less effective than other NSAIDs.[222–223]

SIDE EFFECTS The problem with paracetamol is that it is notoriously toxic to the liver, an effect that lands thousands of people in the UK in hospital each year, kills several hundred and is a major cause of the need for liver transplants.[224] According to Professor Sir David Carter of Edinburgh University, one in ten liver transplants is due to damage caused by paracetamol overdose.[225]

The cortisone dilemma

All of this brings us back to the original 'miracle' painkiller – cortisone and the subsequent steroid-based drugs such as prednisone, prednisolone and betamethasone. Cortisone is a derivative of a hormone produced naturally by the body in the adrenal cortex, which sits on top of each kidney.

Steroid-based drugs were the most commonly prescribed for arthritic conditions back in the 1980s. Since the discovery of cortisone more than 40 years ago, 101 uses have been found for it, including the relief of pain and the treatment of arthritis.

Back in 1948 Philip S. Hench, who later won a Nobel prize, reported miraculous results using cortisone on arthritis suffers disabled by the condition. But the hope that it was a cure for arthritis didn't last long. In one early case, a ten-year-old girl –who had made an amazing recovery from severe arthritis when given cortisone – quickly developed diabetes. When the cortisone was stopped, the diabetes melted away – and the arthritis returned with a vengeance. Even so, 29 million prescriptions for cortisone are written for arthritis each year in the US.

It's still not completely understood exactly how cortisone works. It's known that it brings down inflammation by stopping production of the inflammatory compound histamine. It also suppresses the immune system, which could be good if your immune system is destroying healthy cells as in an auto-immune disease like rheumatoid arthritis. And, in addition, it blocks COX-2, which seems to be the main way it relieves pain.

SIDE EFFECTS The trouble is that once you start taking cortisone, the adrenal glands stop producing it. Given in small amounts, cortisone seems manageable; but in large amounts, particularly over long periods of time, it causes disastrous and even deadly side effects.

'The sad truth is that, like aspirin, cortisone does not cure anything. It merely suppresses the symptoms of the disease,' says Dr Barnett Zumoff of Beth Israel Medical Center in New York City, and formerly of the Steroid Research Laboratory at New York's Montefiore Hospital. Withdrawal from high doses of cortisone must be very gradual to allow the adrenal glands to start producing their own cortisone again. Even so, a full recovery is often not possible, leaving previous cortisone users unable to produce enough to respond to stressful situations such as an accident or operation. Severe adrenal insufficiency can be fatal. Congestive heart failure can also result from long-term use.

Some of the other consequences of taking this drug over a long period of time may not be fatal, but they can certainly be extremely unpleasant. They include obesity, a rounded 'moon' face, a higher susceptibility to infection, slow wound healing and muscle wasting. 'Using it,' says Dr Zumoff, 'is like trying to repair a computer with a monkey wrench.' While cortisone has undoubtedly saved many lives, it is unlikely to cure arthritis if taken over months or years, and may even speed up the disease because it can weaken cartilage and remove minerals from bone.[226]

Painkillers – do the benefits outweigh the risks?

From any rational perspective, it's clear that none of the anti-inflammatories we've described is safe for handling joint pain in the long term. But does their effectiveness outweigh the risks?

A review of 23 trials, including one involving 10,845 patients with arthritic knee pain, published in a 2004 issue of the *British Medical Journal* concludes: 'NSAIDs can reduce short term pain in osteoarthritis of the knee slightly better than placebo, but the current analysis does not support long term use of NSAIDs for this condition. As serious adverse effects are associated with oral NSAIDs, only limited use can be recommended.'[227] What's particularly significant about this review is that the only trial that looked at the long-term effects of NSAIDs versus placebo on pain showed 'no significant effect of NSAIDs compared with placebo at one to four years'.

If you have been on painkillers for some time, all this is worrying, and you might wonder why you weren't told either about the risks or about the alternatives. The answer is that for a long time the truth about the dangers of the COX 2 drugs like Vioxx was deliberately kept from both you and your doctor, and that – as we've seen – doctors get little or no training in nutritional medicine.

The lengths to which drug companies will go to keep the problems with drugs concealed has been covered in Part 1, but let's just look a little closer at the Vioxx case to see the extent of the problem. A *Wall Street Journal* investigation in 2004[228] claimed that an internal document about how to deal with tough questions on Vioxx, which was intended for use by the sales teams that visit doctors, was labelled 'Dodge Ball Vioxx'. In other words, do everything to avoid the question.

The investigation also revealed how the manufacturer of Vioxx, Merck, targeted independent academics who questioned the drug's safety. A Spanish pharmacologist was sued in an unsuccessful attempt to force a correction of a critical article, while a Stanford University researcher was warned that he would 'flame out' and there would be consequences for himself and the university unless he stopped giving 'anti-Merck' lectures.

Yet more details about the way the company suppressed data showing a link between Vioxx and heart attacks emerged in an article published in 2005 in the *New England Journal of Medicine*.[229] In 2000, this journal had published a key trial in favour of Vioxx (nicknamed VIGOR, for Vioxx gastrointestinal outcomes research), which found that the drug caused fewer gastrointestinal problems than an older NSAID. However, when the editor of the journal had been required to testify in one of the ongoing court cases involving Vioxx, he examined the original manuscript reporting the VIGOR trial and discovered 'that relevant data on cardiovascular outcomes had been deleted from the VIGOR manuscript prior to its submission to the journal and that the authors had withheld data on other relevant cardiovascular outcomes'.[230]

So taking painkillers looks a risky business, long-term. If you over-block COX-1 you get intestinal bleeding and kidney problems; if you over-block COX-2 you increase your risk of having a heart attack. Among the most dangerous are aspirin, diclofenac (such as Volterol), ibuprofen (such as Nurofen), ketoprofen and naproxen (such as Naprosyn and Napratec, respectively), and the coxib drugs rofecoxib (Vioxx) and celexib (Celebrex). Paracetamol (or acetaminophen) overdose accounts for over half of the cases of liver failure and death. In some combinations (such as taking aspirin with ibuprofen), these drugs can become even more dangerous.[231] Using them long term when there are other, safer, nutrition-based options seems perverse.

Natural alternatives

Antioxidants, omega-3 essential fats and herbs and spices are important ingredients of a healthy diet. What's less well known is that, judiciously chosen, they're also effective at treating joint pain. This may sound beyond the pale. After all if they were, the experts would be recommending them – right? But as we've seen abundantly now, there are strong commercial reasons why scepticism about this approach remains widespread. And you have to remember that scepticism is quite different from a lack of evidence.

Joint effort – glucosamine

Take one of the best-known non-drug treatments for joint pain, glucosamine. This amino sugar (a molecule combining an amino acid with a simple sugar) is naturally occurring and found in almost all the tissues of your body. It is used to make N-acetylglucosamine which, in turn, is one of the building blocks for the making of cartilage. Daily wear and tear on our joints means that the connective tissue that surrounds them – cartilage, tendons, and ligaments – needs to be constantly renewed, and for that you need a constant supply of glucosamine. When this rebuilding process slows down, the result is degenerative joint diseases such as arthritis.

Although the body can make glucosamine, if you've got damaged joints you are unlikely to make enough unless you are in the habit of munching on sea shells, which is the richest dietary source. Taking a substantial quantity of glucosamine as a nutritional supplement has been shown to slow down or even reverse this degenerative process. There are about 440,000 joint replacements every year in the US, and many could be avoided with the right nutrition. But how does glucosamine do the job?

Cartilage protection

Glucosamine appears to be particularly effective in protecting and strengthening the cartilage around your knees, hips, spine and hands. And while it can do little to actually restore cartilage that has completely worn away, it helps to prevent further joint damage and appears to slow the development of mild to moderate osteoarthritis. As we've seen, traditional NSAIDs prescribed for arthritis actually impair your body's cartilage-building capacity.

In a 2001 study published in *The Lancet*, Belgian investigators reported that glucosamine actually slowed the progression of osteoarthritis of the knee.[232] Over the course of three years, they measured spaces between the patients' joints and tracked their symptoms. Those on glucosamine showed no further narrowing of joints in the knee, which is an indicator of thinning cartilage. Put another way, glucosamine appeared to protect the shock-absorbing cartilage that cushions the bones. In contrast, the condition of the patients taking the placebo steadily worsened.

In a Chinese study of individuals with osteoarthritis of the knee published in 2005, investigators found that participants taking 1,500mg of glucosamine sulphate daily experienced a similar reduction in symptoms as those given 1,200mg daily of ibuprofen. However, the glucosamine group tolerated their medication much better.[233]

Speedier healing

Because glucosamine helps to reinforce the cartilage around your joints, it may hasten the healing of acute joint injuries such as sprained ankles or fingers, and of muscle injuries such as strains. In strengthening joints, glucosamine also helps to prevent future injury.

Back-pain control

Glucosamine strengthens the tissues supporting the spinal discs that line the back. It may therefore improve back pain resulting from either muscle strain or arthritis, and speed the healing of strained back muscles. Glucosamine seems to have similar effects on pain in the upper spine and neck.

Healthier ageing

As your body ages, the cartilage supporting and cushioning all of your joints tends to wear down. By protecting and strengthening your cartilage, glucosamine may help to postpone this process and reduce the risk of osteoarthritis.

Other benefits

In addition, most studies indicate that arthritis sufferers can move more freely after taking glucosamine. Others report increased overall mobility. And several studies suggest that glucosamine may be as effective as NSAIDs in easing arthritic pain and inflammation. In four high-quality 2005 studies that gave glucosamine sulphate versus NSAIDs, the glucosamine worked better in two, and was equivalent to the NSAIDs in the other two.[234] However, it was as well tolerated as the placebo, without the stomach-irritating side effects associated with NSAIDs.

There is some evidence that taking glucosamine in combination with chondroitin, a protein that gives cartilage its elasticity, may be even more effective. In a study funded by the US National Institutes of Health and published in 2005, researchers gave a group of 1,500 osteoarthritis patients a daily dose of either 1,500mg of glucosamine hydrochloride, 1,200mg of chondroitin sulphate, a combination of both supplements, 200mg of the prescription painkiller celeCoxib (Celebrex) or a placebo. Six months later, the researchers found that both celeCoxib and the glucosamine-chondroitin combination significantly reduced knee pain in those with moderate to severe pain, compared to placebo, better than either glucosamine or chondroitin on its own.[235]

This study, however, was widely reported as disproving the power of glucosamine because overall the supplements didn't reduce pain significantly more than the drug – except in those with higher levels of pain.[236] The abstract (the summary at the beginning) and press release failed to point out this last, extremely important positive result.

The trouble with chondroitin is that not all supplements are of the same quality, and hence not similarly utilised by your body. And although there is evidence that chondroitin works, the research does not show that it works better than glucosamine.[237–238] Most of the research has been done using glucosamine sulphate, but the most absorbable form is glucosamine hydrochloride.

The bone builder – sulphur

If you think of building bone as similar to building a house, glucosamine supplies the body's two-by-fours. These are essential for the framework, but you also need nails – and that's where sulphur comes in.

Although not often discussed in a health context, sulphur is involved in a multitude of key body functions, including pain control, inflammation, detoxification and tissue building. Extraordinary results are starting to be reported for pain relief and relief from arthritis in people taking daily supplements supplying 1 to 3g of one of the most effective sources of sulphur, methylsulfonylmethane (MSM).[239] A combination of both glucosamine and MSM is particularly effective.

One trial from 2004, which gave a combination of glucosamine and MSM to its participants, found this combination to be significantly more effective than glucosamine alone.[240] An unpublished double-blind study from 2003 giving 750mg to half a group of arthritis patients and a placebo to the other showed an 80 per cent improvement after six weeks in the first group compared to a 20 per cent improvement in the placebo group.[241]

One possible reason for this remarkable effectiveness is that sulphur deficiency is far more common than realised. A study at the University of California, Los Angeles, School of Medicine found that on 2,250mg of MSM a day, patients with arthritis had an 80 per cent improvement in pain within six weeks, compared with a 20 per cent improvement in arthritis patients who had taken placebos.[242] Foods particularly rich in sulphur include eggs, onions and garlic, but it is also found in all protein foods.

If you have arthritis or joint pain we recommend that you supplement 1,500 to 4,000mg of glucosamine sulphate a day, or glucosamine hydrochloride, together with 1,000 to 2,000mg of MSM. The lower end of the range is enough if you're looking to build joints and prevent their degeneration, while the higher end of the range is for those who have aching joints or a history of joint problems or arthritis, and are looking to maximise recovery.

A DOZEN ANTI-INFLAMMATORY FOODS

- Berries
- Flax seeds
- Omega-3-rich eggs
- Garlic
- Herring or kippers
- Olives
- Red onions
- Mackerel
- Pumpkin seeds
- Salmon
- Sardines
- Turmeric

Omega-3s – fats that fight inflammation

It's a popular misconception that fish oils lubricate your joints. What they actually do is reduce pain and inflammation. This happens because they are converted in the body to anti-inflammatory prostaglandins known as PG3s. These counteract the inflammatory PG2s that NSAID drugs are used to suppress.

It is a story that comes up again and again when comparing drugs and nutritional medicine. All over the body there are chemical accelerators and brakes. We've already seen that COX-1 is involved in producing blood-thickening thromboxane, while COX-2 is part of the pathway that makes the prostacyclin that can reverse that. And the same thing goes on with the chemical chain that produces inflammatory PG3 and anti-inflammatory PG2. But while drugs inevitably create problems when they block part of our system, the food and herbs that we eat don't do that. Otherwise we'd have dismissed them as a poison centuries or millennia ago, and they would never have become part of the human diet.

Good research now shows conclusively that fish oil supplementation can reduce the inflammation of arthritis. A 2002 study giving cod liver oil to osteoarthritis patients scheduled for knee replacement surgery is a case in point. Half the 31 patients were given two daily capsules of 1,000mg high-strength cod liver oil, rich in the omega-3 fats DHA and EPA, and the other half were given placebo oil capsules for ten to 12 weeks. Some 86 per cent of patients with arthritis who took the cod liver oil capsules had no or markedly reduced levels of enzymes that cause cartilage damage, as opposed to 26 per cent of those given a placebo.[243] Results also showed a reduction in the inflammatory markers that cause joint pain among those who took the cod liver oil. An effective amount is the equivalent of 1,000mg of combined EPA and DHA a day, which means two to three of most fish oil capsules.

Talking of fats, there's a special blend of fatty acids called Celadrin that has proven highly effective, both as a cream and in capsules for reducing arthritic pain, in recent double-blind trials.[244–245] Like so many natural remedies it seems to work on many different fronts, but certainly helps damaged cells in inflamed joints to heal more quickly.

Four herbs that kill pain

Turmeric

This bright yellow spice, an ingredient in many curry powders, contains the active compound curcumin which has a variety of powerful anti-inflammatory actions. Trials published in 2003, where turmeric was given to arthritic patients, have shown its efficacy to be similar to that of anti-inflammatory drugs, but without the side effects.[246] In fact, it turns out that this rhizome of the ginger family is what everyone hoped drugs like Vioxx would be. It's a mild COX-2 inhibitor that not does not affect COX-1, is tried and true (in use for hundreds of years with no evidence of any downsides even in high doses of 8g a day), and is even a potent antioxidant.

Astonishingly, an American company tried to get a patent on turmeric in 1995, claiming it was a 'new' discovery for the treatment of inflammation. But the Indian government successfully challenged this on the grounds that the spice had been used for precisely that purpose for generations in India. It has one small downside: it can stain. So keep spillage to a minimum when you cook with it (a heaped teaspoon a day will do the trick). Or you can buy supplements, in which case you'll need about 500mg, one to three times a day.

Boswellia

Frankincense may be the ultimate gift for a friend in pain. More precisely, this very powerful natural anti-inflammatory is called *Boswellia serrata*, also known as Indian frankincense.[247] Not only is it potent; it is also free of any harmful side effects. In one study, where patients initially received boswellic acid and then a placebo later, arthritic symptoms were significantly reduced at first but returned with a vengeance when the treatment was switched over to the dummy pill.[248]

Boswellic acid appears to reduce joint swelling, restores and improves blood supply to inflamed joints, provides pain relief, increases mobility, improves morning stiffness and prevents or slows the breakdown of the components of cartilage. Preparations of boswellia are available in tablet and cream form (the latter being especially useful as a treatment for localised inflammation). With supplements, the ideal dose is 200 to 400mg, one to three times a day.

Ashwagandha

The herb ashwagandha is a promising natural remedy used for hundreds of years as part of Indian Ayurvedic medicine. The active ingredient of this powerful natural anti-inflammatory herb is withanolides. In animal studies, ashwagandha has proven highly effective against arthritis. In one from 1991, animals with arthritis were given either ashwagandha, cortisone or a placebo. While cortisone produced a 44 per cent reduction in symptoms, the reduction with ashwagandha was 89 per cent.[249] Try 1,000mg a day of the ashwagandha root, providing 1.5 per cent withanolides.

Hop extract

Those who think of hops only as an ingredient in beer might be surprised to know it provides one of the most effective natural painkillers of all. This is the extract IsoOxygene, and research in 2004 showed it is one of the top natural COX-2 inhibitors.[250] One study compared the effects of the extract with those from ibuprofen. Two tablets of ibuprofen inhibited COX-2 by 62 per cent, while IsoOxygene achieved a 56 per cent inhibition – so it was almost as good. However, ibuprofen also greatly inhibits COX-1, while IsoOxygene does not. So the hops extract results in fewer gut-related problems. You need about 1,500mg a day.

Unlike drugs, herbs can't be patented and are therefore vastly under-researched and under-marketed. Different combinations of these herbs are likely to be particularly powerful anti-inflammatories and painkillers.

An antioxidant a day . . .

Antioxidant nutrients help reduce inflammation, so if you're arthritic or experience a lot of pain, eat plenty of fruit (especially berries) and vegetables, or consider supplementing an antioxidant formula. A study by the University of Manchester in the UK, published in 2005 and involving 25,000 people, showed that a low intake of the vitamin antioxidants found in fruit and veg significantly increased the risk of arthritis.[251]

So what you want is a combination of the most powerful antioxidants: vitamins C and E, glutathione or N-acetyl-cysteine, lipoic acid and co-enzyme Q10. If you are in constant pain, it could be well worth taking extra amounts of these in supplement form for a while – but ideally, in addition to more fruit and veg, up your intake of fish, seeds and nuts, eggs, onions and garlic.

Certain plant extracts also have powerful antioxidant and anti-inflammatory effects – one of the most exciting being those from olives.

Marvel of the Med

Hydroxytyrosol, an extract from olives, is turning out to be an important anti-inflammatory. Its active ingredient is a polyphenol – a plant chemical that gives some fruit and vegetables their colour. Red grapes and red onions (both of which also contain the natural anti-inflammatory quercitin) contain polyphenols, as does green tea. But with an antioxidant content over ten times greater than that of vitamin C, none of these are as powerful as hydroxytyrosol. You need 400mg of it a day for it to work as an anti-inflammatory.

The polyphenol in hydroxytyrosol isn't the end of the story. Olives and their oil contain another compound called oleocanthal, which is chemically related to ibuprofen. This is the ingredient that gives olive oil a throaty bite, like a slight sting at the back of the mouth, just as ibuprofen does. Researchers at the Monell Chemical Senses Center and the University of the Sciences, both in Philadelphia in the US, found in 2005 that oleocanthal was a potent anti-inflammatory painkiller[252] which partially inhibits the activity of the COX-1 and COX-2 enzymes.

Pain and inflammation can also be triggered in the body when levels of two inflammatory messengers (see page 237), TNF-alpha and interleukin-6, increase. Studies on olive pulp extract have shown that it reduces both of these.[253] However, a combination of olive pulp extract, hop extracts, other herbs such as turmeric and boswellia, and omega-3 fish oils and antioxidants, is perhaps the way forward because it will tackle pain and inflammation on several fronts at once. Ed is a case in point.

> Ed first started getting joint pain in his mid-thirties. He had kept himself fit by playing tennis daily and running, often on hard pavements, before the days of air-filled trainers. By the time he reached his mid-forties, Ed had had surgery on both knees and was suffering from severe arthritis, with ever-increasing pain.

Ed loved playing golf, but his knees just got worse until he could no longer play a round without being in excruciating pain afterwards.

When we met Ed, we told him to take 1.5g glucosamine, plus a range of supplements including essential fats, high-dose niacinamide (500mg), a form of B3, and the B-complex vitamin pantothenic acid (1,000mg), 3g of vitamin C, 400ius of vitamin E and a high-potency multivitamin. Ed transformed his diet, too, with more fish, seeds, fruit and vegetables. By six months, he was virtually pain-free.

'I used to have constant pain in my knees and joints. I couldn't play golf or walk more than ten minutes without resting my legs. Since following your advice my discomfort has decreased by 95–100 per cent. It is a different life when you can travel and play golf every day. I would never have believed my pain could be reduced by such a large degree, and not return no matter how much activity I do in a day.'

Check yourself for allergies

The possibility that allergy might be contributing to your arthritis, persistent headaches or other chronic conditions is well worth investigating. Studies do show that some people experience great benefits on allergy-free diets. In one, from 1992, nine per cent of a group of rheumatoid arthritis patients improved when they were put on an allergy-free diet, and worsened when they stopped the diet. To make sure these results were real, six of these patients were reintroduced to small amounts of non-allergic foods or allergic foods without their knowing which they were taking. Four got noticeably worse on the allergy food rather than the placebo.[254] (For details on food allergy tests, see Resources, page 406.)

John G developed both psoriasis and arthritis in his toes, fingers, ankles and knees at the age of 23. When he turned 40, he couldn't sleep at night from the pain and had to go upstairs on hands and knees. Walking just 100 metres was painful. Holidays were awful. He used to have to think carefully where to park the car when going out so as not to have to walk too far. He saw consultants, read books and took lots of medication, which controlled the pain but had their own side effects – stomach pain and depression. Sometimes he had steroid injections to quell the pain, but it would return later in the day.

Then John heard about food-allergy testing. Although his doctor actively discouraged testing of that type, saying that there was 'absolutely no clinical evidence' that altering diet would improve such a condition, John went ahead and discovered he was allergic to three different foods. He was shocked to discover that the main one was white fish, as everyone had been saying he should cut out red meat and eat much more white and oily fish. Egg white and tea were the other two.

John cut them all out. Gradually the number of painkillers he needed lessened and eventually he stopped taking them altogether. In his own words, 'Life is now pain and tablet-free and I have complete mobility. I am amazed at the difference in my quality of life simply by making such simple adjustments.'

Food or drugs? The verdict

As we've seen, there is no safe and effective painkilling drug, at least in the long term. Nutrients are an entirely different matter. Even glucosamine or omega-3 fats on their own show similar painkilling properties without the side effects. However, the combination of these, plus some of the powerful anti-inflammatory herbs, foods and supplements we've covered here, is a winning formula, without risks, for reducing pain and inflammation.

What works

- Eat a diet high in omega-3s, from oily fish (wild or organic salmon, mackerel, herring, kippers and sardines – tuna steak can also be allowed once a fortnight), flax and pumpkin seeds, and go easy on meat and milk. Also take omega-3 supplements containing 1,000mg of combined EPA/DHA, which usually means two to three fish oil capsules a day.

- Check yourself for food allergies with a proper food allergy test (see Resources, page 406).

- Supplement 1,500 to 4,000mg of glucosamine sulphate a day, or glucosamine hydrochloride, together with 1,000 to 2,000mg of MSM.

- Include plenty of omega-3 rich eggs, red onions and garlic in your diet, all high in sulphur.

- Eat olives, use olive oil and add turmeric to your food (traditional curries and Indian condiments make good use of it, and it is excellent in fish soups or blended with a little olive oil or melted butter and drizzled over cooked vegetables).

- Supplement herbal complexes containing hop extracts, turmeric (or curcumin), boswellia or ashwaghandha.

- Take a good all-round multivitamin with at least 1,000mg of vitamin C.

- Supplement an all-round antioxidant formula if you don't eat at least six servings of fruit and veg a day – but do aim to eat that much.

Working with your doctor

There's plenty you can do yourself to reduce your pain and inflammation, and find out underlying causes such as an identified food allergy. Alternatively, consult a nutritional therapist who will work out your ideal nutritional regime.

If you are on prescribed painkillers or anti-inflammatories, it's wise to let your doctor know that you'd like to use these as little as possible and are going to explore some alternatives. The chances are you take painkillers when you feel the pain, so you'll be the first to know if your need is reduced. Let your doctor know what works for you. They should be delighted if your need for these drugs decreases.

14.

Eradicating Asthma and Eczema
'Puffers' and cortisone creams vs new solutions

LIKE ARTHRITIS, WHICH we looked at in the last chapter, asthma and eczema are inflammatory diseases. Inflammation – pain, redness or swelling – is essentially the body's way of saying something isn't right. In the case of asthma, the airways become constricted by the swelling and it becomes harder to breathe. With eczema, the skin becomes inflamed, red, itchy and dry.

One way of dealing with these conditions is to listen to the body, to discover what's provoking the reaction. But the traditional medical route with either of them is to suppress the reaction with anti-inflammatory drugs – inhalers for asthma, or creams for eczema.

Asthma is very much on the rise in most developed countries. In England, more than one in four children now have asthma, compared to one in 18 back in the 1970s. Asthma is six times more common in children than in adults, partly because some children grow out of asthma, but also because the incidence in today's children is four times higher than it was 30 years ago. In fact, asthma is now the leading cause of school absenteeism for children under 15. In the UK alone over five million people are being treated for asthma, including a quarter of all seven to 11-year-olds – and 1,500 people die of it each year.[255]

Prescriptions for steroid inhalers have risen sixfold over the last two decades. So too has the number of deaths: in the UK alone, one person dies every seven hours from an asthma attack. As you'll see later, the rise in prescription drugs to treat asthma is strongly associated with an increasing risk of having a fatal asthma attack.

Like asthma, the incidence of eczema has increased substantially over the past three decades. Atopic eczema affects one in six school children in the UK and two to three per cent (some say one in 12) of adults.[256] Over a million Australian adults are affected by eczema.[257] The question is, why? Most experts agree that it is likely to be due to changes in diet, lifestyle or environmental factors, with food allergies being very high on the list of contributing factors. Yet few sufferers are informed in any detail about the key contributory factors, or checked out thoroughly for food allergies. Prescriptions for corticosteroid creams or inhalers are routine.

The rise and fall of puffers

In mainstream medicine until recently, the assumption dictating asthma therapy was that the condition was basically an airway-narrowing disease. As a result, medication concentrated on dilating or enlarging the airways with so-called beta-2 agonist drugs (bronchodilators), along with reducing inflammation with inhaled corticosteroids. The combined sales of these in the UK stand at over £600 million – and are on the rise.

Sufferers are advised to take these two types of drugs – delivered direct to the lungs in nebulisers, or puffers – on a daily basis for long-term control. Different variations of these drugs are then used to deal with a sudden serious attack – short-term beta-2 agonists and oral or inhaled corticosteroids.

Corticosteroids

The most commonly prescribed forms of corticosteroids used in puffers are fluticasone (such as Flixotide), beclomethasone (such as Becotide) and budenoside (such as Pulmicorte and Symbicorte). There's no question that they keep the airways open, with best results in doses between 400mg and 1,000mg.[258]

SIDE EFFECTS The long-term use of inhaled corticosteroids doesn't seem to change the progression of the disease, but merely controls symptoms. In children, it has another potential adverse effect – it can stunt or delay growth by as much as an inch a year. Used over years, these drugs can also reduce bone mass, increasing the risk for osteoporosis in later life.[259]

Beta-agonists

Beta-agonists work by stimulating a receptor for adrenalin in the lungs, which has the effect of relaxing the airways. These drugs are used over the short or long term. The most common short-term type is salmeterol; the long-term version is salbutamol. Common brand names are Ventolin, Proventil or Serevent.

SIDE EFFECTS As a study from 2003 has shown, the longer you use these drugs, the less effective they become.[260] There is also evidence that when the short-acting ones are used daily for prevention, they make attacks more severe when they do come. According to the American Academy of Allergy, Asthma and Immunology, the danger of these drugs is that while suppressing symptoms in the short term, they may be part of the reason why deaths from asthma are rising.[261]

The problem seems to be that long-term use may make the adrenalin receptors in the lungs less responsive. In one study published in 2003, adults with asthma who already had heart problems and used three canisters a month doubled their chances of being hospitalised with heart failure, while those who used one canister a month had a 40 per cent increased chance of hospital admission.[262] This constitutes a warning for older asthma sufferers, who have a cardiovascular risk. Other adverse effects are palpitations, tremor and headache.

More and more people are now being prescribed combined inhalers that deliver both a corticosteroid drug and a beta-agonist. The problems with this approach are twofold: when beta-agonists are used excessively, they are associated with an increased risk of a more serious asthma attack.

On top of this, the conventional wisdom that inhalers should be used regularly has been overturned by research from 2005, which shows that you may be better off using them as and when you need them (and as little as possible) rather than having this constant intake of steroids.[263] Knowing that many asthmatics don't use their inhalers regularly as instructed, a group of researchers from the US National Heart, Lung, and Blood Institute's Asthma Clinical Research Network designed a study to see if intermittent users of corticosteroids really were worse off than regular users. They found no difference in rates of asthma or early morning breathing. This controversial finding, published last year in the *New England Journal of Medicine*, will no doubt stimulate more research, but it's certainly worth discussing with your doctor if you are on asthma medication.[264]

The downside of cortisone creams

Cortisone-based creams, usually betnovate (available on prescription), are applied for eczema when the skin flares up. The creams may also contain anti-bacterial drugs. Many eczema sufferers use this anti-inflammatory cream every day, as well as a moisturiser or emollient made out of petrolatum and hydrogenated vegetables oils to stop the skin from drying out and cracking.

Corticosteroid creams

Some cortisone-based creams, such as Cortaid and Cortizone, can be bought over the counter. Higher-dose products that are generally available on prescription include triamcinolone (Aristocort, Kenalog), fluocinonide (Lidex), betamethasone (Valisone, Diprosone, Diprolene), mometasone (Elocon), and clobetasol (Temovate).

In essence, they all work in the same way, by reducing inflammation. They don't have quite the same degree of danger as ingested cortisone, which gradually suppresses the body's ability to make its own.

SIDE EFFECTS Long-term use of cortisone creams isn't desirable because they gradually damage the skin, making it thinner and more prone to drying and cracking. In fact, the changes in the collagen are identical to those seen in ageing. As a result the skin becomes more vulnerable to any infections and heals poorly. It's a vicious cycle; the more you use the creams to help with the problems, the worse they become.

Some of the preparations contain fluorine. Although possibly more effective, the fluorinated preparations such as Lidex are even more likely to cause skin thinning (particularly on the face, armpits, and groin), and they shouldn't be used for prolonged periods on the face or around the eye. Higher-strength glucocorticoids, such as betnovate, in particular, should be spread in a very thin layer, covering only the area requiring treatment. For most conditions, applying the medication once daily will suffice.[265]

Of course, none of these drugs – puffed, popped or put on the skin – do anything to address the underlying causes of the over-inflammation associated with asthma and eczema. And they have considerable long-term side effects. Fortunately, there are natural solutions to both asthma and eczema which, for some, can eliminate the need for medication completely and for most can reduce it significantly.

Natural alternatives

Because asthma and eczema are both inflammatory diseases, the root causes are often quite similar. In most cases this is a combination of exposure to irritants, unidentified allergies, and a predisposition to inflammatory reactions which can be activated by the wrong kind of diet, as well as stress and anxiety. By tackling the root causes, most people find partial to complete relief. This means:

- Checking for airborne, food or chemical allergies

- Ensuring an optimum intake of anti-inflammatory nutrients

- Reducing the use of anti-inflammatory drugs

- Improving air quality and breathing, and reducing stress (for asthma)

- Healing the skin with antioxidant-based creams (for eczema).

The nutritional approach to asthma or eczema is based on the idea that a sufferer's total environmental 'load' – that is, how much pollution, stress and poor nutrition they are dealing with – has exceeded their capacity to adapt to it. While there may be a specific trigger, such as an emotional crisis, exposure to cigarette smoke or eating a food allergen, these can be seen as the final straw rather than the root cause. So the goal becomes to increase a person's adaptive capacity *and* to lessen the total load. Anti-inflammatory drugs, by contrast, merely suppress symptoms.

If you suffer from asthma, the idea of reducing your reliance on bronchodilators might seem daunting; but if you approach the issue by aiming for overall health first, the problem often takes care of itself. John H, for instance, who had suffered from asthma since the age of nine months, is a case in point.

He was on medication all his life and was using inhalers from the age of seven. He was in and out of hospital over 50 times with asthma attacks. On a typical day he had two puffs of both ventolin (beta-agonist) and becotide (steroid) three times a day. But he had noticed that the fitter he got, the less severe his symptoms became.

At 35, John H changed his diet dramatically and went on a low-allergen diet, eliminating milk almost completely. He also learnt a breathing exercise (see page 272). As he says,

'Since I've changed my diet, avoiding foods I'm allergic to, and learnt how to breath using the Buteyko method, I've managed to stop using my bronchoinhalers almost completely. The trick is to find all the factors that contribute and gradually eliminate them.'

In John's case, keeping fit and minimising both caffeine and alcohol makes a difference. He still carries his bronchoinhalers, but 'just in case'.

Identifying hidden allergies: eczema

The two main types of allergies, IgE and IgG, refer to different kinds of antibodies produces by your immune system. IgE or immunoglobulin E antibodies cause the more severe and immediate reactions. These are conventional allergies where, for example, a person's skin flares up if they eat shellfish, or their breathing immediately constricts when they eat a peanut. People with asthma are often found to have higher levels of IgE, making them hypersensitive to certain substances.

You can test your IgE sensitivity and identify specifically what you are reacting to from an IgE blood test. If you have asthma you may already have had this done. If not, ask your doctor or arrange it yourself. These tests are available direct to the public.

However, most eczema and asthma suffers also have IgG-based allergies to foods. These are less obvious, and are sometimes called food intolerances or hidden allergies because they don't cause immediate or severe reactions. Symptoms may not occur for a full 24 hours. Foods that commonly trigger IgG reactions are milk products, gluten cereals (wheat, rye, barley, oats), eggs and yeast. Your doctor is unlikely to offer an IgG allergy test, but you can test yourself using a home-test kit (see Resources, page 406).

The most common food allergy that can provoke eczema, especially in children, is milk. IgG antibodies to milk have been found to be much more common in both children and adults with eczema.[266–270] Other researchers have also found IgG sensitivity to eggs to be far more common in eczema sufferers.[271] But despite the overwhelming evidence of an association with a hidden IgG food allergy, very few eczema sufferers are tested for allergy by their doctors. Those who are are invariably tested for IgE-based reactions, yet these account for only a small fraction of food intolerances. If you have been tested, check which test it was and then have the other one done. Liza is someone who benefited from finding the root cause of her eczematic reactions.

> Liza had used betnovate and other steroid-based creams all her life. After taking an IgG test, she found she was strongly allergic to dairy products and mildly sensitive to gluten and egg white. She was also taking in a lot of caffeine every day – several cups of coffee and a couple of Red Bull drinks. We advised her to take the allergens out of her diet for several months and to cut out the caffeine, which raises levels of the stress hormones adrenalin and cortisol.

You might think that caffeine's adrenal boost would reduce eczema, but substances that reliably indicate inflammation, such as interleukin-6, TNF, C-reactive protein and homocysteine[272] are all raised by caffeine (see page 236 for more details on these substances). A Greek study from 2004 that involved over 3,000 participants found that those consuming

200ml of coffee – two cups – had a 50 per cent higher level of interleukin-6, a 30 per cent higher C-reactive protein and a 28 per cent higher level of TNF compared to non-coffee consumers.[273] We also recommended a vitamin A-based skin cream, which can help to keep the skin healthy once the inflammation calms down.

> One month later, Liza said:

> 'I feel so much better. Nothing like as tired. I have one coffee a week, no headaches, no side effects. No bloating. The milk avoidance itself wasn't so difficult. But I was amazed to find out how many foods had hidden milk, so it took a week to discover what I could and couldn't have. Overall, it's been fine. It's not as hard as it used to be at the beginning. My skin is a lot better. I have no sores or cuts. The vitamin A cream really works very well.'

Three months later, Liza is still eczema-free and has not had to use the betnovate cream once since she went on her allergy-free diet.

Identifying hidden allergies: asthma

Asthma is also strongly linked to either airborne or food allergens. The top suspects are wheat, milk, eggs and soya, while colourings, sulphites and other preservatives and chemical food additives may also be implicated, along with dust mites, mould, animal dander (particles of hair or feathers) and cockroach antigens (proteins from the insects' saliva, eggs and so on).

A German study published in 1998 followed 508 children for their first five years of life to investigate whether having food allergies during early childhood was related to developing an IgE sensitivity in the airwaves later. It found that children with food allergies were three times more likely to suffer from allergic rhinitis and five times more likely to develop asthma.[274] In another trial from 2000, Dr Dan Gustafsson of Orebro Medical Hospital in Sweden noticed a similar link. He followed 94 children with eczema from the age of about 17 months to seven years. He concluded that those children suspected of food allergies in the first three years of life were more likely to develop asthma.[275]

While dairy products are often said to be linked to asthma, and there are several reports of high asthma incidence among dairy farmers and people working in cheese factories, it's important to realise that allergic reactions are highly individualised and need to be checked with proper IgE and IgG tests. When properly tested, few asthma sufferers are found to have both types of allergies.

Once you know what you are reacting to, you need to avoid your allergens. IgE sensitivities last for life, while you can grow out of IgG sensitivities if you avoid the allergens strictly for six months.

Not all are that easy to avoid, however. If you are allergic to dust mites, which live in mattresses and carpets, you'll need to go to war on these creatures by changing your bedding. Ever since central heating became the norm, the incidence of house-dust-mite allergy has gone up hugely, because the bugs love moisture and don't like big temperature changes.

What you'll need to do is either get a new mattress, or wait for a hot, sunny day and put yours out to 'sunbathe'. This will kill the mites. Then cover the mattress in a dust-mite-proof cover, which you can buy from most major department stores, and buy house-dust-mite-proof pillow cases and covers too. Wash sheets and pillow cases frequently in hot water and dry really well. Invest in a bed base that lets the bed air well. Don't make your bed: leave it to 'air' and, ideally, let the room air as well. Ideally, don't have a carpet in the bedroom and don't leave wet towels lying around the place – do your drying in the bathroom. Moulds, which can also trigger off an allergic reaction in some people, will also be less likely to take hold if you follow this regime.

Some asthma sufferers also react to alcohol, especially wine, and some are sensitive to sulphites, which are also found in wine. To minimise chemical exposure, we recommend eating organic whenever possible.

Antioxidants for lungs and skin

It is known that inflamed tissue, be it in the airways or skin, results in more oxidants, so it's sensible to up your intake of antioxidants to counter the inflammation of asthma or eczema. Numerous studies have shown that the lower a person's antioxidant intake, the worse their asthma,[276] and that a high intake of fresh fruit and vegetables – which boosts antioxidant levels – reduces the severity of asthma and eczema.

However, the results of studies in which asthma sufferers were given individual antioxidants are mixed.[277] The antioxidant nutrients that come out top are vitamin C and vitamin A. Vitamin E and selenium have less certain results – some positive, some negative. Zinc supplementation on its own hasn't generally proven positive. What hasn't been tested yet, bearing in mind that nutrients work in synergy – they are team players – is testing out how a combination of these key antioxidants works for asthma sufferers. That's what we would recommend.

The best antioxidant foods

Combating these conditions means eating lots of broccoli, peppers, berries, citrus fruit, apples (all rich in vitamin C), carrots and tomatoes (rich in beta-carotene and the powerful carotenoid lycopene) and seeds and fish (rich in vitamin A, E and selenium). One UK survey of 1,500 asthma sufferers found that people who ate at least two apples per week had a 22 to 32 per cent lower risk of having an asthma attack than those who ate fewer.[278]

Vitamin C is a natural antihistamine, enhancing the action of the enzyme histaminase, which quickly breaks down histamine – the chemical that prompts inflammation during an allergic reaction. That means it will give you instant relief from an asthma attack or eczema flare-up, as long as you take enough. One gram of vitamin C reduces blood histamine by approximately 20 per cent, and 2g reduces histamine by over 30 per cent.[279] There's also evidence that people supplementing 1g of vitamin C a day are able to reduce their need for corticosteroids, and along with that their risk of negative side effects.[280] Another study has found that for every milligram of vitamin E in the diet, there is a drop in the level of IgE in the blood of asthma sufferers.[281] We therefore recommend supplementing 200mg of vitamin E every day.

As far as supplements to optimise antioxidant intake are concerned, we would recommend taking a high-strength multivitamin and mineral, plus 1g of vitamin C with berry extracts (which are high in bioflavonoids) and a good antioxidant formula that provides both vitamins A, C, E, zinc, selenium and glutathione and/or N-acetyl-cysteine. The multivitamin also provides important B vitamins, which help reduce allergic potential.

Switching to antioxidant creams

Eczema sufferers may have a lot of skin damage caused by oxidants, so creams are important. Alternatives to the problematic cortisone creams are products containing the powerful antioxidant vitamins A, C and E. These have proven highly beneficial.[282] In Japanese trials involving a total of around 2,000 patients since the mid-1990s, carried out at Tokyo Medical College Hospital, at Tokyo's Tozawa Clinic,[283] and at Toho University in Chiba, it was found that more than 80 per cent of patients with dry, inflamed eczematic skin responded favourably to home-care treatment with vitamin-based skin creams.

Another trial in patients with facial dermatitis resulted in major improvements, to the point where the people concerned could stop using cortisone creams.[284] The patients were asked to stop using topical steroids and to substitute a moisturising gel or cream containing vitamins A, C, E, beta-carotene and pro-vitamin B5 (panthenol), or an anti-oxidant gel containing tea tree oil.

Topical vitamin A and C are the most potent skin healers. In cream form, vitamin A effectively treats the negative side effects of steroids, encouraging the skin to produce a better water-proofing barrier and significantly reducing the dry skin that arises with eczema. The gentle retinyl palmitate form of vitamin A should be used rather than the acid form. By combining low-dose vitamin A and an antioxidant cream or gel, you can expect to see about an 80 per cent chance of significant improvement of the skin.

It is important, though, to start with low levels, but not too low. If a skin cream provides less than 100iu (33mcg) of vitamin A per gram, it's not worth it. On the label you have to look for retinol palmitate or acetate or retinol. On rare occasions, starting with too high a concentration of vitamin A, for example double or triple this amount, can further aggravate the skin. Skin that has been treated with corticosteroids is severely malnourished, and 'overfeeding' with vitamins would add to the stress. So begin with small amounts of A and C cream on the skin plus the A you'll get from a high-strength multivitamin, and gradually increase the amount. This is best done with the guidance of a skincare therapist used to applying vitamin A-based creams.

Natural anti-inflammatories

We've seen how the swelling of the airways, known as bronchioles, in asthma results from an inflammatory reaction. Steroid inhalers are anti-inflammatories, mimicking the action of the body's own anti-inflammatory adrenal hormone, cortisol.

In the last chapter, we showed how effective a number of natural anti-inflammatories were in reducing joint pain. Many of them are equally effective in reducing inflammation on the skin and in the lungs, including omega-3 fats, MSM, quercetin, zinc, magnesium, ginger and turmeric. Now let's see how they do the job.

The omega-3 connection

A number of studies have found lower rates of asthma in fish eaters,[285] and that the higher the dietary intake of omega-3 fats, the better the ease in breathing.[286] Children with a higher omega-6 to omega-3 fat ratio in their diet also have worse asthma[287] and are more likely to suffer from allergies.[288] Short-term trials to date have shown only modest improvement with omega-3 fat supplementation, and long-term trials are yet to be completed.[289] However, a long-term increase in omega-3 may be more beneficial.

One of the longest trials, published in 2004, conducted at the University of Sydney, Australia, gave 616 children omega-3 fish oil capsules for three years and recommended measures to reduce house-dust-mite exposure. Among the children with a family history of asthma, there was a significant ten per cent reduction in coughing, but not in wheezing.[290] This, of course, is good news but a long way away from a cure. No studies on omega-3 fats have been carried out on eczema sufferers. It's a case of watch this space. Either way, we recommend that you include a food source or supplement of essential fats, both omega-3 and 6, every day.

A small controlled trial in 2006 found that fish oil reduced asthma attacks triggered by exercise, which can affect about 80 per cent of sufferers. Sixteen adults with mild-to-moderate asthma, who had been taking the fish oil for three weeks, found their lung function after exercising improved by 64 per cent, while their use of inhalers decreased by 31 per cent.[291]

As we have already seen, meat and dairy products are high in arachidonic acid, a type of omega-6 fat, while flax seeds and oily fish are high in omega-3s. Foods high in arachidonic acid can encourage inflammation. We would certainly recommend a diet low in meat and dairy and high (that is, three times a week) in oily fish such as sardines, herrings and mackerel. It's a good idea, too, to have a tablespoon of ground mixed seeds, with at least half of those flax seeds, or a dessertspoon of flax seed oil a day, and a daily supplement of 600mg of EPA, 400mg of DHA and 200mg of GLA each day, as the ideal balanced intake.

MSM – the magic molecule

MSM (methylsulfonylmethane), which we have already encountered in Chapter 13, is a non-toxic, natural component of the plants and animals we eat and is also found naturally in breast milk. This molecule contains a highly usable form of sulphur, the fourth most abundant mineral in the human body and part of the chemical makeup of over 150 compounds (all the proteins, as well as sulphur-containing amino acids, antibodies, collagen, skin, nails, insulin, growth hormone and the most potent antioxidant, the enzyme glutathione). Vegans and people on a high-carbohydrate, low-protein diet probably don't get enough MSM. Antibiotic overuse may also contribute to sulphur deficiency by killing off the intestinal bacteria needed to produce essential sulphur-containing amino acids.

Correcting any MSM deficiency is important for eczema and asthma sufferers, as it's particularly effective at damping down allergic responses to food and pollen. MSM also provides the intestinal bacteria with building blocks for the manufacture of major anti-allergy, anti-inflammatory sulphur-containing amino acids, such as methionine and cysteine. Cysteine goes on to increase the production of glutathione, low levels of which are associated with inflammation. Onions and garlic are rich in cysteine.

Along with vitamin C, cysteine is also needed for the production of collagen, the major component of connective tissue. Cysteine itself is very helpful in reducing asthmatic tendencies if supplemented at levels of 400mg or more.[292] MSM helps to bond collagen fibres together, giving elasticity to the skin; it is also very effective in helping the repair of damaged or scarred skin. Although no human studies have shown evidence of this, work with animals has shown faster wound healing when MSM is given with vitamin C.[293]

Asthma sufferers may get real benefits from taking MSM. The sulphur is incorporated into the cells of the bronchial tubes, allowing the cell membranes to become more flexible and enabling the person to breathe more freely. There have been some impressive cases of people with severe respiratory problems being successfully treated with MSM.[294] However, there's a real need for more research on this harmless and potentially beneficial nutrient.

The daily therapeutic dose for MSM ranges from 1,000 to 6,000mg – it can be that high because it's as safe as drinking water. MSM works better if taken with vitamin C. Bear in mind that MSM is not like aspirin or a shot of cortisol. A single, one-time dose of it is rarely effective in lessening symptoms, so you'll have to stick with it for a bit. A reduction in inflammation and other allergic symptoms is usually seen within two to 21 days. One asthma sufferer tried 2g twice a day. Within a few weeks, her breathing became much easier and she was soon able to stop her medication. In her words, 'I can't believe what it has done for me.'

While all the supplement doses given here are for adults, if you have a child with asthma or eczema, the rule of thumb is to divide by body weight. So a 5 stone (about 32kg) child needs roughly half the adult amount, for example 500mg to 2,000mg.

Quercetin – bioflavonoid boon

The bioflavonoids are a group of 4,000 antioxidant and anti-inflammatory chemicals that are found in many plants and have a range of therapeutic effects. Quercetin is one that many nutritional therapists swear by for allergies, reporting that a once-a-day supplement can often reduce allergic symptoms across the board. There have not yet been any double-blind trials of quercetin's benefits, but there is evidence that quercetin can reduce the activity of mast cells – the ones that release the inflammatory chemicals such as histamine, certain prostaglandins, and the inflammatory 'messengers' leukotrienes.[295] That would account for its value in treating allergies.

Quercetin is naturally found in wine, but not beer; tea, but not coffee; and the outer layers of red and yellow onions, but not white onions (see the 'Quercetin-rich foods' table below). For the best effect, you'll need to supplement it, ideally in combination with vitamin C and a high-potency bromelain (the enzyme found in pineapple).

For most people, the effective therapeutic dose is 500mg of quercetin in combination with approximately 125mg of bromelain and 250 to 500mg vitamin C, taken 30 minutes before meals two to three times a day. For maintenance (after your allergic symptoms have been brought under good control), reduce the above dose to once or twice daily, 30 minutes before breakfast and/or again before dinner.

QUERCETIN-RICH FOODS

Food	Quercetin per 100g	Food serving size for 10mg quercetin
Red onions	19.93mg	50g (an onion)
Cranberries	14.02mg	71g (1 cup)
Spinach	4.86mg	206g (three servings)
Apples	4.42mg	226g (two small apples)
Red grapes	3.54mg	282g (two medium servings)
Carrots	3.50mg	286g (two large carrots)
Broccoli	3.21mg	312g (three servings)
Blueberries	3.11mg	322g (large punnet)
Lettuce	2.47mg	405g (four lettuces)
Cherries	1.25mg	800g (two large punnets)
Plums	1.20mg	833g (ten plums)
Blackberries	1.03mg	971g (three large punnets)
Raspberries	0.83mg	1,205g (four large punnets)

Zinc and magnesium – master minerals

Magnesium is the second most abundant mineral in the human body. It works closely with calcium and vitamin B6 to regulate the heart, muscles, brain and immune system. It's also needed for essential fats to work properly, and plays a significant role in the prevention and treatment of various allergy-related conditions, including asthma and eczema. One study from 1980 found that magnesium deficiency produced allergy symptoms in rats.[296] Magnesium supplements have been found to reduce symptoms of asthma, and a recent review showed that intravenous magnesium at the time of an asthma attack halves recovery time and cuts the chances of needing recovery by two-thirds.[297]

Yet despite the fact that it is a proven, cheap and safe treatment, broadly accepted by most doctors, only 2.5 per cent of emergency asthma cases are ever given magnesium.[298] It's another example of how effective nutritional medicine lacks the marketing muscle to be put into practice. What has also been proven is that inhaling magnesium works. A study from 2005 has found that by adding magnesium to beta-agonist drug inhalers, less of the drug is needed.[299] So look out for new inhalers that combine beta-agonists with magnesium. Of course, you could go one step further and have a magnesium-only inhaler, but to our knowledge these are not yet being marketed.

If you're not getting enough magnesium, you may experience symptoms such as constipation, cramps, headaches, insomnia and depression. We recommend eating plenty of green leafy vegetables, nuts, beans, lentils and seeds – especially pumpkin seeds. A small handful of pumpkin seeds (25g) will give you 150mg of magnesium. If you are also supplementing a high-strength multivitamin, that can provide a further 150mg. If you have asthma attacks quite frequently, it's probably worth supplementing an additional 200mg of elemental magnesium in an easily absorbable form (such as magnesium glycinate, citrate or ascorbate) twice daily.

Zinc is another potential star in allergy treatments, turning out to be far more influential in the treatment of food allergy than anyone thought. The mineral is vital for making the essential fatty acids that are known to reduce inflammation, and it is also one of the most important nutrients for the immune system.[300] In animals, zinc deficiency makes the airway constrict, while giving zinc dilates them.[301] It's needed for restoring the delicate linings of the airways and healing the skin. Although zinc on its own certainly isn't a miracle cure, ensuring an optimal intake of zinc is likely to help both asthma and eczema.

Although the RDA for zinc is 15mg per day, doses of 20 to 40mg have had beneficial effects in conditions common among food allergy sufferers, such as acne, dermatitis herpetiformis (an extremely itchy rash associated with coeliac disease), eczema, psoriasis, hyperactivity, eating disorders and learning disabilities. Daily doses of 40mg or higher should not be continued for longer than three months. Zinc also depletes the body of copper, so supplement 1mg of copper with every 10 to 15mg of zinc.

The spice route – ginger and turmeric

Ginger and the yellow curry spice turmeric have long been known to help inflammatory diseases from arthritis to asthma. Ginger, for example, is a common asthma remedy in the West Indies.[302] But exactly why they work has only recently been discovered.

In inflammatory diseases, an inflammation-promoting protein known as nuclear transcription factor kappa B is produced. Ginger and turmeric, along with garlic and pepper, turn it off, thereby reducing inflammation.[303] That's the reasoning behind the seasoning. While we await human trials, animal studies show that curcumin, which is the active ingredient in turmeric, has proven highly effective in reducing asthma symptoms.[304] So we recommend the liberal use of both ginger and turmeric, or taking concentrated supplements, if you suffer from either eczema or asthma. Luckily, they're both tasty additions to curry and relishes in dried form, while fresh ginger is delicious grated with red lentils or sliced in stir fries.

Learn how to breathe

We may worry, and with good reason, about pollution. But it isn't just what you breathe, but how you breathe, that makes a huge difference vis-à-vis asthma. Most of us breathe very shallowly, and breathing that's both deeper and slower can really help reduce asthma symptoms. Breathing techniques are an important part of yoga and t'ai chi, and can help us de-stress – which makes them highly recommended for asthma sufferers. The Buteyko method is a technique for breathing in this way which has been taught to asthma sufferers in the UK over the last decade with great success.

The basic idea behind Buteyko is that asthma sufferers are breathing too fast – more than 12 breaths a minute – causing them to breathe out too much carbon dioxide. This is important because even though we tend to think of CO_2 as just a waste gas, it is also vital for the proper functioning of nearly all body chemistry. A drop in CO_2, for instance, causes both blood vessels and airways to narrow. There are thousands of people who claim to have benefited from the Buteyko method, and many have reported being able to stop taking medication entirely. However, there is still a debate about the evidence.

For instance, in 2003 a double-blind trial with 38 people found that the practice of Buteyko reduced the use of inhaled steroids by 50 per cent and beta 2-agonists by 85 per cent.[305] The authors concluded that it is 'a safe and efficacious asthma management technique'. But a review from 2005 was more cautious: 'Buteyko's theory relating to carbon dioxide levels and airway calibre is an attractive one ... [but] there is currently insufficient evidence to confirm that this is the mechanism behind any effect,' said the authors, who then called for more research to 'establish unequivocally whether [Buteyko] is effective'.[306] (For more details, see Resources, page 405.)

Another system of breathing exercises you may like to try was developed by Frank Goddard, who had suffered from asthma all his life and had been on bronchodilators since they were invented. At the age of 82 he had had enough and, through a combination of optimum nutrition, identifying and eliminating his allergies and certain breathing exercises, he is now both asthma- and drug-free. His lung exercise tube claims to train you to breathe in a way that helps bring oxygen to the brain and reduce the symptoms of asthma (see Resources, page 405).

Having an asthma attack can be frightening. One of the advantages of these breathing techniques is that at the same time as they help relieve symptoms, they calm you down by focusing on the breath.

Food or drugs? The verdict

There's little doubt that the main anti-inflammatory drugs used to treat eczema and asthma, while highly effective in providing relief, particularly in the short term, can make matters worse in the long run and incur risks of a variety of side effects.

It's equally obvious that checking for allergies, upping your intake of antioxidants, essential fats and other natural anti-inflammatories, improving your breathing if you have asthma, and applying appropriate vitamin-based skin creams if you have eczema constitute an approach that at worst, is likely to reduce the need for drugs and at best, will completely relieve symptoms. While there's a lack of good studies to prove the benefits of an all-round nutrition-based approach, there's certainly every good reason to pursue these and see what happens to your symptoms.

What works

- Eat a diet high in oily fish (wild or organic salmon, mackerel, herring, kippers, sardines and tuna steak – tuna may be eaten a maximum of once a fortnight), omega-3 rich flax and pumpkin seeds, and low in meat and milk. Also supplement 1,000mg of the combined omega-3s EPA/DHA, which usually means two to three fish oil capsules a day.

- Check yourself for food allergies with a proper food allergy test (see Resources, page 406).

- Supplement 1,000 to 2,000 mg of MSM and 400mg or more of N-acetyl-cysteine.

- Include plenty of organic free-range eggs (the omega-3-rich type are excellent too), red onions and garlic in your diet, all high in sulphur.

- Eat plenty of fruit and vegetables high in antioxidants.

- Add ginger and turmeric to your food.

- Take a good all-round multivitamin with at least 1,000mg of vitamin C, 150mg of magnesium and 10mg of zinc.

- Supplement an all-round antioxidant formula if you don't eat at least six servings of fruit and vegetables a day, although eating plenty of them is very important. Also supplement 1,000mg of quercetin a day.

- If you have asthma, learn how to breathe using the Buteyko method.

- For eczema, apply vitamin A and C skin creams daily.

Working with your doctor

Many of the recommendations made here to reduce your inflammatory and allergic sensitivity can be put into action without interfering in any way with medical treatment. And they may well reduce the need for it.

For instance, if you have eczema and find that some of the measures we've outlined here are making your skin much less dry, inflamed and sore, you may find that your need for cortisone-based creams becomes lessened. And if you have asthma, and you find these suggestions make your condition much better, it is worth having an informed conversation with your doctor about the value of intermittent versus daily use of bronchodilators.

For both asthma and eczema, one of the most important factors to check for is allergy. Your doctor may be willing to refer you for allergy tests. It is important, however, that you are checked for both IgE and IgG allergies. As few doctors check for IgG-based allergies, you may need to do it yourself using a home-test kit (see Resources, page 406).

15.

Helping Your Heart
Cardiovascular drugs vs alternative heart medicine

MORE PEOPLE DIE prematurely from diseases of the heart and arteries than anything else in the UK – accounting for a third of all deaths before the age of 75. Yet both of these are largely preventable diseases with highly familiar risk factors, such as poor diet, smoking, obesity and lack of exercise. Your risk can also depend very much on where you live. If you are a woman and you live in Scotland for instance, your chances of having a heart attack are eight times higher than if you live in Spain, which shows how big an influence cultural and other local factors can be.[307]

If you've just been diagnosed with some form of heart disease – angina, hypertension (high blood pressure), thrombosis, a stroke or heart attack – your doctor is unlikely to focus on these risk factors. Instead, you'll probably be prescribed a cocktail of drugs to lower your cholesterol, bring down your blood pressure and thin your blood.

You're also likely to get these drugs even if you don't have any symptoms of a cardiovascular problem, but have a measurable risk factor such as high blood pressure or high cholesterol. Drugs to lower these two factors account for the largest slice of drug spending in most countries. In the UK alone they account for well over £2 billion a year,[308] and in Australia over nine million prescriptions were written for statins between May and December 2002, at a total cost of A$570 million.[309] But as we saw in Chapter 2, some experts are very critical of the number of people taking these drugs, accusing the drug companies of lowering the official safe levels of cholesterol and blood pressure to boost sales.

So what are the risk factors for heart disease and stroke that you need to look out for? And, if you have any of them, what's your best course of action? Let's look at these issues now.

Measuring your risk

The main measures used to indicate your level of risk are blood pressure, cholesterol levels, triglyceride levels and homocysteine level.

Blood pressure

This measurement consists of two numbers. The 'systolic', always the higher number, measures the pressure when your heart is contracting to force blood out; the 'diastolic' is the more important because it measures the pressure when your heart is at rest. Blood and other forms of pressure are measured in 'millimetres of mercury' – written 'mmHG' – with the systolic at the top. A normal reading is around 120/76 mmHg; if your blood pressure is above 140/90, you have hypertension and are at much greater risk of heart disease. Every ten-point increase in your diastolic above 76 doubles your risk.

However, you shouldn't rely on just one measure taken at your doctor's surgery. According to a study published in the *Journal of the American Medical Association*, '21% of the patients diagnosed as having borderline hypertension in the clinic were found to have normal blood pressure on ambulatory [while walking about] monitoring.'[310] This is called 'white coat high blood pressure', because anything that makes you nervous – having your blood pressure taken by a doctor in a white coat, for instance – temporarily pushes the pressure up. Insist that your blood pressure is measured a few times over a 24-hour period to get a much more accurate picture.

HOW BLOOD PRESSURE WORKS

Think of your heart as a pump and your arteries as pipes. The arteries are surrounded by muscle cells that can constrict or relax them, and may also become narrower due to 'furring up' and inflammation. Tense arterial muscles or furred-up arteries are the two main causes of hypertension or high blood pressure.

So what is it that makes arterial muscle cells tense? It's all to do with the balance of electrically charged minerals inside and outside the cell. There are two pairs of minerals that move between a cell's interior and exterior: a sodium and potassium pairing, and a calcium and magnesium pairing. The more sodium inside your cells and the less potassium, the higher the tension, which raises your blood pressure. Similarly, the more calcium inside your cells and the less magnesium, the higher your blood pressure.

You can control your blood pressure either by decreasing sodium (that is, eating less salt) and increasing potassium (such as through eating more vegetables), or by boosting your intake of magnesium or stopping calcium from getting into cells. This last option is what a calcium-channel blocker drug does (see page 289).

There's one other vital factor in this pump/pipe system: the amount of liquid or blood in the system. If the amount of blood goes down, so does your blood pressure. The organ that controls the

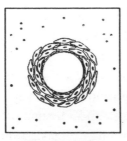 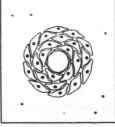 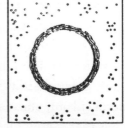

| Normal calcium and magnesium | Normal calcium and low magnesium | Normal calcium and high magnesium |

How magnesium controls blood pressure

amount of blood is the kidneys. By extracting water, and other substances including minerals, from your blood, the kidneys control blood pressure. If you force the kidneys to work harder – which is what diuretics do – your blood pressure comes down. But you also lose more valuable minerals such as magnesium and potassium.

You'd think that drinking more water would raise blood pressure, but the reverse is true. Normally, the kidneys have no problem removing excess water. But when there's a lack of water, the body does everything it can to reserve it for your body cells. Sodium levels inside cells go up, because sodium can hold water inside cells. Consequently, your blood pressure goes up. Also, tiny blood vessels are shut down to conserve more fluid. As a consequence, blood volume goes up, further raising blood pressure. This is why it's so important to drink enough water.

So: water, potassium and magnesium-rich foods lower blood pressure. Sodium raises it. You also need the right balance of calcium to magnesium. Most people have too much of the former and not enough of the latter.

Cholesterol level

Confusingly, your level of cholesterol is measured in two different units – 'milligrams per decilitre', written mg/dl, which is only used in the US; and 'millimoles per litre', written mmol/l and used by everyone else. A millimole is a certain number of molecules. There are three cholesterol readings you can have: your total cholesterol, your LDL ('bad') cholesterol and your HDL ('good') cholesterol. You want to have a low LDL cholesterol (ideally below 2.7mmol/l or 100mg/dl), a high HDL cholesterol (ideally above 1.5mmol/l or 60mg/dl), and a total cholesterol of not less than 3.9mmol/l or 150mg/dl and not more than 5.2mmol/l or 200mg/dl. Of these, raising your HDL is the most important.

As a rough indicator, with every 1.3mmol/l point increase in your total cholesterol above 5.2mol/l, you double your risk of death from cardio-vascular disease. With every 1.3mmol/l increase in LDL, you double your risk, and with every 0.5mmol/l decrease in HDL below 1.5mmol/l, you double your risk.

Triglyceride level

Triglycerides are fats found in the bloodstream, and this measurement reflects the level of those. Triglyceride levels are raised when a person is regularly eating foods high in fat and sugar or drinking a lot of alcohol. Your trigylceride level should be below 1mmol/l or 89mg/dl. As a rough indicator, every 0.56mmol/l increase doubles your risk.

Homocysteine level

If you're at risk of cardiovascular disease, or have a family history of heart disease or stroke, it is essential that your doctor checks your homocysteine level. We've encountered homocysteine in a number of contexts in this book, as this blood amino acid is an important indicator of a number of degenerative diseases, from Alzheimer's to cardiovascular problems. And it is more and more widely researched: a simple visit to Medline, the online library of medical research run by the US National Institutes of Health, shows no fewer than 11,000 studies on it. There's no question that having a raised homocysteine level is a significant and independent risk factor for cardiovascular disease.

Fortunately, homocysteine is easy to measure in the blood and even easier to lower – with B vitamins. Yet, if your level is slightly raised (five points) you'll increase your risk of a heart attack by 42 per cent, of deep vein thrombosis by 60 per cent and of a stroke by 65 per cent, according to a meta-analysis of 92 studies in the *British Medical Journal*.[311] 'These results provide strong evidence that the association between homocysteine and cardiovascular disease is causal,' says lead author David Wald, Clinical Research Fellow in Cardiology at the Wolfson Institute of Preventive Medicine at Barts in London.

To put this into context, the average adult in Britain has a homocysteine level of around 11 mmol/l. The ideal is below six. So the average doubles the risk. If your homocysteine level is 16, that's around four times the risk. The highest we've seen is one patient whose homocysteine score was 119.

There is one study, published in 2001, that shows a raised homocysteine level is a better predictor of cardiovascular problems than a stroke victim's age (each additional year adds only a 6 per cent risk), blood pressure, cholesterol level or whether or not they smoked.[312] It involved 1,158 women and 789 men aged 60 years or older who had already taken part in studies investigating homocysteine levels as a predictor for stroke. After seven years, those who had had a homocysteine score above 14 units had an 82 per cent increased risk of total stroke, compared to those with less than 9.2 units.

There are other important measures, such as your platelet adhesion index and your fibrinogen levels, which both measure the stickiness of your blood; lipoprotein (a) level, which is a highly significant risk factor; and C-reactive protein level, which indicates inflammation in the arteries. A comprehensive cardiovascular screening could include these important risk factors as well. (see Resources, page 406.)

How is your heart health?

Check yourself out on this simplified cardiovascular questionnaire.

- [ ] Is your blood pressure above 140/90?
- [ ] Is your pulse above 80?
- [ ] Is your cholesterol above 5.5?
- [ ] Is your cholesterol/HDL ratio above five?
- [ ] Is your homocysteine level above nine?
- [ ] Do you get out of breath climbing up stairs or inclines?
- [ ] Do you sometimes get chest pains?
- [ ] Do you smoke more than five cigarettes a day?
- [ ] Do you exercise less than twice a week?
- [ ] Are you overweight?

☐ Do you have cardiovascular disease?

☐ Does your mother, father, or any brothers or sisters suffer from cardiovascular disease or high cholesterol?

☐ Do you eat less than three servings of fruit and vegetables most days?

☐ Do you eat fried food, meat or other high fat foods most days?

☐ Do you rarely take vitamin supplements?

☐ Do you consider your lifestyle stressful?

Score 1 for every 'yes' answer. If you answered yes to:

Less than 4: you have few in indicators of risk. The ideal score is '0' and therefore it is best to address any 'yes' answers if possible.

5 to 8: you have a high risk of cardiovascular disease and need to take action to change your diet and lifestyle to reduce your risk.

More than 8: you are in the very high risk category for cardiovascular disease and should both see your doctor and a nutritional therapist to actively reduce your risk with dietary changes as well as supplements.

The cardiovascular drugs

There are several categories of heart medications, each designed to affect the different aspects of cardiovascular health that are measured. The main ones are:

- Cholesterol-lowering drugs, including statins

- Blood-pressure-lowering drugs, including thiazides (diuretics), beta-blockers, ACE inhibitors, calcium-channel blockers, and nitro-vasodilators

- Blood-thinning drugs to make clotting less likely, such as warfarin (coumadin) and aspirin.

If you have cardiovascular disease, or are at a high risk of developing it, the chances are you're on more than one of these medications already. All of them interfere with some aspect of your body's chemistry and none is necessary if you address the underlying causes of heart disease.

Statins and cholesterol-lowering drugs

About a third of all money spent on cardiovascular drugs is spent on statins. The big brands include simvastatin (Zocor), atorvastatin (Lipitor), pravastatin (Pravachol), rosuvastin (Crestor) and fluvastatin (Lescol). If you've had a heart attack or have significant cardiovascular risk, research published in 2003 shows that statins can reduce your risk of a heart attack by up to 60 per cent, and your risk of stroke by 17 per cent.[313] However, the risk reduction is minimal in the first year you take it. If you haven't had a heart attack but your cholesterol level is above 5mmol/l, you'll probably be prescribed a statin.

At first sight, this might seem like a wise precaution. But not everyone agrees. If you haven't had a heart attack, taking statins 'does not significantly reduce all causes of mortality or the overall risk of serious illness', according to Dr John Abramson of the clinical medical faculty at Harvard Medical School. As we saw in Chapter 2, there is a darker side to statins that you are unlikely to hear about from standard medical sources.

Overall, statin medication can be expected to lower LDL cholesterol by an average of 3.8mmol/l if taken for several years. Statins, however, are not very effective at raising HDL cholesterol, which is the more important indicator of reducing your risk (see the 'Cholesterol – the good, the bad, and the best' box below) and the one that can be most influenced by changing your diet.

CHOLESTEROL – THE GOOD, THE BAD, AND THE BEST

Your cholesterol is broken down into total cholesterol, LDL (bad) cholesterol, and HDL (good) cholesterol. You want your LDL cholesterol to be low (ideally below 100mg/dl or 2.7mmol/l), your HDL cholesterol to be high (ideally above 60mg/dl or 1.5mmol/l), and your total cholesterol to be between 100mg/dl or 3.9mmol/l and 200mg/dl or 5.2mmol/l.

Your HDL cholesterol is the most predictive of cardiovascular risk, and so is the most important measure. In fact, the best predictor of all is your total cholesterol/HDL ratio. This is your total cholesterol score divided by your HDL score. The result should be below four, indicating that at least a quarter of your cholesterol is in the 'good' HDL form, which means that your body will be able to clear excess cholesterol from your arteries.

It doesn't matter if your total cholesterol level is elevated if a high percentage of it is in HDL form. Ideally, your total cholesterol/HDL ratio should be three or less. A ratio of five or more is not good, while a ratio of eight or more is bad.

If you're male, aged 50 to 75, and have had a heart attack, a stent inserted, a coronary bypass or an angioplasty, statins will probably reduce your risk. If you're an otherwise healthy woman with raised cholesterol, they probably won't.

Why statins can be bad for your heart

Besides the fact that a large number of people have to take a statin for just one of them to benefit (see Chapter 2), there's another problematic feature of statins that comes up time and again with drugs: in the process of blocking something to reduce one set of symptoms, they also block something else that is vital for healthy functioning. Your doctor is unlikely to mention that as well as blocking LDL cholesterol, statins also reduce production of an enzyme known as Co-enzyme Q10 (CoQ10), which is, ironically, essential for heart health. A deficiency in CoQ10 has been associated with fatigue, muscle weakness and soreness, and heart failure.[314]

Just how serious these problems are is still unclear, not least because the major trials of statin drugs deliberately excluded those with class 3 and 4 heart failure – the more serious forms – which are a major effect of CoQ10 deficiency.[315] Another side effect reported on statins is transient amnesia. NASA astronaut Duane Graveline was prescribed statins after a heart attack. After six weeks on the drug he lost his memory for six hours.

Later, he lost it completely for 12 hours.[316] Although this side effect is quite rare, there are many other reports of memory loss from statins. (For more on CoQ10, see Chapter 15, page 298.)

SIDE EFFECTS Other symptoms associated with statins include dizziness, headache, extreme fatigue, swelling of the ankles, muscle aches, fatigue, and suppressed immunity.

> They certainly don't suit everybody. Feona is a case in point. With a cholesterol level of 8.5mmol/l, she was prescribed Lipitor. 'I only took one tablet and woke up at 3 am with pins and needles, which gradually crept up my arms and across my face and tongue. Next morning I felt as if someone had punched me in the right shoulder.'
> So instead, Feona opted for the natural approach – diet, exercise and stress control – and managed to lower her cholesterol to 4.4mmol/l.

Unbelievably, statins are now available over the counter at UK pharmacies, although Britain is still unique in this respect.

Blood-pressure-lowering drugs

Of all the cardiovascular medicines, more prescriptions are written out for blood-pressure-lowering drugs than for any other kind – around 40 million a year,[317] in fact. These drugs fall into five main categories, described on the following pages, but all of them produce similar reductions in blood pressure – a drop of around 5.5mmHg in diastolic blood pressure. In fact, there has been a big debate in the last few years about whether the newer, expensive ACE inhibitors are actually any better than the older, very cheap diuretics, following a major trial published in 2002 that found no difference between them.[318] (For more on this, see Chapter 2, page 46.)

Whatever their relative merits, all these blood-pressure-lowering drugs come with considerable risks, a fact that has been known by doctors for years. One of the first proper controlled trials, for instance, was done over 20 years ago on the diuretics. Nicknamed MRFIT (Multiple Risk Factor Intervention Trial), it involved 12,800 men at high risk of heart attack because they smoked and had high cholesterol and high blood pressure. The trial compared 'usual care' with the aggressive use of diuretics and found that even though diuretics did lower blood pressure, not only was there no reduction in risk of death among those being more aggressively treated, those with borderline hypertension (below 150/100) had a higher risk of death.[319]

Thiazides

These drugs are diuretics that essentially work by telling your kidneys to make you urinate more, as less liquid in the blood equals less pressure. They include chlorothiazide (Diuril), benzthiazide (also called triamterene and benzthiazide in the UK, with the brand name Dytide or Exna) and cyclothiazide (Anhydron, Fluidil). Of course, as soon as you increase the flow of urine, a number of vital minerals get washed out of the body as well so you can end up with too little potassium and magnesium. Some types of drugs spare potassium, including spironolactone and triamterene, but not the vital heart mineral magnesium. Also, lowering the amount of fluid in the blood causes the body to retain more sodium. So this kind of approach is fighting against the body's design and makes no sense over the long term.

SIDE EFFECTS Kidney damage, fatigue, muscle cramping, faintness and an increased incidence of gallstones. Long-term use may increase cholesterol and risk of heart irregularities and blood-sugar levels, so they're especially bad news for both full-blown and borderline diabetics.

The longer you are on these drugs, the greater the risks become. Since blood pressure can be relatively easily lowered by dietary and lifestyle changes, it makes sense to do these first before incurring all the potential hazards of these medications. As an editorial in a 1991 issue of the *British Medical Journal* stated:

> Treatment of hypertension is part of preventive medicine and like all preventive strategies, its progress should be regularly reviewed by whoever initiates it. Many problems could be avoided by not starting antihypertensive treatment until after prolonged observation. Patients

should no longer be told that treatment is necessarily for life: the possibility of reducing or stopping treatment should be mentioned at the outset.[320]

ACE inhibitors

These drugs block an enzyme (known as angiotensin converting enzyme) that is necessary for the production of a substance that causes blood vessels to tighten. As a result, they relax blood vessels, lowering blood pressure. ACE inhibitors have names that usually end in 'pril', such as captopril, ramipril, and trandolapril.

SIDE EFFECTS There are plenty of them with these drugs: a dry and persistent cough, headache, diarrhoea, loss of taste, nausea, unusual tiredness, dizziness, light-headedness or fainting, skin rash with or without itching, fever and joint pain. ACE inhibitors are contraindicated if you are pregnant, and not suitable for those with kidney or liver problems. They can cause excess potassium accumulation, the symptoms of which are confusion, irregular heartbeat, nervousness, numbness or tingling in hands, feet, or lips, shortness of breath or difficulty breathing, and weakness or heaviness of legs. Contact your doctor immediately if you experience fever and chills, hoarseness, swelling of face, mouth, hands, or feet, sudden trouble with swallowing or breathing, stomach pain, itching, or yellow eyes or skin.

Even so, these are probably the safest of the blood-pressure drugs on offer.

Beta-blockers

These drugs counter our normal stress response by preventing the heart from reacting to stress. This lowers blood pressure. Beta-blockers can sometimes help people with congestive heart failure by reducing tachycardia – that is, rapid heartbeats.

SIDE EFFECTS There are real concerns about these drugs for anything other than short-term use or for people who have had heart attacks that have resulted in erratic heartbeats due to damage to the heart's left ventricle – beta-blockers can reduce the risk of sudden cardiac death in these cases. These drugs also deplete CoQ10, but to a much lesser extent than statins.

The *Physician's Desk Reference*, which is the book American doctors refer to on drugs, warns of the dangers of long-term use:

> Cardiac Failure. Sympathetic stimulation is a vital component of supporting circulatory function in congestive heart failure, and a beta-blockade carries the potential hazard of further depressing myocardial contractility and of precipitating more severe failure.
>
> Patients Without a History of Cardiac Failure. Continued depression of the myocardium with beta-blocking agents over a period of time can, in some cases, lead to cardiac failure.
>
> Adverse Reactions – Cardiovascular. Shortness of breath and bradycardia (heart rate below 60) have occurred in approximately 3 of 100 patients. Cold extremities, arterial insufficiency of the Raynaud type, palpitations, congestive heart failure, peripheral oedema, or hypotension have been reported in 1 of 100 patients.

So, if you've had cardiac failure these drugs could make it worse. If you haven't, long-term use could induce it.

That's not the end of the side effects, however. There is a host of less severe ones, including a decreased sex drive, insomnia, fatigue, dizziness and nausea.

If you want to come off beta-blockers, be aware that you mustn't go cold turkey: this could precipitate angina, high blood pressure or even a heart attack. It is better to wean yourself off them. The elderly, pregnant women and people with kidney or thyroid disease should be especially cautious about taking beta-blockers, and use the lowest dose possible to get their blood pressure under control – or follow the non-drug options outlined later in this chapter.

Calcium-channel blockers

The relaxation and tension of muscle cells depends on the balance between calcium and magnesium inside and out. One highly effective way to reduce blood pressure is to eat more magnesium (see page 295).

But calcium-channel blockers, like all the other hypertension drugs, block just one element in a carefully balanced system – in this case, the cell's ability to take up calcium.

The action of these drugs, which include verapamil, diltiazem and nifedipine, is bad news. Cells need calcium even if depriving them of it does lower blood pressure. A study in a 1995 issue of *Circulation*, the journal of the American Heart Association, showed that patients on one of the calcium-channel blockers – nifedipine – were more likely to die. As the paper said, 'High doses of nifedipine were significantly associated with increased mortality,' adding, 'Other calcium antagonists may have similar adverse effects.'[321] Norvasc is a newer version of this drug.

SIDE EFFECTS These include potassium loss, elevated serum cholesterol, headaches, dizziness, nausea, oedema, hypotension and constipation. Calcium-channel blockers also appear to affect the liver and interfere with carbohydrate metabolism and may not be suitable for diabetics for this reason.

Blood-thinning drugs

If you have blood that is prone to clotting, the abnormal heart rhythm known as atrial fibrillation, or you've had a heart attack or ischemic stroke (that is, one involving a clot), you are very likely to be prescribed blood-thinning drugs. They're also used in medical emergencies and may be given in the short term if you are having an operation.

A stroke is essentially an injury to brain cells resulting from a disruption to blood flow. There are three main types of stroke. The first two are ischemic, while the third results from bleeding in the brain.

- Thrombotic strokes occur when a blood clot forms within the brain, blocking blood flow. They account for about 40 to 50 per cent of all strokes.

- Embolic strokes result from the formation of a blood clot elsewhere in the body that breaks off, travels to the brain and blocks the finer blood vessels there. These account for around 20 per cent of all strokes.

- Haemorrhagic strokes, as the name suggests, result from a haemorrhage or uncontrolled bleed in the brain. This type occurs much less frequently, and accounts for about ten to 15 per cent of all cases, but it is usually far more devastating in effect.

Warfarin/Coumadin

Warfarin, sold as Coumadin in the US, is usually prescribed following an ischemic stroke. Unfortunately, warfarin increases the risk of having a haemorrhagic stroke.

The case of Israel's former prime minister, Ariel Sharon, may be a tragic illustration of this. On 18 December 2005, Sharon had a minor ischemic stroke from which he had no lasting ill-effects. His doctors gave him large doses of blood thinners, which stopped the blood from clotting.

According to a British cardiologist, as reported by the BBC, 'blood-thinning treatment would alleviate his condition as diagnosed but could prove "catastrophic" if Mr Sharon had suffered an undetected haemorraghic stroke, or "small bleed" in his brain.' According to a report in the British newspaper, the *Guardian*, 'Doctors in Israel have admitted making a mistake when treating Israeli prime minister Ariel Sharon for a minor blood clot. The anti-coagulants may have caused the serious haemorrhagic stroke, which has put him in a coma for months.'[322] As this book goes to press, there is little hope for a meaningful recovery.

Warfarin is also given to those with atrial fibrillation, which worsens blood flow, because it can reduce risk of an embolic stroke by thinning the blood. Warfarin works by interfering with the formation of vitamin K, the body's natural blood-clotting agent, in the liver, and the dose is managed by frequent blood tests to measure the time taken for blood to clot. This is known as the INR or international normalised ratio.

A normal INR is between 0.8–1.2. If you are taking warfarin because you're at high risk of a stroke or heart attack, your dose will be managed to achieve an INR of between two and three in most cases to prevent your blood from clotting too much. It's a fine balance because under-clotting carries its own risks.

Heparin

This drug is very similar to warfarin but can only be administered by injection, whereas warfarin is usually taken orally. It works faster and is usually prescribed with warfarin. Then, as warfarin starts to work, the patient is weaned off it.

Aspirin

Aspirin has an antiplatelet effect – it inhibits the hormone-like substances prostaglandins that encourage blood platelets to stick to each other and form blood clots. There is no similar measure of effectiveness to determine dose. In women over the age of 65, approximately 100mg of aspirin has been shown to prevent stroke, but the overuse of aspirin causes thousands of death a year from gastrointestinal bleeding.

SIDE EFFECTS The major side effect of the blood-thinning drugs is excessive bleeding, such as eye and brain haemorrhages, blood in the urine, and bleeding gums. Warfarin can also cause hypersensitivity, hair loss, rashes, diarrhoea, 'purple toes', liver dysfunction, nausea and vomiting.[323] Aspirin causes gastrointestinal bleeding, as we've seen, and should be avoided if you have gut problems, a history of haemorrhagic stroke, bleeding ulcers, haemorrhoids, bleeding into the eyes or diabetes.

Note that you should never take warfarin and aspirin at the same time.

Natural alternatives

If you are on one or more of these drugs, it's highly likely they are going to unbalance various complex systems in your body, possibly putting you at risk for a number of other problems in the future. The same applies if you're reasonably healthy but have been given statins due to your age or your cholesterol level. Wouldn't it make sense, therefore, to make a serious effort to bring down your risk levels in ways that didn't have this very real drawback?

There's now evidence that several foods, nutrients and spices can all help to protect you against heart disease, strokes and circulation problems. Together they are likely to be far more effective, and certainly much safer, than today's drugs. Backed up with the necessary lifestyle changes – not smoking, reducing alcohol and regular exercise – many people find rapid improvements in cholesterol, blood pressure and other indicators of risk. And they find they need less, and even no, medication. For people not on medication, these same nutritional and lifestyle changes can help make sure they never need it.

A combination of the following is far more likely to give you a healthy heart than the usual mix of drugs:

- Plant sterols and soluble fibre for lowering LDL cholesterol

- Niacin for raising HDL cholesterol

- Mineral-rich foods for lowering blood pressure

- Antioxidants to protect arteries from damage

- B vitamins to lower homocysteine

- Herbs and spices to reduce blood clotting

- Omega-3 fish oils for both lowering overall risk and speeding up recovery.

While some of these natural solutions have major effects on cholesterol or blood pressure, say, we recommend all of them even if you only have high blood pressure, or only high cholesterol. That's because they affect your whole system in a positive way.

> Andrew O is a case in point. When he had his cholesterol measured it was 8.8. He was put on statins and, six months later, it was 8.7. He was also gaining weight, feeling tired and stressed, and not sleeping well.
>
> With help, Andrew changed his diet and started taking supplements very close to those we recommend here. Three weeks later, he had lost ten pounds (about 4.5kg), his energy levels were great, he no longer felt stressed and he was sleeping much better. And his cholesterol level had dropped to a healthy 4.9.

One note of caution: vitamin E and omega-3 fish oils both help thin the blood, so if you're on blood-thinning medication such as warfarin, you'll need to work with your doctor to see how best to proceed with supplementing these. See page 310 for more on this.

Bring down 'bad' cholesterol with plant sterols

If you've ever bought a pint of soya milk, you might have seen the words 'lowers cholesterol' on the label. This is because soya is a particularly rich source of hormone-like substances called plant sterols. Seeds, nuts, beans and lentils also contain high levels of them. In the average Western diet, these foods are relatively rare, so most of us consequently fail to get enough plant sterols in our diet.

Plant sterols aren't the only plant-based cholesterol busters. Other plants, such as oats, barley, aubergines and okra, contain soluble fibre that does the job as well.

Two studies have now shown that eating these foods is more effective at lowering high cholesterol than taking a statin.[324] The latest, published in 2006 in the *American Journal of Clinical Nutrition*, put 34 patients with high cholesterol on a low-fat diet for a month, a low-fat diet plus statins for a month, or a diet high in plant sterols for a month. Each patient had to do each diet for a month, although they were assigned in random order. On the high plant sterol diet, they ate the equivalent of 2.5g of plant sterols, in:

- 50g of soya (a glass of soya milk, or a small serving of tofu, or a small soya burger)

- 35g of almonds (a small handful of almonds)

- 25g of soluble fibres from oats and vegetables (the equivalent of five oat cakes, plus a bowl of oats and three servings of vegetables)

Statins, as we've seen, are relatively ineffectual at raising 'good' HDL cholesterol, but do lower 'bad' LDL cholesterol. Both statins and the plant sterol diet significantly lowered LDL cholesterol to the same degree, but nine of the volunteers (26 per cent), achieved their lowest LDL cholesterol while on the plant sterol diet, not the statins.[325]

In the words of Professor David Jenkins, who led this study, 'People interested in lowering their cholesterol should probably acquire a taste for tofu and oatmeal.' There's no question that plant sterols do have this effect, which is why increasing them in your diet is an easy and safe way to keep your cholesterol at a safe level. There's also evidence, from a study published in 2005, that the more soya you eat, the lower your blood pressure.[326]

Vitamin B3 – better than statins

Since we're talking about cholesterol, you might be surprised to find that taking niacin or vitamin B3 is the most effective way to raise HDL cholesterol levels. This kind of cholesterol is the stuff that can remove unwanted or damaged cholesterol from your arteries and, according to a recent review in the *New England Journal of Medicine*, niacin increases levels of HDL by 20 to 35 per cent.[327]

Niacin also lowers LDL cholesterol by up to 25 per cent. One of the authors of this study was cardiology expert Roger Blumenthal, an associate professor and director of the Ciccarone Center for the Prevention of Heart Disease at The Johns Hopkins University School of Medicine and its Heart Institute in Baltimore, Maryland. Statins, by comparison, only raise HDL by between 2 and 15 per cent.

Niacin also reduces your levels of two other markers for raised risk of heart disease – lipoprotein A and fibrinogen. So, why aren't doctors prescribing it?

It's a good question. The lack of prescriptions certainly has nothing to do with a lack of research. Medline, the database of research for the US National Institutes of Health, quotes over 40 positive studies from the last five years recommending niacin over statins, or with statins to further improve their cholesterol-lowering effect.[328] We recommend 1,000mg a day to lower raised LDL cholesterol and raise a low HDL cholesterol.

SIDE EFFECTS 'No-flush niacin', or niacin inositol hexanicotinate, is the kind we advise you to take. This is because, at a dose of 1,000mg a day, other forms of niacin can produce a blushing sensation, or tingling, itching or a hot-flush sensation for up to 30 minutes. This isn't to everybody's liking – although it's entirely harmless.

If you can't get hold of no-flush niacin at the moment but want to take niacin, you can reduce the flushing by starting with a low dose of 50 to 100mg per day, then double the dose each week until an effective level is reached. The flushing becomes less intense after a week or two of this. Note that niacinamide, another form of niacin, doesn't help lower cholesterol.

Niacin can also cause blood-sugar fluctuations, so diabetics should be cautious about using it in high doses. However, a recent randomised controlled trial reports that of 148 diabetic patients, only four discontinued niacin because of inadequate glucose control.[329] Finally, niacin is best taken with high-dose homocysteine-lowering nutrients (see page 304), as there is some evidence that niacin may otherwise slightly raise homocysteine levels.

Simple ways of lowering blood pressure

As you saw in 'How blood pressure works' (page 278), instead of lowering blood pressure with a calcium blocker or a diuretic, the logical alternative is to drink enough water, eat more fruit and vegetables high in both potassium and magnesium, and eat more seeds high in magnesium, while avoiding salt.

Magnesium ensures that the muscle cells both in the arteries and heart don't get too tense, improving heart-muscle function and blood pressure. In fact, it has been shown to lower blood pressure by about ten per cent,[330] as well as reduce cholesterol and triglycerides,[331] thus substantially lowering the risk of death from cardiovascular disease. Unfortunately, a lot of us are deficient in magnesium – the average intake in the UK is 272mg, while an ideal amount is probably 500mg, especially if you have high blood pressure. The richest source of this mineral is dark green vegetables, nuts and seeds. We recommend you supplement 300mg a day; a good multivitamin can provide 150mg.

Although increasing your potassium does lower blood pressure, it isn't worth supplementing potassium because the amount you'd get is just a fraction of what you would manage to pack away by eating your greens (a serving will do it). Drinking more water – eight glasses, or one to two litres, a day – also helps because a lack of water makes the sodium level inside cells go up, which raises blood pressure.

Patients with high blood pressure have long been advised to cut out salt, but there is one kind that may even be helpful. It's a special sea salt called Solo, which has 61 per cent less sodium, but more potassium and more magnesium, than regular salt. A study in the *British Medical Journal* found it reduced high blood pressure.[332] This is because potassium and magnesium are good news as far as the arteries and your blood pressure are concerned.

The power of antioxidants

As we'll see in Chapter 18, which discusses 'vitamin scares', a lot of confusion has been created about the role of antioxidants such as vitamins C and E in reducing the risk of developing heart disease. Certainly your doctor is unlikely to recommend that you supplement them. But there is no doubt that oxidising free radicals, from such sources as smoking or eating fried foods, not only damage artery walls but also the cholesterol in the bloodstream. Plaques can then form on blood vessel walls, and oxidised cholesterol will accumulate at the site. This growing wound on the artery wall encourages inflammation and blood clots.

Antioxidants work by disarming the harmful oxidants, with vitamin E being particularly useful in this context. Technically known as d-alpha tocopherol, vitamin E is a fat-soluble antioxidant and, as such, can help to protect fats such as cholesterol.

The best way to get all-round antioxidant protection is to eat a diet rich in natural antioxidants and take a multi-antioxidant supplement. The best protective foods are shown opposite. These not only contain vitamin A, C and E, but also contain many other key antioxidant nutrients such as proanthocyanidins, lycopene, glutathione, cysteine and more. So, the golden rule is to eat at least five to six servings of fresh fruit and vegetables a day and make sure your diet in naturally multicoloured. Green, red, yellow and blue foods such as broccoli, strawberries, avocados and blueberries all provide a varied and rich supply of anti-oxidants to fight off the oxidants that invade your arteries. Going for an antioxidant 'rainbow' alone has been shown to cut stroke risk by a quarter.[333]

TWELVE OF THE BEST ANTIOXIDANT-RICH FOODS

The total antioxidant power of a food can be measured using a scale called the oxygen radical absorption capacity (ORAC). These foods came out on top.

Per 100g

- Blueberries   2,234
- Blackberries   2,036
- Kale   1,770
- Strawberries   1,536
- Spinach, raw   1,210
- Raspberries   1,227
- Tenderstem   1,183
- Plums   949
- Alfalfa sprouts   931
- Spinach, steamed   909
- Broccoli   888
- Beetroot   841

Vitamin E

The evidence for a protective effect from antioxidant supplements is strongest for vitamin E and C. A large-scale controlled trial on vitamin E, carried out by Professor Morris Brown and colleagues at Cambridge University ten years ago, showed a 75 per cent decrease in heart attack in a group of 2,000 patients with heart disease, compared to those on placebo.[334] These results are approximately three times better than the protection offered by aspirin. Brown said,

This is even more exciting than aspirin. Most people in our study were already taking aspirin. The average benefit from taking aspirin is in the order of 25 to 30 per cent reduction. Vitamin E reduced the risk of heart attack by a massive 75 per cent.

This was the third large-scale trial of vitamin E's benefits. In one, published in 1993 in the *New England Journal of Medicine,* 87,200 nurses were given 100iu (67mg) of vitamin E daily for more than two years.[335] A 40 per cent drop in fatal and non-fatal heart attacks was reported amongst the subjects, compared to those not taking vitamin E. In the other study, published the same year, 39,000 male health professionals were given 100iu (67mg) of vitamin E for the same length of time and had a 39 per cent reduction in heart attacks.[336] A ten-year study involving 11,178 people aged 67 to 105 found that those supplementing vitamin E had a reduced risk of death from all causes of 33 per cent, and a 47 per cent reduction in death from a heart attack.[337]

However, not all studies have been positive. One trial gave 800ius (536mg) of vitamin E to those at risk and found no decrease in mortality rates. Some studies have even suggested that vitamin E, in large doses, might slightly increase risk. A possible reason is that these more recent studies have involved very sick patients likely to be taking statins, which interfere with the effects of vitamin E by reducing availability of co-enzyme Q10, but more research needs to be done. To date, the evidence suggests that vitamin E is more effective if taken *before* you are at risk. (For a more detailed discussion of this issue, see Chapter 18.)

So provided you are not on a statin and include co-enzyme Q10 in your supplement programme, the chances are that vitamin E is still protective, even after a heart attack, at levels up to 400mg. You should, however, speak to your doctor before taking more than 300mg of vitamin E if you are on blood-thinning medication, as vitamin E does have a blood-thinning effect.[338] (See page 310 for more on combining cardiovascular drugs with natural blood thinners.)

Co-enzyme Q10

Co-enzyme Q10 is an antioxidant made by the body that helps heart and all muscle cells to become more efficient. After the age of 40, your levels of this enzyme begin to gradually decline, falling off precipitously in your eighties – a drop that comes at just the time when congestive heart failure becomes more common. CoQ10's positive effects on heart health is documented in over 100 clinical studies.[339] It is, however, very hard to get enough from food (see the 'Foods rich in co-enzyme Q10' box opposite).

FOODS RICH IN CO-ENZYME Q10
(milligrams per 100 grams)

FOOD	AMOUNT	FOOD	AMOUNT
Meat		**Beans**	
Beef	3.1	Green beans	0.58
Pork	2.4 – 4.1	Soya beans	0.29
Chicken	2.1	Aduki beans	0.22
Fish		**Nuts and seeds**	
Sardines	6.4	Peanuts	2.7
Mackerel	4.3	Sesame seeds	2.3
Flat fish	0.5	Walnuts	1.9
Grains		**Vegetables**	
Rice bran	0.54	Spinach	1
Rice	——	Broccoli	0.8
Wheatgerm	0.35	Peppers	0.3
Wheat flour	——	Carrots	0.2
Millet	0.15		
Buckwheat	0.13	**Oils**	
		Soya oil	9.2

A six-year study of people with congestive heart failure, conducted at the University of Texas in the US, found that 75 per cent of a group on CoQ10 survived three years, while only 25 per cent of a similar group on conventional medication lived that long.[340] In over 20 properly controlled studies published in the last two years, CoQ10 has repeatedly demonstrated a remarkable ability to improve heart function and is now the treatment of choice in Japan for congestive heart failure, angina and high blood pressure, especially among older people.

Angina is usually caused by blockages in the tiny arteries that feed the heart muscle cells with oxygen; sufferers feel severe pain in the heart area when exerting themselves. In one study from 1986 at Hamamatsu University in Japan, angina patients treated with CoQ10 were able to increase their tolerance to exercise and had less frequent angina attacks.[341] After only four weeks on CoQ10, the patients were able to halve the other medication they were taking. In another trial, from 2004, researchers demonstrated that CoQ10 treatment increased the capacity of elderly people to sustain a cardiac workload by 28 per cent.[342]

CoQ10 is also excellent for lowering high blood pressure. In a joint study by the University of Austin, Texas, and the Centre for Adult Diseases in Osaka, Japan, 52 patients with high blood pressure were treated either with CoQ10 or a placebo.[343] There was an 11 per cent decrease in blood pressure for those on CoQ10, compared to a two per cent decrease for those on a placebo. In another trial, from 2001, 60mg of CoQ10 given twice daily for 12 weeks helped promote normal blood pressure levels by reducing systolic blood pressure.[344] A controlled clinical trial published in 2002 meanwhile showed that supplementation with 200mg of CoQ10 a day helps to promote normal blood pressure levels.[345]

CoQ10, at a daily dose of 90mg, has also been shown to reduce oxidation damage in the arteries, thereby protecting fats in the blood such as LDL cholesterol from becoming damaged and contributing to arterial blockages.[346]

We recommend taking 30 to 60mg a day for prevention, and 90 to 120mg a day if you have cardiovascular disease, together with 200mg vitamin E. CoQ10 in an oil-based capsule is more readily absorbed by the body.

Vitamin C

Vitamin C is another antioxidant that lowers high blood pressure and the risk of a heart attack. A number of studies have shown that the higher a person's vitamin C status, the lower their blood pressure. One double-blind study from 1991 gave 1,000mg of vitamin C or a placebo to participants, and found significant reduction in the systolic blood pressure, but not the diastolic. The team, at the Alcorn State University in Mississippi, concluded that 'vitamin C supplementation may have therapeutic value in human hypertensive disease'.[347] Another study, from 1992, gave 2g to participants and found a 10 point drop in systolic blood pressure in only 30 days.[348]

The capability of vitamin C to lower blood pressure at a daily level of 1 to 2g, as well as cholesterol levels, has been demonstrated in other studies as well. It's also protective. A review of studies on antioxidant intake from 2004 found that those supplementing in excess of 700mg of vitamin C a day cut their risk of developing cardiovascular disease by a quarter.[349]

Supplementing both vitamins C and E were found in a study from 1996 to cut the overall risk of death by 42 per cent and the risk of death from a heart attack by 52 per cent.[350] Vitamin C also lowers another marker for cardiovascular disease, lipoprotein(a).

We recommend supplementing 400mg of vitamin E and 4g of vitamin C, plus other antioxidants every day if you have cardiovascular disease, and half this amount if you don't.

Note that if you are taking a blood-thinning drug, limit your daily intake of vitamin E to 300mg – or speak with your doctor about reducing the drug and increasing blood-thinning nutrients. This is easily done by taking an all-round antioxidant supplement, plus a high-strength multi-vitamin and mineral, plus 1,000mg of vitamin C. Since vitamin C is rarely supplied in sufficient amounts in multis, you will need to take a good high-strength antioxidant formula and additional vitamin C. When choosing a vitamin E supplement, it is better to select one that has mixed tocopherols, including d-alpha tocopherol, gamma tocopherol and tocotrienols.

The homocysteine-lowering Bs

There's no question that having a raised homocysteine level is a significant and independent risk factor for cardiovascular disease.

What's still open for debate is how best to lower it and then what level of risk reduction you can achieve by doing it. The body only makes high levels of homocysteine if you don't have enough vitamin B2, B6, B12, folic acid, zinc, magnesium or TMG, which is found in root vegetables. Of these nutrients, the most powerful for preventing homocysteine accumulation, which damages the arteries, are the vitamins folic acid, B12 and B6, in that order. The current consensus is that lowering your homocysteine level by 25 per cent should result in about a ten per cent drop in coronary heart disease risk and about 20 per cent lower stroke risk.[353] One in ten people inherit a genetic tendency to raised homo-cysteine, and for them, higher intakes of these vitamins, especially 'methyl' folic acid or methylcobalamin (B12), are needed.

There have been four studies. The 2005 VISP trial showed a clear 21 per cent reduction in stroke, coronary disease or death in those given higher doses of vitamin B12.[352] A survey in the US and Canada, published in 2006, has shown a clear reduction in deaths from stroke in those countries since folic acid fortification of foods such as pasta and bread was introduced, compared to countries such as the UK, which don't fortify food with folic acid.[353]

Next came the HOPE 2 trial, published in the *New England Journal of Medicine* in 2006, which gave supplements of B6 (50mg), folic acid (2.5mg) and B12 (1mg) to patients with vascular disease or diabetes. This study, widely reported as negative because there was no significant reduction in overall cardiovascular events, did show a clear and significant effect of the vitamins on stroke risk, reducing it by 25 per cent (although there was no reduction in heart-attack risk).[354]

The last trial, known as NORVIT and also published in the *New England Journal of Medicine* in 2006, gave B vitamins to patients immediately following an acute heart attack. They were found to make no difference in cardiovascular deaths.[355] This may be because the risk of another cardiovascular event after a heart attack may have little to do with long-term risk factors.

While the results of these last two trials are somewhat disappointing, they don't mean that taking large amounts of B vitamins to lower homocysteine *won't* prevent heart disease from developing in the first place. They just mean that, in people with vascular disease, or who've had an acute heart attack, taking B vitamins alone is unlikely to make much difference.

These trials also looked at the effects of relatively small changes in homocysteine, of 3 or 4 mmol/l or 15 to 25 per cent. Better results might be achieved by giving the right levels of all the homocysteine-lowering nutrients – vitamin B2, B6, B12, folic acid, zinc, magnesium and TMG – which are easily available in homocysteine nutrient formulas.

At 73, Valda had suffered from high blood pressure for over 30 years, as well as a touch of arthritis. Her doctor had prescribed an ACE inhibitor and an aspirin for her, to take every day. They had helped a bit, but her blood pressure was still high – averaging 150/80. She decided to have a homocysteine test.

Valda's score was 42.9, putting her in the very high risk category. She went on a homocysteine-lowering diet and supplement programme. After two months she retested and her homocysteine score had dropped to a healthy 5.1. This level of reduction would equate to more than halving her risk for a stroke and, at least, cutting her risk of a heart attack by a third.

Her blood pressure has also dropped and stabilised at 132/80 and she no longer needs medication. Her arthritis has improved with much less joint pain and she feels better in herself.

Apart from a reduced risk of heart disease, there are many other benefits associated with lower homocysteine. It is linked with a decreased risk of death from all causes. Most people also report more energy, better mood, better concentration and less pain.

But as with so many of the natural treatments we've outlined in this book, the homocysteine 'cure' is neither patentable nor profitable. It involves simple, undramatic changes in your diet and lifestyle (see the 'Nine ways to lower your homocysteine' box below). All you need to do is test your homocysteine level, which you can now do with home-test kits (see Resources, page 406) or through your doctor, and then – along with our other recommendations – take the required number of homo-cysteine-lowering nutrients (see 'The best homocysteine-lowering supplements' box overleaf).

NINE WAYS TO LOWER YOUR HOMOCYSTEINE

- Eat less fatty meat, and more fish and vegetable protein
- Eat your greens
- Have a clove of garlic a day
- Cut back on tea, and especially coffee
- Limit your alcohol
- Reduce your stress
- Stop smoking
- Correct oestrogen deficiency (see page 168)
- Supplement homocysteine-lowering nutrients every day.

THE BEST HOMOCYSTEINE-LOWERING SUPPLEMENTS

These are guidelines for the amount of homocysteine-lowering nutrients to supplement depending on the level of homocysteine in your blood after testing. If your level is below six, a high-strength multivitamin should do the trick. If your homocysteine is above six, it is best to supplement a homocysteine formula – shown as number of tablets, spread throughout the day – to lower your level to below six. If you're supplementing these nutrients separately, you can also do that using the guide below.

NUTRIENT	GOOD	LOW	HIGH	VERY HIGH
	<6	6–9	9–15	Above 15
Homocysteine formula	–	2	4	6 per day
Folate	200µg	400µg	1,200µg	2,000µg
B12	10µg	500µg	100µg	1,500µg
B6	25mg	50mg	75mg	100mg
B2	10mg	15mg	20mg	50mg
Zinc	5mg	10mg	15mg	20mg
TMG	500mg	750mg	1–1.5g	3–6g

Heart of the matter – omega-3s

Omega-3 fish oils are a must for anyone with cardiovascular risk. A 2004 review of ten randomised controlled trials showed that fish oils decrease the blood fats known as triglycerides by an average of 29 per cent, lower cholesterol by 12 per cent, lower the bad LDL cholesterol by 32 per cent and increase HDL by ten per cent.[356] They also offer anti-inflammatory benefits.[357] Basically, they work a lot better than statins and have a range of other beneficial effects.

The strongest evidence for the effectiveness of omega-3s lies in their ability to reduce the risk of a heart attack if you've already had one. Eating only one serving of oily fish a week cuts your likelihood of having another heart attack by a third. As a study published in 1999 showed, supplementing omega-3 fish oils also cuts your risk of dying from cardiovascular disease by 21 per cent.[358] In the *British Medical Journal* in 2004, a review of the many studies that consistently show benefit from omega-3 rich fish oils concludes: 'Omega-3 fatty acids from fish and fish oils can protect against coronary heart disease. There is evidence to support the use of fish or fish oil supplements after myocardial infarction.'[359]

A Japanese study from 2005 gave over 9,000 people the omega-3 EPA (1.8g a day) with statins and compared that with 9,000 people receiving only statins. After four and a half years, those taking the fish oils had 19 per cent less incidence of cardiac death, heart attacks or other serious cardiovascular problems.[360]

As we've seen, fish oils also help to thin the blood, so if you're already on blood-thinning medication you should consult your doctor before taking them so that he or she can closely monitor your international normalised ratio or INR – that is, how well your blood coagulates.[361] (See page 290 for a fuller discussion of this issue.)

However, it's not all plain sailing for omega-3s vis-à-vis heart health. A review in the *British Medical Journal* published in 2006 looked at 12 studies (nine showing a benefit, one no effect and two a very small negative effect), and didn't find a clear reduction in mortality.[362] So don't put all your fish in one basket.

As we've seen, fish oils contain two kinds of omega-3s – EPA and DHA. It's the EPA particularly that seems to reduce risk of both heart attacks and strokes. A serving of oily fish, such as a piece of organic salmon, can provide around 3g of omega-3 fats. Of this perhaps a quarter, 800mg, is EPA. You should aim for around 400mg of EPA a day, minimum. That's either two high-potency omega-3 fish oil capsules a day, or half a serving of an omega-3 rich fish such as sardines, herring or mackerel. Having three servings of fish a week and an omega-3 fish oil capsule providing around 200mg of EPA a day is a good place to start. If you already have cardiovascular disease, you might want to double this.

Heart-healthy herbs and spices

Garlic

This mainstay of world cuisines reduces blood platelet 'stickiness' – their ability to cohere – and promotes healthy blood pressure, cholesterol and triglyceride levels. Even one clove of garlic a day can reduce a high cholesterol score by nine per cent, according to a review of numerous studies made by Stephen Warshafsky at the New York Medical School in 1993.[363] A report from the Royal College of Physicians in London, published the following year, confirmed these findings, showing an average cholesterol reduction of 12 per cent from garlic supplements.[364]

Garlic is especially powerful in combination with omega-3 fats. One trial from 1997 reported that the combination of a garlic concentrate (900mg a day) and fish oil resulted in a substantial reduction in cholesterol, LDL cholesterol and blood-fat levels.[365] Like the statin drug Crestor, garlic has been shown to reduce the plaques that clog up our arteries. (The only difference was that Crestor got front-page headlines in almost every national newspaper – and no one mentioned garlic!)

To enjoy its benefits, you can eat two cloves of garlic a day or simply take two garlic capsules.

Turmeric

The curcumin in the yellow spice turmeric is a powerful antioxidant, and as a 2005 study shows it reduces platelet stickiness and relaxes arteries.[366] Another study from the same year showed that combined with garlic, it's even more potent.[367] Either supplement 400 to 600mg curcumin twice daily or use this spice liberally when cooking (it's great with curries and couscous salads, with spicy fish or chicken dishes, or mixed with olive oil and drizzled over vegetables). Ginger also has a similar effect.[368]

Ginkgo biloba

This extract from the ginkgo tree has been shown in a 2005 study to inhibit platelets in the blood from sticking to each other.[369] It's certainly a useful addition to a cardiovascular disease prevention strategy.[370] We recommend taking 20 to 40mg of a standardised extract a day.

SIDE EFFECTS Some people experience mild gastrointestinal problems or occasional, mild headache when taking ginkgo. If you are on warfarin, the addition of gingko may further decrease blood clotting, so you may need to lower the dose of the drug.[371] However, you must consult your doctor about combining these two, or taking aspirin, since they will need to more closely monitor your blood's ability to clot by testing.

A note on natural blood-thinners

As we've mentioned, a number of supplements that are highly beneficial for the heart also thin the blood. Garlic, gingko and fish oil are generally not recommended if you're taking blood-thinning drugs: there have been some isolated reports of bleeding on gingko and long-term aspirin therapy. It is also wise to limit your intake of vitamin E if you're on one of these drugs.

However, it has to be said that you can't have it both ways. If these nutrients do substantially thin the blood, and they do, they are obviously preferable to blood-thinning drugs. So, perhaps the caution should read: 'Do not take warfarin or aspirin if you are supplementing large or combined amounts of omega-3 fish oils, vitamin E, gingko biloba and garlic.' But since the effect of these nutrients is less immediate and less quantified, they shouldn't be used in the short term after a medical crisis. They could be used to reduce the need for anti-coagulant drugs once your condition and your INR (see page 290) are stable – although if you are on warfarin, you should stick to food sources of these nutrients, not concentrated daily supplements.

It is vital to discuss all this with your doctor to ensure they monitor your INR as you increase the nutrients, so that they can reduce the drugs accordingly.

Take heart – shifting diet and lifestyle

On top of the risk reductions you can expect from the recommendations above, improving your diet can also dramatically lower your risk of dying from, or ever having, cardiovascular disease.

For example, limiting your consumption of saturated fat, red meat and alcohol can reduce your risk by 50 per cent, while reducing your sodium intake can lower your risk by 25 per cent. Conversely, increasing your intake of fresh fruits and vegetables can cut your risk of heart disease by 30 per cent. Along the same lines, increasing your level of aerobic activity and decreasing your stress levels can both cut your risk for cardiovascular disease in half. But the big risk reduction involves cigarettes. Simply quitting smoking reduces your risk by an astounding 70 per cent!

> Feona and Andrew, whose cases we've already encountered, and Mike, all went on a low-GL diet, ate more fruit, vegetables, fish and garlic, cut back on alcohol, started exercising more often and took supplements. Feona took magnesium plus B vitamins and Mike took B vitamins, magnesium and omega-3 fish oils. They both increased their intake of plant sterols. Andrew also took 'no-flush' niacin at 1,000mg a day.
>
> Feona's cholesterol level dropped from 8.5 to 4.4 mmol/l over two years. Mike's dropped from 6.5 to 5.1 in five weeks. Andrew's dropped from 8.7 to 4.9 in three weeks. They all feel fantastic as a result.

Food or drugs? The verdict

The combined strategy of changing your diet, improving your lifestyle, and taking the right supplements is likely to be far more effective than taking prescribed drugs for both preventing and reversing cardiovascular disease, without the side effects. If you are on medication and take these steps to reduce your risk, and thereby achieve normalisation of the biochemical markers for cardiovascular disease, there should be no need to continue taking cardiovascular medication.

However, do not, and we repeat, DO NOT, change any prescribed medication without first consulting your doctor.

What works

- Exercise every day, stop smoking and lose weight if you need to.

- Eat plenty of soya (as tofu or soya milk, for instance), almonds, seeds, oats and beans and loads of vegetables to get plenty of the cholesterol busters plant sterols and fibre, as well as folic acid and magnesium.

Also use turmeric and ginger liberally in your cooking and have at least one, if not two, cloves of garlic every day – or a garlic capsule. Avoid sugar, deep-fried foods and salt, except for Solo sea salt. Cut back on meat, cheese and other high-fat foods and avoid alcohol in excess.

- For omega-3 fats, think fish. Have three servings a week of oily fish such as mackerel, wild or organic salmon, herrings or sardines, and a daily omega-3 fish oil capsule providing around 200mg of EPA a day, or double this if you have cardiovascular disease. This is the equivalent of 1,000mg of omega-3 fish oil twice a day, depending on the potency of the supplement.

- Get your B vitamins to lower homocysteine. To know how much you need to take, check your homocysteine level (either ask your doctor or go for a home-test kit – see page 406 of Resources) and supplement accordingly. In any event, make sure you are supplementing 50mg of B6, 400mcg of folic acid and 250mcg of B12 (if you are over 50), as well as eating plenty of greens and beans. Have 1,000mg of 'no-flush' niacin (B3) if your cholesterol level or LDL level is high, or HDL level is low.

- To ensure your diet is antioxidant-rich, eat lots of fruit and vegetables, fish and seeds and also supplement 200mg of vitamin E (400mg if you have cardiovascular risk and are not on a statin), together with 30 to 60mg of CoQ10 (double this if you have cardiovascular disease or are taking a statin) and 2g of vitamin C (double this if you have cardiovascular disease). Don't take individual antioxidant nutrients on their own. They are team players. Consider also supplementing 20 to 40mg of gingko biloba and 400 to 600mg of turmeric extract.

- In addition to eating plenty of vegetables, nuts and seeds, especially pumpkin seeds, supplement 150mg of magnesium every day and double this if you have cardiovascular disease.

In practical terms, a supplement programme to prevent or reverse cardiovascular disease might look like this:

	For prevention	For treatment
High-strength multivitamin	2	2
Vitamin E 200mg	1	
Vitamin C 1,000mg	2	2
Omega-3 fish oil	1	2
CoQ10 30mg	1–2	2–4
Homocysteine-lowering B vitamins	1	3
		(if homocysteine is high)
Ginkgo biloba 20mg	1	2

Working with your doctor

Obviously, if you've had a heart attack or have very high blood pressure, we're not suggesting you throw your drugs away. Let your doctor know you want to pursue nutritional and lifestyle changes to minimise your need for medication. It's a good idea to establish the goal that would make it no longer necessary for you to have medication, for example, a cholesterol measure below five, or blood pressure below 130/85. As you start to incorporate the nutritional changes we recommend into your life, you can monitor the effect.

If you're on blood-thinning drugs such as aspirin or warfarin, speak to your doctor before taking concentrated supplements of omega-3 fish oils, gingko biloba or vitamin E above 300mg since they may want to monitor your INR and platelet adhesion index and consider reducing the drug accordingly. (See also page 307.)

As your vital heart statistics improve, your doctor will want to reduce your medication accordingly. You can always consult a nutritional therapist to help devise a plan of action for you.

Supplements for preventing and reversing cardiovascular disease

These are the ideal levels of nutrients to supplement to reduce your cardiovascular risk.

Nutrient	Daily dosage
Vitamin C	2,000mg
Vitamin E	200mg
Niacin	1,000mg
Magnesium	300mg
Vitamin B6	50mg
Vitamin B12	500mcg
Folic Acid	1,000mg
TMG	1,000mg
Garlic	2 cloves or 2 capsules
Ginkgo biloba	20–40mg
Curcumin	400–600mg
CoQ10	Prevention: 30–60mg
	Treatment: 90–120mg
Omega-3 fatty acids	2,000mg (giving 400mg EPA)

16.

Solving Attention and Learning Problems
Ritalin vs making kids smarter

SOME CHILDREN JUST can't seem to sit still. With a short attention span and volatile moods, they get into fights and disrupt the class at school. These are classic signs of a syndrome known as ADHD, or attention deficit hyperactivity disorder, diagnoses of which are very much on the rise. Children with the condition have a hard time at school and at home, performing badly and repeatedly getting into trouble. They're often shunted from school to school.

Now affecting an estimated one in ten boys and one in 30 girls in the UK and, according to a recent estimate in *The Lancet*, as many as eight to ten per cent of children worldwide,[372] ADHD is often blamed on poor parenting or schooling. But there is a variety of other possible causes: heredity, smoking, alcohol or drug use during pregnancy, oxygen deprivation at birth, prenatal trauma, environmental pollution, allergy and inadequate nutrition.

The symptoms of ADHD usually begin early, by the age of three or four, and can persist into adulthood for around half of sufferers. In our experience, children and adults with ADHD often have one or more nutritional imbalances that, once identified and corrected, can dramatically improve their energy, focus, concentration and behaviour.

Does your child have ADHD?

It can be difficult to draw the line between normal high spirits and abnormally active behaviour. Check yourself or your child out on the questionnaire below. There are three parts to the diagnosis.

Attention Deficit

At least five of the following symptoms must have persisted for at least six months to an extent that is unusual for your child's age and level of intelligence.

- [ ] Fails to pay close attention to detail or makes careless errors during work or play

- [ ] Fails to finish tasks or sustain attention in play activities

- [ ] Seems not to listen to what is said to him or her

- [ ] Fails to follow through instructions or to finish homework or chores (not because of confrontational behaviour or failure to understand instructions)

- [ ] Disorganised about tasks and activities

- [ ] Avoids tasks like homework that require sustained mental effort

- [ ] Loses things necessary for certain tasks or activities, such as pencils, books or toys

- [ ] Easily distracted

- [ ] Forgetful in the course of daily activities.

Hyperactivity

Your child must have exhibited at least three of the following symptoms for at least six months to an extent that is unusual for their age and level of intelligence.

☐ Runs around or climbs over a lot of things. (In adolescents or adults only feelings of restlessness may occur)

☐ Unduly noisy in playing, or has difficulty in engaging in quiet leisure activities

☐ Leaves seat in classroom or in other situations where remaining seated is expected

☐ Fidgets with hands or feet or squirms on seat.

Impulsivity

At least one of the following symptoms must have persisted for at least six months to an extent that is unusual for your child's age and level of intelligence.

☐ Blurts out answers before the questions have been completed

☐ Fails to wait in lines or await turns in games or group situations

☐ Interrupts or intrudes on others, such as butting into other children's conversations or games

☐ Talks excessively without appropriate response to social restraint.

If your child has these symptoms, both at home and at school; if they are getting in the way of their normal development; and if there's no other explanation – such as stresses or psychological issues – then they should be checked for potential ADHD.

But here's an important caveat. In truth, every child is different and there's no clear evidence that ADHD even is a single condition. It may be a blanket term for an increasingly common set of symptoms. Some children have problems with words (dyslexia), some children are physically poorly co-ordinated (dyspraxia), some can't sit still (hyperactive and impulsive), and some can't concentrate (attention deficit).

The rise of Ritalin and other ADHD drugs

Sadly, many hyperactive children are not tested for nutritional imbalances or food or chemical sensitivity. Nor are they treated nutritionally or given counselling or family therapy. Instead, they're more likely to be put on stimulant drugs such as Ritalin (methylphenidate), which acts like an amphetamine. They might also get a slow-acting form of Ritalin, called Concerta, or a variation on that theme called dextroamphetamine, which is marketed as Adderall or Dexedrine.

You might wonder how an amphetamine could calm a hyperactive child down. One theory is that these children don't have enough of the neurotransmitter dopamine in the part of the brain that is supposed to filter out unimportant stimuli. The theory is that the drug inhibits the breakdown of dopamine, giving them a short-term ability to focus, which is why it is usually given on the way to school.

The number of children with hyperactivity and/or ADHD continues to rise and might affect as many half a million children (one in 20), in the UK, according the National Institute for Health and Clinical Excellence (NICE) – although some research from 2003, based on surveys, suggests it affects one in 40.[373] The actual incidence of diagnosed ADHD is much lower, around one in 200, as many children with hyperactivity and/or ADHD are not diagnosed. Prescriptions of Ritalin, however, have risen 180-fold – from 2,000 in 1991 to 259,000 in 2004. The drug is currently given to seven million schoolchildren in the US, nearly one in five.[374]

This is all good news for drug-company sales. The bill for this class of drug now stands at over $3 billion per year in the US. In 2004 in Britain the number of prescriptions for methylphenidate (Ritalin and Concerta) atomoxetine and dexamfetamine had almost doubled to 418,300, costing almost £13 million.[375]

The lowdown on Ritalin

While there is no question that some children and adults regain control on drugs such as Ritalin, there is little evidence that they are particularly effective for most. In September 2005 a massive review of 2,287 studies on ADHD drugs was published by the Oregon Evidence-based Practice

Center at the Oregon Health and Science University in the US. It concluded that although 27 different drugs are prescribed for ADHD, 'the evidence is not compelling that the drugs improve the thinking or quality of life of adults or help with adult anxiety or depression'.

Children often take these drugs for a long time but, the report said, there was 'no evidence on long-term safety … in young children or adolescents'. Finally, it found that the available evidence was of little use to clinicians trying to decide which of the 27 drugs might be useful for particular patients because very few comparisons between the drugs had been done as to how they affected academic performance, quality of life or social skills.[376]

Shocking as this might be, it should have come as no surprise to the experts; five years earlier, a study by the Agency for Healthcare Research and Quality, part of the US Department of Health and Human Services, found that studies of ADHD drugs were of such poor quality that they could find 'no evidence to support the claims made about [them]'. And as far back as 1998, the US National Institutes of Health concluded that there was no evidence of any long-term improvement in scholastic performance on Ritalin.[377]

ADHD or bipolar disorder?

For some children, the effect of these drugs can be devastating. It is now known that some children diagnosed with ADHD actually have bipolar disorder or manic depression, causing them to switch from states of mania and hyperactivity to crying spells and depression. Something in the order of one in seven children with mood problems fits the diagnosis of bipolar disorder.[378] Drs Janet Wozniak and Joseph Biederman from Harvard Medical School found that 94 per cent of children with mania as a symptom met the criteria for a diagnosis of bipolar disorder.[379] The trouble is that bipolar disorder is almost never diagnosed in children.

This is bad news, because the last thing a bipolar child needs is stimulant drugs such as Ritalin. Dr Demitri Papalos, associate professor of psychiatry at Albert Einstein College of Medicine in New York City, studied the effects of stimulant drugs on 73 children diagnosed as bipolar and found that 47 of these children were thrown into states of mania or psychosis by stimulant medication.[380] His excellent book, *The Bipolar*

Child, co-authored with his wife Janice Papalos, helps to differentiate between those suffering from bipolar disorder and ADHD. These are the differences they've observed:

- Children with bipolar disorder essentially have a mood disorder and go from extreme highs of mania, tantrums and anger into extreme lows. Some may go through four cycles in the year, while for others these cycles can happen in a week. This rapid cycling is rarely seen in adults.

- Bipolar children also have different kinds of angry outbursts. While most children will calm down in 20 to 30 minutes, bipolar children can rage on for hours, often with destructive, even sadistic, aggressiveness. They can also display disorganised thinking, language and body positions during an angry outburst.

- Bipolar children have bouts of depression, which is not a usual pattern of ADHD. They frequently show giftedness, perhaps in verbal or artistic skills, often early in life. Their misbehaviour is often more intentional, while the classic ADHD child often misbehaves through their own inattention. A bipolar child can, for example, be the bully in the playground.

Ritalin: a catalogue of side-effects

Given that Ritalin is a drug prescribed extensively for children, the official range of possible harmful side effects listed by the US Food and Drug Administration (FDA) is very alarming. It includes increased blood pressure, heart rate, respiration and temperature; appetite suppression, stomach pains, weight loss, growth retardation, facial tics, muscle twitching, insomnia, euphoria, nervousness, irritability, agitation, psychotic episodes, violent behaviour, paranoid delusions, hallucinations, bizarre behaviours, heart arrhythmias and palpitations, tolerance and dependence, psychological dependence – even death. Some of these symptoms do not go away when the child stops taking the drug.

Ritalin can cause addiction in much the same way as cocaine, by promoting levels of dopamine. Using brain-imaging techniques, Dr Nora Volkow of the Brookhaven National Laboratory in Upton, New York, has shown that Ritalin occupies more of the brain cells responsible for the high experienced by addicts than smoked or injected cocaine. The only reason Ritalin has not produced an army of addicted schoolchildren, she concludes, is that it takes about an hour for Ritalin in pill form to raise dopamine levels in the brain, while smoked or injected cocaine does this in seconds.[381] There are now growing reports of teenagers and others abusing Ritalin by snorting or injecting it to get a faster rush.

Dr Joan Baizer, Professor of Physiology and Biophysics at the University of Buffalo in New York state, has shown how Ritalin, long considered to have only short-term effects, can initiate changes in the brain structure and function of rats that remain long after the therapeutic effects have dissipated.[382] This in turn could lead to a greater susceptibility to drug dependence in later life.

A growing incidence of reports of heart attacks, strokes and hypertension in both adults and children who have taken ADHD medications, including 25 deaths, has prompted the FDA to issue a 'black-box warning' on all ADHD stimulant medication.[383] 'The issue of drug treatment of attention deficit disorder in children has been a controversial one without this issue of cardiovascular risk too,' said Arthur Levin, the consumer representative for the FDA's Drug Safety and Risk Management Advisory Committee. 'It adds another concern.' The few previous long-term studies of ADHD medications had not examined the potential for cardiovascular risks of the treatments.

Yet more drugs

Ritalin-type drugs aren't the only ones given to children diagnosed with ADHD. They have also been treated with SSRIs – which as we've already seen are now not recommended for children because of an increased suicide risk. So a new range has been developed known as NARIs (standing for noradrenalin reuptake inhibitors), which target another neurotransmitter in the brain – noradrenalin.

Already, however, problems with NARIs are emerging. In 2005 the FDA advised doctors to be cautious about prescribing one called Strattera (atomexetine) – which has already been given to 2.5 million American children with ADHD – because of evidence that it also increased risk of suicidal thoughts.[384] The agency advised that those taking it 'should be closely monitored for clinical worsening, as well as agitation, irritability, suicidal thinking or behaviours, and unusual changes in behaviour, especially during the initial few months of therapy or when the dose is changed'.

There is also a growing trend to prescribe more than one drug to children diagnosed with behavioural problems. No one really has any idea of what the effect might be. 'It's not uncommon to find a child on an anti-depressant, a mood stabilizer, and a sleep agent all at the same time, but there's no research to see how these drugs interact with each other,' says Dr Joseph Penn, a child psychiatrist with the Bradley Hasbro Children's Research Center in Rhode Island in the US. In a ten-year study looking at prescribing practice, Penn and his colleagues conclude that there are almost no studies or published research that justify prescribing multiple medications for psychiatric disorders in children.[385]

The natural alternative

Here, again, is the central irony. Tens of thousands of our children are being prescribed drugs that have been shown, via good scientific evidence, not to work very well and even to be fairly dangerous. It does seem extraordinary that compared with the hundreds of millions of dollars spent developing and marketing these products, a mere pittance is available to investigate non-drug approaches.

Although it is unlikely that ADHD is purely a nutrient-deficiency disease, most children with this diagnosis are deficient and do respond very well to nutritional supplements. The combination of the right vitamins, minerals and essential fats can truly transform children with learning and behavioural difficulties. Adrian is a case in point.

> When Adrian was three years old, his parents brought him to the Brain Bio Centre in London because they were concerned about his loss of speech development. They had already put him on a diet free of dairy and gluten, and were pleased to see that his eczema had disappeared and his asthma had improved dramatically. Tests showed he was very low in magnesium, selenium and zinc and also in essential fats. He was given supplements of

fish oils and a multivitamin and mineral. Within days, Adrian started talking again and is now developing normally.

There are four nutritional solutions that have been well proven to make a difference to learning, behaviour and concentration. These are:

- Sugar-free and low-GL diets (see Chapter 8, page 143)

- Essential fats, especially omega-3s

- Vitamins and minerals

- Allergy- and additive-free diets.

Let's examine the evidence.

Cut out sugar

If you feed your child rocket fuel – that is, a diet high in sugar and caffeine – don't be surprised if their behaviour is out of control. Sugar, stimulants and refined carbohydrates aren't good for anyone. Even so-called 'normal' children can become uncontrollable after a sugarfest.

Glucose is the main fuel for the brain as well as the body, and refined sugars are swiftly converted to glucose. If your child's regular diet is full of refined carbohydrates, such as biscuits and white bread, stimulants, sweets, chocolate, fizzy drinks, juices and little or no fibre, every meal or snack will send their blood-glucose levels soaring, only to crash soon after until the next 'fix'. The result? Their blood glucose will be on a permanent rollercoaster ride – shooting up and dipping down.

So it's not surprising that levels of activity, concentration, focus and behaviour will also fluctuate wildly, which is exactly what is seen in children with ADHD. The usual calming effect sometimes observed after sugar consumption may well be the initial normalisation of blood-sugar levels from a blood-sugar low, which has been causing feelings of tiredness and an inability to concentrate.

And it seems that the research bears this out. Dietary studies do consistently reveal that hyperactive children eat more sugar than other children,[386] and reducing dietary sugar has been found to halve disciplinary actions in young offenders, as we'll see in more detail on page 371.[387] Other research has confirmed that the problem is not just sugar. If a child is eating a poor diet anyway, is getting lots of pure refined sugar as well and, on top of that, has a metabolism that can't handle glucose well, they are likely to experience many of the symptoms of ADHD. A study of 265 hyperactive children found that more than three-quarters displayed abnormal glucose tolerance,[388] meaning that their bodies were less able to handle sugar intake and maintain balanced blood sugar levels.

Ensure essential fats

We've already seen the remarkable range of health benefits essential fats, and omega-3s in particular, have to offer. They also clearly have a calming effect on many children with hyperactivity and ADHD, as we'll see in a moment. It's notable in this context that children diagnosed with ADHD also often have symptoms of essential fatty acid deficiency, such as excessive thirst, dry skin, eczema and asthma.

Omega-3 deficiency may be a reason why four out of five ADHD sufferers are boys – males have a much higher essential fat requirement than females. They may not absorb them as well, or convert them as easily into the specialised forms of omega-3 fats, called EPA and DHA, that help the brain communicate. According to a study from 1981, they may also be less efficient at converting DHA into prostaglandins, which are also important for brain function.[389]

So it is particularly interesting that the vital process of turning essential fats into forms that can by used by the brain can be blocked by precisely those foods that cause ADHD-type behaviour in some children – wheat and dairy (see 'Just an allergy', p. 324). The task of converting the fats is performed by certain enzymes, and for them to do their job properly they need a good supply of certain vitamins and minerals, including vitamin B3 (niacin), B6, C, biotin, zinc and magnesium. Zinc deficiency is common in ADHD sufferers.

In 1995, researchers at Purdue University in Indiana, in the US, showed that children with ADHD didn't get enough of these vitamins and minerals from their diet to allow the enzymes in question to work effectively. As a result, they had lower levels of essential fats – the omega-3s EPA and DHA, and the omega-6 arachidonic acid – than children without ADHD.[390] But this wasn't proof that giving these fats to children would actually make a difference.

Now, thanks to the ground-breaking research of pioneer researchers such as Dr Alex Richardson and colleagues from the University Lab of Physiology and Mansfield College, Oxford and Madeleine Portwood from Durham, we have proof based on a series of double-blind trials of the benefit from supplying extra essential fats to children with learning and behaviour problems.

One such trial, published in 2002, involved 41 children aged eight to 12 years who had ADHD symptoms and specific learning difficulties. Those who got essential fat supplements were both behaving and learning better within 12 weeks.[391] In a controlled trial from 2005, at a school in Durham, 117 children with learning, behaviour and psychosocial difficulties got either a supplement of omega-3 and omega-6 or a placebo for three months. Those in the group given the omegas more than doubled their gain in reading age, and more than tripled their gain in spelling age over the three month study, compared to those children getting the placebo.[392]

IQ-boosting vitamins and minerals

We know that academic performance improves and behavioural problems diminish significantly when children are given nutritional supplements. To date, 12 double-blind studies on vitamins and IQ have been carried out, and ten out of 12 show a clear improvement.[393] Of the other two, one was too short (lasting only a month) and the other did show a trend towards improvement.

While improving mental performance is not quite the same thing as reducing the symptoms of ADHD, one study at the University of Reading investigated why supplements boosted children's IQs. It found that children were able to work faster and concentrate for longer and so were able to answer more questions.[394] These are all improvements that you would expect to help children with ADHD.

The two minerals these children are most commonly deficient in are zinc, as we've mentioned, and magnesium. And what are the classic symptoms of magnesium deficiency? Excessive fidgeting, anxious rest-lessness, insomnia, co-ordination problems and learning difficulties, despite having a normal IQ. Sound familiar?

A Polish study from 1997 that examined the magnesium status of 116 children with ADHD found that magnesium deficiency occurred far more frequently in them than in healthy children (95 per cent of children with ADHD were deficient), and they also noted a correlation between levels of magnesium in the body and the severity of symptoms. Supplementation of 200mg of magnesium for six months improved their magnesium status and significantly reduced their hyperactivity, which worsened in the control group who did not receive magnesium supplementation.[395]

A classic example of how effective magnesium can be in helping restless, hyperactive children is the story of Andrew W. When he was three years old, his sleep-deprived parents brought him to the Brain Bio Centre in London. Andrew was hyperactive and seemed never to sleep. Not surprisingly, he was pretty grumpy most of the time. We recommended that his parents give him 65mg of magnesium daily in a pleasant-tasting powder added to a drink before bed. Two weeks later, Andrew's mum phoned to say that he was sleeping right through every night and had been transformed into a delightful child during the day too.

A similar story can be told for zinc. A trial from 2005 involving 209 children aged ten to 11 in North Dakota in the US found remarkable improvement in mental performance after supplementing with zinc.[396] The children first performed a series of tests that measured attention, memory, problem-solving and hand-to-eye co-ordination. Then they were given a supplement of either 10mg (the RDA) or 20mg of zinc, or a placebo, for three months. Those who got 20mg, compared to the placebo, showed dramatic improvements – three times faster on word recognition and six times the score on attention and vigilance. Those getting the RDA amount of zinc showed no significant improvement.

You don't have to give supplements to children to improve the way they behave, however. Changing diet alone can have a powerful effect. That has been extensively investigated by Dr Stephen Schoenthaler of the Department of Social and Criminal Justice at California State University.

In Schoenthaler's many placebo-controlled studies involving over a thousand long-term young offenders, he has found that improving their diets improved their behaviour by between 40 and 60 per cent. Blood tests for vitamins and minerals showed that around a third of the young people involved had low levels of one or more vitamins and minerals before the trial, and those whose levels had become normal by the end of the study demonstrated a massive improvement in behaviour of between 70 and 90 per cent.[397]

Just an allergy?

But even though a change of diet and supplements can make a big difference, the effect isn't as great as what can be achieved by identifying food sensitivities in the child diagnosed with ADHD, and cutting out whatever is causing the problem.

In one study, ADHD children turned out to be seven times more likely to have food allergies than other children. Dr Joseph Bellanti of Georgetown University in Washington DC found that 56 per cent of hyperactive children aged seven to ten tested positive for food allergies, compared to less than eight per cent of 'normal' children.[398] So what was most likely to cause problems?

A separate investigation in 2001 by the Hyperactive Children's Support Group in the UK found that 89 per cent of ADHD children reacted to food colourings, 72 per cent to flavourings, 60 per cent to MSG, 45 per cent to all synthetic additives, 50 per cent to cow's milk, 60 per cent to chocolate and 40 per cent to oranges.[399]

Other substances often found to induce behavioural changes in children are wheat, dairy, corn, yeast, soya, citrus, peanuts and eggs.[400] Associated symptoms that are strongly linked to allergy include nasal problems and excessive mucus, ear infections, facial swelling and discoloration around the eyes, tonsillitis, digestive problems, bad breath, eczema, asthma, headaches and bedwetting. So if a child has several of these allergic symptoms and ADHD-type behaviour, it is more likely that allergy has been a cause of the behaviour.

A PIECE OF THE PUZZLE – ANTIBIOTICS

In most cases, the reason children lack certain nutrients is because of their diet. But there could be another reason – the overuse of antibiotics. In a 1997 study of 530 hyperactive children versus children without ADHD, Dr Neil Ward of the University of Surrey found that a significantly higher percentage of those with ADHD had taken several courses of antibiotics in early childhood compared to those children who had not.[401] Further investigations in 2001 revealed that those who had had three or more antibiotic courses before the age of three had significantly lower levels of zinc, calcium, chromium and selenium.[402] Antibiotics kill off the beneficial bacteria in the gut, which are involved in extracting minerals from food.

There's also a link between antibiotics and allergies. For example, children given antibiotics for ear infections often have an underlying allergy which is causing excessive mucus, which then blocks the Eustachian tube from the nose to the ear, leading to an infection. The antibiotics then irritate the gut, making the child more susceptible to allergies, triggering more mucus and another infection. It's a vicious cycle.

Up to 90 per cent of hyperactive children benefit from eliminating foods that contain artificial colours, flavours and preservatives, processed and manufactured foods, and 'culprit' foods identified by either an exclusion diet or blood test.[403] Child psychiatrist Professor Eric Taylor from the London-based Institute of Child Health was sceptical of the reports from parents that their children responded to chemical-free diets designed to eliminate their allergens, so in the early 1990s he and his colleagues designed a study to rigorously test this proposition.

They placed 78 hyperactive children on a 'few foods' diet, eliminating both chemical additives and common food allergens. During this open trial, the behaviour of 59 of the children (76 per cent) improved. The researchers then secretly reintroduced the foods and additives that had provoked reactions for 19 of the children. The children's behaviour rapidly became worse and so did their performance in psychological testing.[404]

Combining vitamins, minerals, and essential fats while eliminating allergens can be remarkably effective at relieving the symptoms of ADHD. Eight-year-old Richard is a case in point.

> Diagnosed with ADHD, Richard was 'out of control' and his parents were at their wits' end. Richard had also been constipated his entire life. Through biochemical testing at the Brain Bio Centre, they found that he was allergic to dairy products and eggs and was very deficient in magnesium. By looking at his diet they saw that he was eating far too much sugar on a daily basis.
>
> He was given a low-sugar, low-GL diet, free of dairy and eggs, and was also given magnesium and omega-3 supplements. Within three months, his parents reported that Richard had calmed down considerably and had become much more manageable. His constipation had also cleared completely.

And finally . . .

There are a couple of other things that can help some ADHD children. It may be worth testing for excess toxic minerals (with a hair or blood test) to check that they don't have excessive amounts of copper, cadmium, mercury or aluminium in their system, because these can deplete the body of essential nutrients such as zinc and affect behaviour.

The other is to try a stimulating brain nutrient called DMAE (sold as Deanol in the US). The children who might benefit from this are those suffering from what is called 'reward deficiency syndrome',[405] which manifests as a constant need for stimulation. What seems to be happening is that either they don't produce enough of the motivating neurotransmitter dopamine (from which adrenalin and noradrenalin are made), or don't respond strongly enough to their own dopamine.

Ritalin appears to increase dopamine levels, at least in the short term, so for these children, the drug can seem a miracle cure. But in the long term, the concern is whether it causes 'down-regulation' – making a child less sensitive to the increased dopamine – so they need even more stimulation. As was found in a 2001 study, several months off Ritalin seems to undo much of the damage, but does not effect a full regain in sensitivity.[406] This could lead to a child off Ritalin seeking dopamine stimulation from other substances.

Food or drugs? The verdict

There have been far too few direct comparisons of these two approaches – drugs versus nutrients – but in one of them the nutritional approach came out very significantly ahead. The director of the Autism Research Institute in San Diego, Dr Bernard Rimland, collected data on ADHD children's response to a nutritional plan. He looked at 191 ADHD children who had switched their way of eating, then calculated what's called the 'relative efficacy ratio' – the number helped vs the number harmed. If twice as many are helped, the ratio would be two.

Rimland then made the same calculation for children treated with a number of different drugs (see chart below), and found that about as many ADHD sufferers are made worse by medication as are helped. The drug regime was given a ratio of one. In stark contrast, the ratio for the nutritional approach was 18.[407]

VITAMINS VS DRUGS – WHICH WORK BEST?

Medication	Total	No. helped	No. worsened	Relative efficacy ratio
Dexedrine	172	44	80	0.55
Ritalin	66	22	27	0.81
Mysoline	10	4	4	1.00
Valium	106	31	31	1.00
Dilantin	204	57	43	1.33
Benadril	151	34	25	1.36
Stelazine	120	40	28	1.43
Deanol/DMAE	73	17	10	1.70
Mellaril	277	101	55	1.84
All drugs	**1,591**	**440**	**425**	**1.04**
Vitamins/minerals	**191**	**127**	**7**	**18.14**

In fact, the best drug was Mellaril, not Ritalin. However, neither of these drugs was as effective as vitamin B6 and magnesium or the brain nutrient DMAE, which was also twice as effective as Ritalin.

In a more rigorous open trial from 2003, involving 20 children diagnosed with ADHD, ten were treated with Ritalin and ten with a comprehensive combination of dietary supplements for four weeks. Upon completion, the children were given an extensive battery of tests to measure changes in their attention and concentration. On virtually every test, the children on the supplements had made significant improvements compared to those on the drugs.[408]

Given the long list of side effects, not all of which are reversible, it is extraordinary that the drug approach is still more popular than a nutritional approach. While there is much you can do yourself, ADHD is a complex condition requiring supervision and treatment by a qualified practitioner who can devise the correct nutritional strategy for your child.

What works

- Sort out your child's blood-sugar levels. Children with hyperactivity and ADHD seem particularly sensitive to sugar, so remove *all* forms of refined sugar from the diet and any foods that contain it. Replace them with wholefoods and complex carbohydrates (brown rice and other whole grains, oats, lentils, beans, quinoa and vegetables), which should be eaten 'grazing'-style throughout the day. Processed 'juices' should also be avoided because these deliver a large amount of sugar very quickly.

- Further improve their blood-sugar balance by making sure carbohydrates are eaten with protein (half as much protein as carbohydrates at every meal and snack). Two easy examples are eating nuts with fruit, or fish with rice.

- Help your child get enough omega-3s. Children rarely eat enough rich sources of these, so give more oily fish (salmon, sardines, mackerel, wild or organic salmon, or tuna steaks – but this last only every fortnight to once a month because of mercury content) and seeds such as flax, hemp, sunflower and pumpkin or their cold-pressed oils. Most ADHD children will also need supplements of omega-3 and omega-6. They should contain at least 200mg of EPA, plus 100mg of

DHA – the most potent forms of omega-3 – plus 50mg of GLA, the most potent form of omega-6.

- Make sure they have enough minerals and vitamins. Give them a daily multivitamin providing sufficient B vitamins, zinc and magnesium, and keep a filled fruit bowl, raw crudités and the like to hand for snacks, along with substantial portions of veg and fruit at meals.

- Supplement probiotics, such as *Lactobacillus acidophilus* and *Bifidobacteria*, especially following antibiotics to restore the balance of gut flora.

- Get rid of toxic effects. Arrange a food-allergy test and hair-mineral analysis test through a nutritional therapist to determine if food allergies and/or heavy metal toxicity are an issue.

Working with your doctor

As well as working with your doctor, we advise consulting a nutritional therapist with experience of treating hyperactive children. They can assess your child's ideal diet and supplement requirements, as well as testing for food allergy. Your child will need to follow the plan for a minimum of three to six months before either of you see any really substantial results, but their hyperactivity may start to calm and their concentration increase very quickly. As children start to feel better and behave better, the positive feedback they receive from their parents and teachers can encourage them to stick to their nutritional programme over the long term, and that's what matters for their well-being as well as their progress.

In the meantime, keep your doctor, paediatrician or child psychiatrist informed of what you are doing and, as your child improves, discuss decreasing the dose of any stimulant medication with them, with the ultimate aim being to stop.

Part 4

Changing the System

17.

The Medicines Act: Catch-22
How non-drug medicines that work are banned

WHEN PEOPLE BEGIN to realise that there is a safer, better and ultimately cheaper form of medicine than the drug their doctor has prescribed for them, they usually begin asking some serious questions. Why wasn't I told about this? Why didn't my doctor give me this option? Why do doctors only use drugs when they could use the nutrition-based approach as well?

If you are one of these people, you might also be wondering what it would be like to go for an approach that focuses more on treating the underlying causes of your disease. You might also start thinking about what changes might be needed to make such a system widely available.

In this final part of the book we explore what needs to happen to bring about just such a medical revolution, and what you can do to help. But first we need to discover the obstacles to change, and how pharmaceutical medicine gained legal control in the first place. If you're surprised by our use of the word 'legal', you should know that the law as it stands renders effective nutritional medicine illegal, and also makes it hard for people to learn the truth about nutrients.

Creating a medical monopoly

Forty words published in 1968 gave the pharmaceutical industry a near-monopoly on medicine in the UK, in exchange for a yearly payment of millions of pounds. The words may vary elsewhere, but the basic principle has been applied around the world.

Those 40 words are contained in the UK Medicines Act (now called the EU Health Products and Medicines Directive), which drew a line in law between a food and a medicine and at a stroke eliminated nutritional medicine as a serious competitor. The act defines a medicine as either:

'Any substance or combination of substances presented for treating or preventing disease in human beings'

or

'Any substance or combination of substances which may be used in a human being with a view to restoring, correcting or modifying physiological function.'

In its broadest sense this means that water, which clearly 'modifies physiological function' and 'restores' the body's water balance, could be deemed a medicine. So too could any vitamin that 'cures' the many diseases that are caused by nutritional deficiencies. But the act also forbade any manufacturers to claim that any substance cured or could treat disease without having first been granted a medical licence. Even the phrase 'An apple a day keeps the doctor away' is a medical claim about apples, and so is illegal to have on display in a greengrocer's without a licence. Although legislators rarely push the application of the Medicines Act to such extremes, you can see the power and far-reaching consequences of this act.

The Medicines Act and its equivalent in other countries set out the requirements for licensing drugs. It is a costly one involving hundreds of thousands of pounds to produce the required dossiers and cover licence fees to a country's regulatory agency – whether the UK's Medicines Healthcare Products Regulatory Agency (MHRA), the US Food and Drug Administration or the Australian Therapeutic Goods Administration – as well as hundreds of millions, in the case of drugs, for research to show they are effective and safe. Although the process is designed to protect the public, it can, as we've seen with SSRIs and Vioxx, go badly wrong.

For a pharmaceutical company with a man-made patented drug, it's money very well spent. Having a licence means that you can claim to treat or prevent a condition and if it is patented, you alone can market it. Sales of drugs for common disorders can run into the billions, as we've seen.

But for natural products which can't be patented, there is little financial incentive to pay for a licence. Take the case of vitamin C, proven to prevent colds at doses of 1,000mg or more a day. A company could pay for the licence that would allow it to make such a claim, but without a patent it couldn't stop anyone else from selling vitamin C and making the same claim. The first company that tried to go down the licensing route with a nutrient was Scotia, which invested millions of pounds into research on evening primrose oil. But the company underestimated the regulatory hurdles, and was unable to get the licences it needed.

Essentially, it's a case of put up or shut up. You can buy apples, fish or vitamin supplements but no greengrocer, fishmonger or vitamin manufacturer can claim they prevent, treat or cure any disease, even if they do, simply because the licence is prohibitively expensive.

This is a double-bind of the sort brilliantly captured by Joseph Heller in his famous novel, *Catch-22*, about the absurdities of life on an American air base off Italy during the Second World War. The 'catch-22' of the title is a regulation stating that if you were insane you didn't have to fly on bombing missions, but if you requested to be excused from a mission on the grounds of insanity you were clearly sane and were ordered to fly.

Any nutrient that can be shown to be an effective treatment becomes a medicine, so it becomes illegal to sell it without a licence which is too expensive and financially not worth it unless you can patent the product, which you can't do if it's a nutrient. A classic catch-22.

Black hole for natural medicines

This is exactly what happened to an amino acid called S-adenosyl methionine, or SAMe for short. It's in food, it's in your body – in essence, it's a vital, natural substance that helps your brain work. In July 1999 the magazine *Newsweek* reported: 'It's effective against depression. It hasn't been found to cause the side effects associated with prescription anti-depressants . . . and it tends to work more quickly.'[1] Dr Teodoro Bottiglieri, formerly of the UK Institute of Psychiatry but now working in the US, where laws on nutritional medicine are less restrictive, agrees. 'SAMe is one of the most effective, safe nutrients for treating depression,' he says.

In fact, it's so effective that last year, EU officials ruled that it was a medicine! No one can afford to apply for a licence because SAMe is unpatentable – it's a natural substance – and so it has vanished from sale. It has disappeared down the black hole designed to remove potentially threatening natural medicines. That's why we didn't discuss SAMe in the chapter on depression – because you can't get it. It is illegal to sell SAMe in Europe, even though there are over 100 double-blind trials showing that it is a highly effective anti-depressant. Catch-22.

In fact, if a health food shop or vitamin company made a claim about almost any non-drug product mentioned in this book – from omega-3 fats to antioxidants – it could trigger a ban, because it's illegal to make such claims, whether true or not, about products you are selling. SAMe isn't the only non-drug product to fall foul of this double-bind. Recently, during a meeting with the MHRA, we were told that the more evidence they see that glucosamine works for relieving the pain of arthritis, the more likely they are to classify it as a medicine. The Medicines Act is effectively a gagging order on the truth about natural medicines, and a tragedy for medicine and for you.

Of course, the official and worthy purpose of this licensing system is to protect the public from false or misleading claims. More specifically, it is meant to provide it with tried and tested pharmaceutical drugs, as opposed to 'unproven' non-drug medicines. However, as this book has shown, for many foods and nutrients the proof is there. The producers simply lack the resources to gain a permit to say that, while year after year the so-called safe, licensed medicines are killing more people than road-traffic accidents.

So what are the changes that need to be made so that people can be told about unlicensed, unpatentable treatments that have been shown to be effective and safe?

Unravelling Catch-22

One move in the right direction would be to follow a legal change made in the US over a decade ago. In 1994, the American pharmaceutical industry lost its virtual monopoly on medicine with the passing of the Dietary Supplements Health Education Act, known as DSHEA (pronounced 'deshay'). The DSHEA acknowledged that non-drug treatments could be beneficial, and that people had a right to be informed about them. This extract from the introduction to it gives some idea of the intentions behind the act and makes a number of the points we have been making in this book.

Congress finds that:

- the importance of nutrition and the benefits of dietary supplements to health promotion and disease prevention have been documented increasingly in scientific studies . . .

- there is a link between the ingestion of certain nutrients or dietary supplements and the prevention of chronic diseases . . .

- clinical research has shown that several chronic diseases can be prevented simply with a healthful diet . . .

- healthful diets may mitigate the need for expensive medical procedures, such as coronary bypass surgery or angioplasty . . .

- preventive health measures, including education, good nutrition, and appropriate use of safe nutritional supplements will limit the incidence of chronic diseases, and reduce long-term health care expenditures . . .

- there is a growing need for emphasis on the dissemination of information linking nutrition and long-term good health . . .

- consumers should be empowered to make choices about preventive health care programs based on data from scientific studies of health benefits related to particular dietary supplements . . .

- dietary supplements are safe within a broad range of intake, and safety problems with the supplements are relatively rare . . .

- legislative action that protects the right of access of consumers to safe dietary supplements is necessary in order to promote wellness . . .

DSHEA allowed people selling foods and nutritional supplements to say what the vitamins actually do and how they can positively affect the mind or body, without falling foul of the licensing requirements that had been in force before. It made it clear to the American regulatory body, the FDA, that restricting the public's access to safe food-based medicines was not in the public's interest.

However, it has proved to be no legislative panacea. The pharmaceutical industry still retains a stranglehold on doctors – as described in Part 1 – and attempts are constantly being made to water the DSHEA down or even repeal it. Even under its protection, manufacturers still have to fight tooth and nail to be able to say anything that sounds as if it is suggesting that food could be medicine.

For instance, one of these foods is tomatoes, which contain the antioxidant lycopene. Research has shown that lycopene can reduce the risk of prostate cancer. The FDA has put out a statement saying that 'very limited and preliminary research' indicates that eating between half a cup and a full cup of tomatoes or tomato sauce (the equivalent of three or four tomatoes) a week could reduce the risk of prostate cancer.

The FDA has ruled that companies selling lycopene supplements are not, however, allowed to claim that they are good for reducing the risk of prostate cancer. But one of these companies – American Longevity – is suing the FDA on the grounds that its ruling against lycopene 'greatly misleads the American consumer', and claims that its First Amendment right to commercial free speech has been violated.

So it can still be difficult to tell the truth about foods or nutrients in the US, but it is certainly easier than it is in Europe. In Australia the law is also highly restrictive and until recently, France and Germany forbade the sale of vitamins much above RDA levels. The UK's Food Standards Agency (FSA) still recites the mantra that 'you can get all the nutrients you need if you eat a well-balanced diet', despite a growing mountain of research, some funded by the agency itself, showing that this simply isn't true.

For instance, one study showed that among older people, the amount of vitamin B12 needed to correct mild deficiency, which is very common in people over the age of 60, is above 640mcg – that's more than 500 times the RDA.[2] Another found that the folic acid contained in supplements was twice as effective at improving blood levels and lowering dangerous levels of the amino acid homocysteine as that contained in vegetables such as broccoli.[3] Largely focused on safety, the FSA also has yet to address the point, accepted a decade ago by DSHEA, that it may well be far less safe *not* to supplement vitamins and minerals.

What's clearly emerging from all this is an attitude, common among regulators and in the medical profession, that supplements are best treated as if they were drugs. This stance is very obvious during the occasional highly publicised scares about the safety of vitamins. Every now and then a piece of research is published suggesting either that taking a particular vitamin or mineral is ineffective, or that it is positively dangerous. These claims are invariably given wide media coverage and people are left with the impression – to give two recent examples – that beta-carotene gives you cancer, or that vitamin E is not effective in reducing the risk of heart attacks. (These are covered in detail in the next chapter.)

Even though from any rational perspective it is clear that the scale of the dangers posed by pharmaceutical drugs is several orders of magnitudes greater than any possible harm from supplements, these scares contribute to the notion that supplements are potentially dangerous and so need to be hedged about with restrictive legislation. No one is suggesting that supplements should be free of any kind of control – anything, even salt and water, can be harmful if handled in a foolish way. But there needs to be a sense of proportion and any controls need to be based on reliable science.

That is a huge concern, given the prevailing mindset of some researchers. What is particularly worrying about the supplement scares, discussed in the next chapter, is how unscientific the negative research is – either actively distorted or based on a lack of understanding of how vitamins and nutrition work. It is this that needs to be changed, and in the rest of this part we will outline what a more rational medical system might look like and how you could contribute to creating it.

18.

The Bad Science behind Attacks on Vitamins
Why vitamins are a health essential

'TAKING MULTIVITAMINS COULD be a waste of time and money'
(*Daily Mail*, 19 May 2006)
'Too much vitamin C can bring on pre-eclampsia, women told'
(*The Times*, 30 March 2006)
'High dose vitamin E death warning' (*BBC News*, November 2004)
'Vitamin pills could cause early deaths' (*Daily Mail*, October 2004)
'Over-use of vitamins may lead to cancer' (*Financial Times*, May 2003)

These are a few examples of headlines that have appeared in recent years, seemingly on the basis of good evidence that, especially in medical circles, have contributed to a sense of distrust and wariness about the value of taking vitamins, minerals and supplements.

A survey of doctors found, for example, that 41 per cent of doctors in Britain think it's common for people to overdose on vitamins,[4] despite the fact that the authorities have only received 11 adverse event reports connected to vitamins and minerals in the last 11 years. Compare that with the hundreds of thousands of such reports for drugs, most of which are commonly prescribed by doctors every day. Because of this misconception, doctors often caution against taking even something as basic as a multivitamin.

For example, doctors often tell pregnant women to 'take folic acid but don't take any other supplements', despite the fact that in order to obtain the benefits of folic acid – lower homocysteine and improved methylation, which reduce the risk of DNA damage and birth defects – it is also necessary to take vitamin B6, B12 and zinc. In truth, a pregnant woman would be far better protected by an all-round multivitamin. One study found 35 per cent lower risk of birth defects among women taking a multi.[5]

But is there good reason for the caution? Is it time to abandon the notion of vitamins as a panacea? Is this once nice idea now disproven, discredited and potentially harmful? Or is this yet more propaganda in a fiercely competitive medical marketplace that is intended to kill off the competition?

Before we go close up on the evidence to separate fact from fiction, it's worth looking at the big picture where safety is concerned by examining the comparative risk from various sources. The chart below, created from Australian statistics, puts things into perspective.

Tobacco tops the risk score with 6,333, immediately followed by 'preventable adverse effects of medical care' in hospitals (2,333) and then

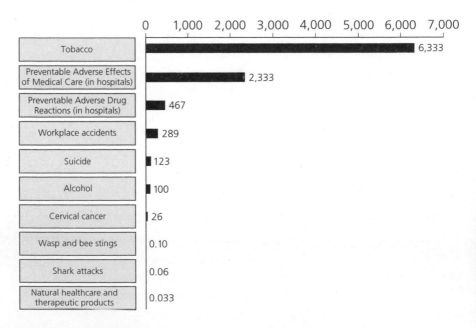

Relative risk of deaths from various hazards

'preventable adverse drug reactions in hospital' (467). At the bottom, below 'wasp or bee stings' (0.10) and shark attacks (0.06), comes 'risks from natural healthcare and therapeutic products' (0.033).

This explains one of the key factors missing from the vitamin death scares – case histories. However alarming the headlines may be, you never hear of any actual person who is said to have died from taking, say, vitamin E – far less that someone's family is now suing the vitamin manufacturers. That's because there isn't anyone who's suffering in this way. There has never been a death thought to have been caused by a vitamin supplement, or a multivitamin, as far as we know, anywhere in the world – *except* for the deaths of young children who swallowed handfuls of their mother's sugared, brightly coloured iron pills. We know because journalists wanting to put the spin on a scare story often call up looking for cases, so we have researched this.

Nutritionists from the Institute for Optimum Nutrition (ION) treat an estimated 50,000 people per year and have a system for reporting adverse reactions. Many of these people are taking supplements. Occasionally we hear reports of people who get a headache on a certain supplement, perhaps nausea if they take too many, or diarrhoea on large doses of vitamin C. Once we heard of a woman who got tingling in her hands on a high dose of vitamin B6. But all of these symptoms disappear on stopping or reducing the amount of vitamins taken.

So whatever the risk of vitamins, we are not talking about anything immediate or acutely life-threatening, unlike some of the side effects reported from taking Vioxx or SSRI anti-depressants. Certainly, none of the risks from supplements would stand up in a court of law. No vitamin company, as far as we know, has ever been sued for apparently causing harm. By comparison, as we've seen in Part 1, the number of court cases against pharmaceutical companies in the US runs into tens of thousands.

Almost all the claims that people have been harmed by vitamins involve large-scale trials of sick people, almost always on medication, some of whom are also given a single vitamin as well. The final analysis then shows that those taking the vitamin appear to have a slightly increased, rather than a decreased, risk of death. Let's examine the evidence behind three of the most common scare stories.

The beta-carotene scare

Carrots are one of the richest sources of beta-carotene, an antioxidant nutrient found in most orange-coloured foods. It's been well researched – 7,000 studies in all, 2,000 of which relate to cancer.

There's no doubt that eating foods rich in beta-carotene reduces risk of cancer. The World Cancer Research Fund, which reviewed hundreds of studies, concludes that carotenoids – antioxidants found in fruit and vegetables, of which beta-carotene is one – are highly protective. (Others among many include lycopene, which is found in tomatoes, and lutein and zeaxanthin, both found in green veg. Collectively, they are probably more protective than any one in isolation.) For example, for lung cancer the WCRF says: 'Overall, the extensive data show a weak to strong decrease in risk with higher dietary intakes of carotenoids.'[7]

There's also no doubt that having a higher beta-carotene level in your bloodstream is good news. Last year a ten-year study of several thousand elderly people in Europe, conducted by the Centre for Nutrition and Health at the National Institute of Public Health and the Environment in the Netherlands, found that the higher the beta-carotene level, the lower the overall risk of death, especially from cancer. Eating probably the equivalent of a carrot a day (raising blood level by 0.39mcmol/l) meant cutting cancer risk by a third.[8]

All this good evidence has led to trials over the past 20 years in which people have been given beta-carotene supplements, sometimes in combination with other antioxidant nutrients. Many have proven protective. For example, research on 1,954 middle-aged men showed beta-carotene as having a protective effect against lung cancer.[9]

That's the good news. But what about the bad news that tends to make the headlines and stick in people's memories, such as the ones that found an increased risk of cancer with beta-carotene? If you analyse the studies this scare is based on, you find that the claim boils down to the fact that one smoker out of a thousand who takes beta-carotene on its own and takes no other antioxidant supplement, and keeps on smoking, will have a slightly raised risk of cancer. This is how a very minor risk is whipped up into something alarming.

A study by the National Cancer Institute in the US gave smokers beta-carotene and reported a 28 per cent increased incidence in lung cancer in those who continued to smoke.[10] Of course, the press had a field day, with headlines such as 'vitamins cause cancer'. A closer look at the figures, however, shows a rather different picture. In fact, the difference between those getting beta-carotene and those getting the placebo was not big enough to reach 'statistical significance'; it was only what is known as a 'trend'. That's important because it means that the result could have occurred by chance.

The actual figures were 50 cancer cases out of some 10,000 in the placebo group and 65 cases out of 10,000 among those getting beta-carotene. Put another way, this means that for every five cases of cancer out of a thousand people taking the placebo, there were 6.5 cases out of a thousand among those taking the beta-carotene supplement. And remember, both groups involved people who had smoked for years and probably had undetected cancer before starting the trial.

But how could such a result be seen as increasing cancer risk by 28 per cent? This, again, is the difference between absolute risk and relative risk that we discussed in Chapter 4. This way of interpreting results is also regularly used in drug trials to make a very small benefit look much more impressive. Here 64 divided by 50 equals 1.28, or an increased *relative* risk of 28 per cent. It sounds dramatic put this way but, as we've seen, it is actually not even statistically significant. The *absolute* risk, remember, is six cases per year in 1,000 for smokers taking beta-carotene, as compared to five cases in 1,000 for smokers on a placebo.

As if this distortion was not unscientific enough, there was another set of findings in the research paper that never made it into the summary, let alone the newspaper headlines. Hidden in the body of the paper, which almost nobody ever reads because they depend on the summary, was the finding that among those who gave up smoking during the trial and took beta-carotene, there were 20 per cent *fewer* cases of lung cancer. Again, this was not statistically significant, but if one 'trend' is worth reporting, surely another is. Unless you assume that beta-carotene makes moral distinctions, giving smokers cancer while protecting those who give up, the implication of this finding is that there is something about smoking that makes it harder for beta-carotene given alone to have an effect.

And this points up another shortcoming of the trial. Besides being scientifically careless – highlighting a negative 'non-significant' finding and ignoring a favourable one – the researchers were also obviously ignorant of basic nutritional principles. This is a serious failing if you are trying to test supplements. Unlike drugs, which often combine in a harmful way, nutrients, especially antioxidants, usually reinforce each other's effects. As we'll see time and time again, giving an individual nutrient on its own, as if it were a drug, to sick people without changing their diet or lifestyle, bears no relationship to the nutritional medicine approach to disease.

The importance of giving antioxidants together showed up in the other study that contributed to the 'beta-carotene-causes-cancer' scare. This time, male smokers were given either vitamin E, vitamin E plus beta-carotene, or beta-carotene on its own. The first two groups showed no significant change, but the beta-carotene-only group showed an increased risk.[11] Once again, giving beta-carotene on its own to smokers shows up as very slightly raising the risk of cancer.

More recent research has shown this too. A review of all studies giving beta-carotene versus a placebo, and involving over 100,000 people, concluded: 'For people with risk factors for lung cancer no reduction (or increase) in lung cancer incidence or mortality was found in those taking vitamins alone compared with placebo.'[12]

So, all this fuss about beta-carotene boils down to a non-significant, tiny increased risk of lung cancer, only in smokers or people at risk, if given on its own. The chances are it means absolutely nothing. In the worst-case scenario it means that, out of a thousand smokers supplementing beta-carotene on its own, just one might get lung cancer earlier. For people not 'at risk', not smoking and not supplementing beta-carotene on its own, the evidence for beta-carotene's protective effect remains highly positive overall. One large study involving 13,000 people between the ages of 35 and 60 to investigate the effects of a pill containing a cocktail of antioxidants (beta-carotene, vitamin C and E) found a highly significant 31 per cent reduction in the risk of all cancers in men, plus an overall 37 per cent lower death rate.[13]

Another found this combination of antioxidants highly protective against colon cancer, but there was no such effect among those who were heavy drinkers and smokers and only took beta-carotene. In fact, for these people there was a very slight increased risk.[14] The British *Daily Mail* had a field day with this story, running a headline that read 'Vitamin pills could cause early death' with a subheading that read: 'vitamins, taken by millions, could be causing thousands of premature deaths'. But you try finding a heavy drinker and smoker who pops beta-carotene on its own! Talk about a needle in a haystack.

So if you look at these beta-carotene and cancer studies with a detached scientific eye, they don't actually form the basis for a scare story at all. Instead, they tell you something useful about how antioxidants work and how best to use them. Antioxidant nutrients are team players, as the diagram below illustrates. Their job is to disarm dangerous oxidants, generated by combustion, from a lit cigarette to frying bacon. They do this by passing the oxidant through a chain of reactions involving vitamin E, C, beta-carotene, co-enzyme Q10, and others you may be less familiar with, such as glutathione and lipoic acid. On their own, these could do more harm than good, by generating more of these radicals (see figure below). This is probably what's happening to beta-carotene among smokers.

So our advice would be not to supplement beta-carotene on its own if you are a heavy smoker or drinker – and to stop smoking and excessive drinking! But even among smokers, a high dietary intake of beta-carotene

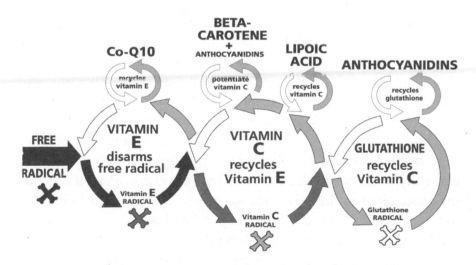

How antioxidants disarm an oxidant or 'free-radical'

is not associated with increased risk.[15] So, keep eating the carrots and supplementing all-round antioxidant supplements or multivitamins, as many other studies shows that this combination results in a clear reduction of cancer risk. In relation to cancer, the true danger is not increasing your intake through diet and supplements.

Twisting the statistics

Besides using vitamins in an inappropriate way and ignoring results that don't suit a particular case, another way of creating scares about supplements is to conduct what is called a 'meta-analysis' or 'systematic review' in a highly selective way. A meta-analysis is a standard way of discovering the real value of a treatment by combining a number of studies and then using statistics to tease out benefits or problems that may not show up in the individual trials. Done carefully, this can be very useful but its effectiveness depends heavily on which trials you choose to include and how you do your statistics.

A good example of how not to do it is a systematic review of antioxidants and gastrointestinal cancers that was published in the prestigious medical journal *The Lancet* in 2004.[16] The abstract – the summary at the beginning and the only bit most people read – says: 'We could not find evidence that antioxidant supplements can prevent gastrointestinal cancers; on the contrary, they seem to increase overall mortality.'

Apparently another blow for supplements, leading to another round of negative headlines in the press. However, a bit of investigation, including contacting the lead author of the paper that was crucial in producing the negative result, revealed a quite different picture. He told us that he was horrified at the way his results had been distorted.

The authors of the review in *The Lancet* looked at seven trials which, they said, were of high enough scientific quality to be included – that is, they had 'high methodology'. The first hint that the selection might not have been entirely impartial was that they excluded at least one major trial that showed benefit; this had been published by the US National Cancer Institute,[17] so should have shown 'high methodology'.

Even so, six of the trials in the review showed benefits from antioxidants. That left just one that came up with an apparently negative result.[18] However, the statistical analysis gave it so much weight that the findings from this one study were enough to outweigh the other six and show that antioxidants increased mortality.

When we looked at this key study, however, it didn't seem to be negative so we contacted the lead author, Dr Pelayo Correa from the pathology department at the Louisiana State University Health Sciences Center in New Orleans, and asked about the increased risk he had supposedly found. He was amazed, he said, because his research, far from being negative, had shown clear benefit from taking vitamins.

His study, published in the *Journal of the National Cancer Institute*, had involved giving people with gastric cancer either beta-carotene, vitamin C or antibiotics to kill off the stomach bacterium *Helicobacter pylori*. All three interventions produced highly significantly improvements, causing substantial regression of gastric cancer. Correa and his colleagues had concluded: 'dietary supplementation with antioxidant micronutrients may interfere with the precancerous process, mostly by increasing the rate of regression of cancer precursor lesions, and may be an effective strategy to prevent gastric carcinoma'. No evidence of increased mortality there.

In fact, as Correa told us, there was no way the study could show anything about mortality. 'Our study was designed for evaluation of the progress of precancerous lesions,' he said. 'It did not intend, and did not have the power, to study mortality and has no value to examine mortality of cancer.'[19] Without this study the main conclusion, widely reported in the media, that antioxidants may increase gastrointestinal cancer, becomes completely invalid.

But the distortion 'scientific medicine' is capable of didn't stop there. The paper in *The Lancet* did find a highly significant and consistent reduction of overall risk (expressed as 'p.00001' – meaning that if you ran the trials 100,000 times you get the same result 99,999 times) in four trials giving selenium supplements. These positive results, however, were dismissed on the basis of 'inadequate methodology' in three out of four studies. It's this kind of distorted selection and statistical analysis that, after extensive promotion to the media, adds another brick to the wall designed to keep food medicine out of the mainstream.

Vitamin E – good or bad for your arteries?

Another big scare story concerned vitamin E. Long thought to be protective against heart disease, recent studies have reported that this is a mistake and that high-dose supplementation might even increase the risk of a heart attack. This generated headlines such as: 'High dose vitamin E death warning'. However, the truth behind the headlines is similar to the beta-carotene saga, with a twist.

As with beta-carotene, almost 50 years of research into vitamin E has shown that the higher your intake, the lower your risk of a heart attack. The real heroes, although they are rarely mentioned these days, are Drs Wilfred and Evan Shute who, back in the 1940s and 1950s, treated 30,000 patients with heart disease with an incredibly high success rate. But this was before the days of double-blind trials, so this research is not considered valid today. However, since then there have been numerous studies showing that giving supplements of vitamin E to reasonably healthy people seems to prevent heart attacks.

In one, published in the *New England Journal of Medicine*, 87,200 nurses were given 67mg of vitamin E daily for more than two years. A 40 per cent drop in fatal and non-fatal heart attacks was reported compared to those not taking vitamin E supplements.[20] In another study, 39,000 male health professionals were given 67mg of vitamin E for the same length of time and achieved a 39 per cent reduction in heart attacks.[21] This is what is called ' primary prevention' – preventing a disease from developing.

Then a 'secondary prevention' study, giving vitamin E to people with cardiovascular disease to prevent further problems, came up trumps. The study, carried out by researchers at the UK's Cambridge University Medical School in 1996, gave some 2,000 people vitamin E or a placebo. Those given vitamin E had a 75 per cent reduced risk of a non-fatal heart attack but, interestingly, no reduced risk of death from fatal heart attacks. The research showed vitamin E to be almost four times as effective as aspirin in reducing heart attacks.

All was looking good with vitamin E until 2000, when a large-scale double-blind trial of around 20,000 people with cardiovascular disease were given vitamins (600mg of vitamin E, 250mg of vitamin C and 20mg of beta-carotene) or placebos. This trial was part of a much larger study testing the effects of statin drugs. It found no difference in those taking the vitamins versus the placebos, but statins performed well in comparison. Then, things got worse for vitamin E.

An American study, the HOPE (Heart Outcomes Prevention Evaluation) trial, published in the *New England Journal of Medicine*, hinted at a slight increased risk of heart attack in heart patients who were on medication and taking vitamin E.[22] The trial was extended for a further two and a half years and, in 2005, the results of what was called the HOPE2 trial were published in the *Annals of Internal Medicine*, showing a slight increased risk of heart attack in heart patients who were on medication and taking vitamin E. This prompted a review of all trials in which vitamin E had been given to people with cardiovascular disease.

The results showed that vitamin E, in higher doses, seemed to increase mortality, while at lower doses, seemed to decrease mortality.[23] The overall conclusion was that 'vitamin E supplementation did not affect all-cause mortality' in other words, the same number of people overall died in the group that took vitamin E as did in the group that didn't. But as with beta-carotene, there was a group that did slightly worse (those on a high dose, above 268mg), and a group that did slightly better (on a low dose, below 268mg).

Either way, though, the results looked pretty damning. The effect of taking vitamin E, for these people, was not that greatly positive or negative – and certainly not as positive as the preventive power of giving vitamin E to reasonably healthy people. The question is why, and why the difference between the high and low doses? The answer may be linked to the other drugs that the patients were taking – specifically the statins which, it is well known, have an effect on the same antioxidant network that is central to the functioning of beta-carotene. It is an effect that is very familiar to statin manufacturers, who supported the trial and who would benefit if their product was shown to be more effective than vitamin E.

So how does the connection work? The first thing to notice about these trials is that not only were the majority of the people taking part very unwell – with either advanced cardiovascular disease or diabetes or both – but most were, on an average, taking five drugs, including statins.

As you will have read in Chapter 15, statins not only block the enzyme that makes cholesterol, they also block the enzyme that makes Co-Enzyme Q10 (CoQ10) – and vitamin E can't work as an antioxidant without it. Vitamin E is a fat-based antioxidant, sacrificing itself to disarm an oxidant from, for example, burnt fat. In the process, the vitamin E becomes oxidised and dangerous. CoQ10 helps to recycle oxidised vitamin E so it can fight another battle.

So, giving a large amount of vitamin E to someone on a statin drug, without giving co-enzyme Q10, would be expected to increase oxidation, not decrease it. In other words, statin drugs could make high-dose vitamin E worse for you. You'd be naïve if you thought that the makers of statins aren't aware of this. They have already patented the combination of statins plus CoQ10, potentially to issue a 'new improved' statin perhaps when the existing patent runs out, or a safer statin if the press gets bad.

Nutritionists are taught *never* to give high-dose vitamin E (above 250mg) to a person on statins without also giving 90mg or more of CoQ10. Yet, that is exactly what these trials have done. Once again, a supposedly scientific trial is set up to test the effectiveness of a supplement and then conducted in a way that shows no understanding of the way supplements work. Or if you take a cynical view, with a clear and hostile knowledge.

The *raison d'être* for giving vitamin E, a powerful fat-based antioxidant, is to decrease oxidation. The big question these trials raise is 'Was vitamin E reducing oxidation, as would be predicted?' This can be measured with a blood test but, unfortunately, this wasn't done in these trials, even though it's a relatively simple and obvious thing to do. So we don't really know if vitamin E was increasing or reducing oxidation, and, if so why. The drug's effect of depleting CoQ10 is certainly a major contender. Until that measurement is done, there are simply not enough facts to make a final verdict on high-dose vitamin E for those with cardiovascular disease.

However, based on what we know already, supplementing something like 50 to 200mg of vitamin E, which is five to 20 times the RDA, seems to be nothing but good news. This kind of level, and possibly more, may also be good for people with cardiovascular disease, but possibly only if taken with CoQ10 if you're on statins – although more research is needed to reach any definitive conclusions.

The other important point to make is that these trials aren't comparing a drug-based approach with a nutritional approach. They are designed on the assumption that the drugs are essential, and therefore patients get drugs plus a placebo or drugs plus vitamins. For all we know, the cocktail of blood-thinning, cholesterol-lowering, artery-relaxing drugs they are on might render the nutrients unable to make much difference. It is also entirely possible, as we saw in Chapter 15, that a combination of diet, supplements and lifestyle that can also thin the blood, lower cholesterol and relax arteries might render the drugs unnecessary.

The vitamin C scandal

One of the most powerful vitamins of all, capable of seriously reducing the need for drugs, is vitamin C. Unsurprisingly, it too has been consistently attacked on scientifically spurious grounds. Myths about vitamin C include that it promotes cancer; makes kidney stones; increases risk for heart disease; doesn't work for colds; and can't be absorbed in high doses. As a result, many doctors still believe that if you take vitamin C supplements you're just making expensive urine and possibly raising your risk of diarrhoea. It is true that vitamin C in large amounts of around 5g a day does give you diarrhoea. The cure is simple – take less. So where did these myths come from and what is the truth behind them?

The one about the inability to absorb vitamin C can be found in the official publication by the UK Department of Health on the RDA of vitamin C, which is 60mg – roughly what you'd find in an orange. The book makes reference to three studies that gave volunteers increasing amounts of vitamin C and measured the levels in the blood (plasma).[24] The charts overleaf are reproduced from this government publication.

The first chart implies that vitamin C levels 'plateau' above 80 to 100mg. The data (the dots and triangles) shows no evidence of a plateau in plasma levels, as the daily amount of vitamin C increases, nor is there any actual data beyond 80mg.

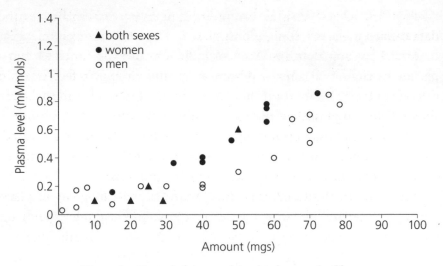

Vitamin C and the mythical 'plateau' effect

As you can see, the more vitamin C consumed, the higher the plasma level. But that's not what the publication says. Instead, it says 'Vitamin C plasma levels approach an upper plateau (with an intake) between 70 and 100mg per day.' The publication shows this data with the 'line of best fit' added (see below), implying that you can't absorb more than, say, 80mg.

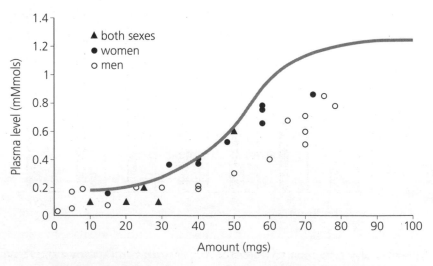

Vitamin C intake levels with 'line of best fit' added

This 'line of best fit' is an invention. It bears no resemblance to the data carried out in these simple studies. You'll notice, for example, that there isn't any actual data beyond 80mg. So how can you conclude that a plateau of vitamin C is reached between 70 and 100mg? In fact, vitamin C levels in blood plasma continue to rise up to at least 2,500mg a day, as shown below in published research.[25] This isn't a difficult test to run.

OK, you might say, even if high doses of vitamin C can be absorbed, what's the point? Aren't you just risking side effects such as kidney stones? Let's deal with that old chestnut here and now.

According to Professor Allen Rodgers from the University of Cape Town in South Africa, who is one of the world's leading experts on kidney stones, the answer is simply 'No'. At the Kidney Stone Research Laboratory at the university, he conducted a controlled trial in which volunteers were required to ingest 4g of vitamin C per day for five days. Urine samples were collected before, during and after the ingestion period. These were rigorously analysed for a host of independent risk factors, all of which are regarded as powerful indicators of the risk of kidney-stone formation. The results showed that these risk factors were

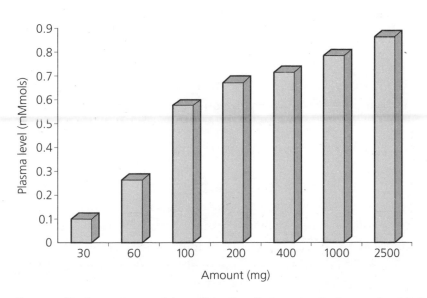

What really happens to blood levels of vitamin C above the RDA intake

not altered. He concluded that ingestion of large doses of vitamin C does not increase the risk of forming kidney stones.[26]

So why the scare? Professor Rodgers explains:

> The widespread belief that vitamin C causes kidney stones is based on the well established metabolic conversion of ascorbic acid (vitamin C) to oxalic acid and the observation that oxalic acid levels in urine are elevated after vitamin C ingestion. Oxalic acid is a key component of calcium oxalate stones – 70 per cent of all kidney stones contain this substance. Obviously, an elevated urinary oxalic acid level is undesirable. However, while metabolic conversion does indeed take place, it is insignificant. The apparently higher levels of oxalic acid in the urine that have been previously reported arise from the fact that ascorbic acid which is excreted in the urine undergoes a chemical conversion to oxalic acid while it is in a test-tube prior to analysis. In our study, we simply put a preservative in our urine collection bottles to prevent this conversion. Previous studies failed to take this precaution and hence reported erroneously high oxalic acid levels in their urine specimens. Vitamin C doesn't cause kidney stones.

So, now you know you can absorb it and it won't give you kidney stones, but what's the point of upping your intake of vitamin C?

Apart from being remarkably non-toxic even in massive amounts, vitamin C really does help get rid of infections – from colds to AIDS – and is profoundly anti-cancer. So don't stop taking it.

Who fuels the fire of vitamin scares?

In the last 30 years, virtually every major vitamin discovery that has any potential to eat into drugs sales has been successfully squashed. Doctors prescribe folic acid for pregnancy, iron and B12 for anaemia, calcium for osteoporosis and a few are now prescribing omega-3s for cardiovascular disease – and that's about it. None of these is much of a threat to the major 'blockbuster' drugs (see Part 1). As any strategist will tell you, one way to dominate the market is to kill the competition. This is done by creating scares through deviously designed studies, publishing negative studies and using the press to fuel scare stories. After all, nothing sells better than bad news.

Maybe that's all it is. Over-cautious regulators and headline-grabbing PR. A classic case of this was a press release issued by the UK Food Standards Agency in May 2003, announcing an extensive review of vitamin safety by the Expert Group on Vitamins and Minerals (EVM). 'Vitamins can damage your health' was the gist of the headlines in *The Times*, *Telegraph* and *Guardian*, picking up on statements in the FSA's press release that 'chromium in the form of chromium picolinate may have the potential to cause cancer'; 'vitamin C above 1,000mg could cause abdominal pain and diarrhoea'; 'high intakes [of B6] over a long period can lead to loss of feelings in arms and legs'.[27]

Let's look at the last two of these statements. There is some truth to them, but we need to see how serious the claims really are. Vitamin B6, if taken on its own in amounts of 1,000mg, can cause neuropathy (that is, numbness, pain, tingling and other sensations in the nerves), but who takes this much? That's ten of the highest-dose B6 pills a day, and no nutritionist would ever advise it. Vitamin C in large amounts can cause diarrhoea. So can curry. You just have less. These aren't life-threatening side effects.

The effect of chromium, on the other hand, sounds really serious. In truth, this apparent risk was based on a test-tube study that hinted at increased DNA damage, versus numerous human trials that failed to find any suggestion of such effect. The FSA's committee of experts weren't too worried, and concluded: 'the significance of such results is unclear' but the press release hyped it up into 'chromium picolinate may have the potential to cause cancer' ... and the newspapers went further. The *Telegraph* stated said the FSA 'wants to ban chromium picolinate because of its potential cancer-causing properties'. Worrying stuff and enough to cause a massive decrease in sales of chromium supplements.

Now wind forward to December 2004 and you'll hear a very different story from the FSA.[28] 'The Committee on Mutagenicity reviewed the genotoxicity [harmfulness to DNA] of chromium and chromium picolinate. The Committee concluded that the balance of the evidence suggested that chromium picolinate was not genotoxic. For those people who wish to supplement their diet with chromium, the maximum upper level recommended by the FSA is 10mg a day. There is no need to avoid chromium picolinate.' Not only is chromium now in the clear, but the maximum upper level allowed in a supplement is 10mg – that's 10,000mcg. The average person consumes less than 50mcg and the high-dose chromium supplements contain 200mcg. In other words, the FSA think it's safe to take 50 chromium pills a day!

So much for the scare. How many drugs would be safe if you took 50 a day? And how many drugs would be damned by one inconclusive piece of evidence? All too often vitamins and minerals, the stuff we've evolved to need, are guilty until proven innocent, while drugs are innocent until thousands of people have died.

The other side of the coin is to ask whether it is safe *not* to take supplements, in this case chromium. As we saw in Chapters 8 and 10, chromium has well-supported benefits in treating diabetes and depression, so this unfounded scare might have had dire consequences for diabetics or depressed people who stopped taking chromium quite unnecessarily. There is a downside and a real cost resulting from scaring people off good medicine.

Despite the fact that no one has ever died from taking a multivitamin, and that every major survey yet undertaken has shown that those who supplement their diet live longer, feel better and are less likely to get sick, vitamin scares aren't about to stop. A few may be valid, but the vast majority are not. Unless you live and breathe this subject as we do, it isn't easy to know when you really need to be concerned. We'll help you sort out the wheat from the chaff if you subscribe to our free e-news (see www.foodismedicine.co.uk). Armed with a more in-depth analysis, plus your own common sense, you'll be in a better position to judge for yourself.

There are a number of other things that you can do to keep yourself better informed and to work towards changing the law, which we deal with in the final chapter. But before that, in the next chapter we look at the way vitamin scares have had a direct effect on health regulations in Europe. If you care about being able to use nutritional medicine in the most effective way, it's worth knowing what the legislators have in store, because the new developments could make it even harder to practise nutritional medicine and make some of the key nutrients less available .

19.

Too Safe Can Mean Sorry
Why the 'precautionary principle' may be damaging your health

ARE YOU WORRIED about the return of nuclear power or the possible dangers of genetically modified crops, or is it the level of pesticides in mothers' milk that keeps you awake at night? Whatever the large-scale hazard people are most agitated about – and there is certainly no shortage of them – in a rational world, very few would be worried that widespread damage was being done to people's health by vitamin, mineral and food supplements.

However, if you have just read the previous chapter on vitamin scares, you will be aware that there are many misconceptions about supplements; and because they are rarely corrected, officials in charge of health and safety regulation in the European Union are gradually constructing a framework for controlling vitamins based on assumptions that would be more appropriate to an outbreak of salmonella or the disposal of toxic waste. If you are not in Europe, these developments are still very likely to affect you because EU regulations are bound to have a powerful impact on official thinking elsewhere in the world.

The key idea behind the new regulations is a rather obscure concept from risk assessment theory known as 'the precautionary principle'. But before going into exactly why this very large regulatory hammer is being used to crack such a healthy nut, let's just backpedal briefly and explain how we got here.

Many people would agree that it makes sense to have some sort of regulations and control of food supplements. How much should you take? What is the safe upper limit? But the starting point for this should be that minerals, vitamins and other supplements have been used for decades without any indication they are causing large or even small-scale health problems. As we've seen, your chances of being seriously harmed by a supplement are smaller than those of being stung by a bee or wasp. Not that this stopped the EU, in 2002, from issuing a directive that at first threatened to drive about 75 per cent of currently used supplements off the market (see 'The big EU guns trained on food supplements' box below).

THE BIG EU GUNS TRAINED ON FOOD SUPPLEMENTS

Food Supplements Directive
You may recognise this one. Issued in 2002, its aim was to restrict the number of supplements that could be sold in the EU to those on a 'positive' list. It has been the object of extensive lobbying and a court case. Current consensus is that it is not going to outlaw as many as was first feared.

The Human Medicinal Products Directive
This replaced the Medicines Act (see Chapter 17) and, like it, can be used to classify a supplement as a medicinal product, which effectively makes it unavailable if it proves too effective.

The EU Nutrition and Health Claims Regulation
This new piece of legislation kicks in at the end of 2006. This one will have control over any and all claims made about a food product. The claim is that it will provide consumers with accurate and meaningful information while allowing supplement manufacturers to use serious and scientifically substantiated claims as a marketing tool. Critics fear it will ignore good evidence and reduce the number of claims that can be made.

> *The European Food Safety Authority (EFSA)*
> This is the body charged by the Supplements Directive with strict regulation of supplements to protect public health. The principles it will be using to assess risk assume supplements have no intrinsic health benefit.

But what's at stake here isn't just how safe supplements are. The threat of heavy-handed legislation comes at a time when almost every week brings fresh evidence of both the key role food plays in chronic diseases and the very low level of nutrients many people are getting.

To take just two recent examples: food-related ill health now costs Britain's NHS an estimated £6 billion pounds a year – that is, four times the cost of treating smoking-related disorders.[29] Now, look at the other example – that there is little difference in the 'nutritional profile' of children who have school dinners and those who don't.[30] The problems with school dinners in the UK – all too often, burgers or highly processed pizzas, fizzy drinks and other junk foods – have now been well aired in the media. But that children bringing a packed lunch from home are eating just as badly as those getting school meals is evidence of a major nutritional problem that may well lead to chronic conditions such as diabetes.

In a rational health system, we would be making a serious attempt to tackle these problems in the most direct way – by applying knowledge of nutrition and supplementation. Instead, yet more drugs for diabetes are recommended. In 2005, one of these turned out to double the number of strokes, according to data that the FDA had felt justified licensing it.[31] And meanwhile, tiers of European bureaucracy are being used to assess the safety and dose levels of supplements, using a risk assessment system developed to handle such intrinsically toxic substances as pesticides, the results of which will have repercussions in international law on nutrients.

This is happening because the Food Supplements Directive instructs the European Food Safety Authority (EFSA) to assess the 'potential of vitamins and other nutrients' to cause 'hazard, risk and adverse health effects'. And this is where the 'precautionary principle' comes in. It's a technical way of saying 'better safe than sorry', and the rule is that if there is any information suggesting there just might be a problem – and we've seen how misleading studies on vitamins can be – then a 'high level of health protection' has to be applied. Keeping salmonella levels to a minimum obviously makes sense, but is it really appropriate to apply such caution to vitamins?

One reason for thinking it is not is that vitamins have a very large 'therapeutic index': the size of the dose that can cause serious harm is many times greater than the dose normally taken. The RDA for vitamin C, for instance, is 60mg but a recent report found that there were no observable harmful effects at 3g,[32] which is 50 times that. Other than loose bowels, there are no harmful effects at 30g – 500 times the RDA. In contrast, the recommended adult dose for paracetamol is 500mg–1g, while the toxic dose is 6–10g, less than ten times the safe amount.

But there is a more serious problem with applying the better-safe-than-sorry approach to supplements. The precautionary principle assumes that the hazard you are warding off has no intrinsic benefit. That's fine with salmonella or industrial PCBs – no one feels better from a daily dose of either, after all. The technical term for this is that the 'opportunity costs' of banishing salmonella are zero. But is that a sensible assumption to make about vitamins? In fact, as we saw in Part 3, there are all sorts of situations where giving relatively high doses of vitamins can have a very beneficial effect. Tightly limiting their availability will actually have high opportunity costs.

Some have suggested that this new legislation – the EU Nutrition and Health Claims Regulation – could be beneficial. One of its stated aims is to protect us from the misleading claims of junk foods masquerading as healthy ones. It also says that it will make it legal to make claims about nutrients reducing the risk of a disease, providing that there is the evidence to back it up. However, other observers are not so optimistic.

First of all, the cost of gathering the evidence according to the standards set by the Health Claims Regulations will be considerable, ruling out small companies. Then, claims will have to based on 'reasonable science'; but exactly what this means is not specified. If the poor-quality research used to discredit vitamins, described in the previous chapter, is allowed, the outlook is not good. Next, the claims have to be approved by the EFSA, which is more concerned with safety than health promotion. It certainly doesn't have a positive remit to actively encourage optimum nutrition or the new kind of medicine that we propose. Nor is it designed to consider how unsafe it is *not* to encourage the promotion of food as medicine – the opportunity cost.

But even if the EFSA allows a claim under the Health Claims Regulations, this can be over-ruled by the all-powerful Human Medicinal Products Directive, which can declare a food to really be a medicine. The directive also still absolutely outlaws any claim that a diet or nutrients prevent, cure or treat a condition, even if it's undeniably true.

In the end, the new arrangements are most likely to be a closed shop. Experience has shown that the sort of regulatory bodies involved are at best suspicious of supplements, believing in myths such as 'the well-balanced diet provides all the nutrients you need', and swayed far more by big industry politics than cutting-edge science. One very plausible scenario is that under the guise of reasonable science, the door to accepting food as medicine could become even more firmly shut than ever.

And this is why campaigning for a more rational approach to supplements is so important. If the nutritional approach is going to fulfil its potential contribution to our health, then the regulators will have to take into account the benefits of supplements when assessing their risk. Just how to achieve this, and how you can make a difference right now, is covered in the last chapter. If you think you're too small – as the Dalai Llama once said – try sharing a room with a mosquito. But first, the next chapter paints a picture of the kind of new medicine that you will be fighting for.

20.

The Medicine of Tomorrow
Our vision for the future – how it could be

MRS VIGDIS OALAAN hadn't felt really well for some time. Looking after four children and being nearly fifty years old, she was overweight and both her cholesterol and blood-pressure levels were raised. Her doctor had given her a cholesterol-lowering statin and a diuretic to bring her blood pressure down, but she still felt terrible. 'I felt tired most of the time and although I knew I should lose weight and take some more exercise it seemed such an effort. Sometimes it seemed as if food was the only thing that cheered me up.'

Drug-based medicine didn't have much more to offer Mrs Oalaan. She could have asked for an SSRI anti-depressant and even something like Xenical to block fat absorption in her gut for weight loss, but the chances of that combination with their range of adverse drug reactions giving her the energy and feeling of well-being she craved was vanishingly small. Her doctor dispensed general advice about losing weight and eating well, but nothing more.

What she wanted was something that would tackle her underlying problems, not treatment that had a good chance of creating a whole new set of symptoms to deal with. She wanted something that was safe and effective, and would actively help her to turn her life around. In short, she wanted good medicine.

Luckily for Mrs Oalaan, she lived in Oslo, which has one of four pioneering clinics in Norway that offer not just a nutritional approach but active and specific help to support patients making the lifestyle changes that go with it – changes that are often difficult to begin with.

The first thing Mrs Oalaan discovered was that she had diabetes. 'My regular doctor had told me to "live like a diabetic" but he never gave me any concrete advice,' she said. 'In fact it wasn't that big a surprise because both my parents had died of it in their sixties.' What the clinic offered was something very specific. She was told to exercise, cut out high-glycemic food, and eat a low-GL diet (see page 143) with more protein and vegetables.

But that was just the beginning. Rather than being left to battle with the challenge of implementing the big changes involved on her own, she had a team of experts to help her. Several nutritional therapists worked at the clinic, as did a lifestyle coach and a psychologist who was available for people who had particular emotional problems with making the changes. There was a gym available nearby with fitness instructors to help with a personal programme, while nurses also ran seminars on the links between nutrition and health and you could take cooking classes to give you ideas about the foods that fitted the new regime. Within a few months, Mrs Oalaan no longer needed her blood pressure and cholesterol-lowering pills, and her blood-sugar readings showed she was no longer diabetic.

This is the way the new food-based medicine can work. Dr Fedon Lindberg,[33] who established these Norwegian clinics, with new ones due to open in Finland and Spain, is one of a number of doctors who are showing what this approach can do. At the moment they are all privately run, not least because the kind of inbuilt hostility we explored in the last section means that this approach is not currently available on, say, the UK's National Health Service. In the US, however, treatment at the clinic of another one of these pioneers is covered by one of the largest insurance groups – Kaiser Permanente. After initial scepticism, they accepted the simple financial logic: patients treated in this way cost less because they are healthier.

In just a few years, the four clinics Lindberg has opened have treated 12,000 patients, most of them with diabetes and weight and heart problems. His crucial insight is that it's no good telling people to change; you have to help them through it. 'Compliance is a key issue for any type of treatment,' says Lindberg, 'and making lifestyle changes is like trying to write with the opposite hand. You can do it but it takes time and effort and you have to have a reason.'

Many of the patients who have been overweight for long periods find the hardest thing is to start exercising, which is why having a gym on site with several instructors is a key part of the regime. 'If you start going to a normal gym to get fit,' says one of the team of physiotherapists, Linda Andersson, 'and you miss a few sessions, no one cares. But here as soon as someone doesn't turn up twice we are on the phone asking what is happening and how we can help.'

So what do we do?

The notion that poor diet and lifestyle is at the root of many of our chronic diseases is hardly disputed by anyone. The big question is what to do about it. Conventional medical wisdom has it that in an ideal world, everyone would eat healthily and exercise and all would be well. But in fact, people don't, and getting them to change their diet and lifestyle is too hard and too expensive to be worth it. Hence the need for ever-increasing quantities of drugs to try to keep the problem under control.

But Lindberg has shown that in a few years, it's possible to make major changes in the way thousands of people approach their health using straightforward common-sense techniques. Critics complain that the evidence for non-drug approaches is weak. There are two reasons for this, and both relate to the way drug companies dominate the medical agenda. The first is that there is a serious lack of funds to do such research; as the next chapter shows, several recent reports have called for that to change.

The second is the power of pharmaceutical PR. If a new drug has been found to be effective, doctors get to hear about it fast. Reprints of the relevant journal article are run off for widespread distribution, it is presented and re-presented at international conferences, and an army of salespeople bring doctors the good news. Contrast what happens with equally positive findings for the benefits of a lifestyle approach. It is published in a journal, then maybe a couple of newspaper stories pick up on it and that's it.

So let's look briefly at a couple of impressive bits of evidence. Lindberg's nutritional approach is based on the Mediterranean diet, which involves eating minimally processed foods – fruits, vegetables, pulses, whole grains. It's also both low-GL and strongly anti-inflammatory.

In 2004 a very large-scale trial, involving over 74,000 people, found that the more closely you followed it, the more your risk of dying early dropped off. In more technical terms – there was a statistically significant reduction of mortality of eight per cent for every two points you get closer to the Mediterranean diet, on a scale from zero to ten. So adopting the diet full-scale would result in a drop of 40 per cent in premature deaths.[34] If that were a drug, doctors would be going all out to prescribe it.

So the diet works, but what about the claim that it is too hard to get people to change? At around the same time as the trial above, a large American study found that treating 2,390 patients who had high blood pressure, high cholesterol and raised blood sugar with just 12 weeks of exercise, counselling and nutrition training was effective in enabling a significant proportion of them to bring down all these markers to safe levels without use of any drugs.

Over 60 per cent achieved their blood-pressure targets, 23 per cent hit the cholesterol target and 39 per cent got their blood sugar under control. 'Our conclusions refute the notion that intensive lifestyle intervention is not worth the effort,' says lead author Neil Gordon, Clinical Professor of Medicine in the Emory University School of Medicine in Atlanta, Georgia. 'Unlike single drug therapy, it favourably impacts on multiple cardiovascular risk factors and it is generally less expensive than most medications.'[35]

And that's far from the only positive study. A smaller one involving 337 volunteers taking a 40-hour, four-week course on 'making healthful lifestyle choices and ways to improve exercise levels and nutrition' led to improvements in markers for heart disease. The authors concluded that the programme 'has the potential to dramatically reduce the risks associated with common chronic diseases in the long term'.[36]

The powerful effect of simply being told the facts of nutrition came across very clearly in a magazine article written by journalist David Aaronovitch.[37] Having reached an 'elephantine' 252lb (114kg), he went off to the Pritikin Longevity Center in Miami, Florida, where the diet on offer is low-fat and high-carbohydrate but with the same emphasis on fresh food and exercise. He ate unfamiliar meals, worked out in the gym and watched his weight drop off, while his energy and disease markers improved dramatically. But in the end, what seemed to make the biggest impact was his realisation of just how a poor diet can mess up your various metabolic systems.

'As I listened I felt tears creep into my eyes,' he wrote. 'I really hadn't realised all this. Sure, people had said, "you eat too much salt" and I'd only recently begun to cut down, but I didn't know just how dangerous it was. My doctor had simply recommended losing weight and then put me on beta-blockers, which, I also found out, made me more likely to gain weight and more likely to develop diabetes.' Aaranovitch had actually learnt something that made sense of how he felt, and that was impossible to ignore. When he got back home, it was his new-found knowledge and diet prescription that was the key to keeping him healthy, not a drug prescription.

Your perfect diet and lifestyle

An even stronger feeling of not having been told the truth about the power of nutrition is one that is common among the clients at another pioneering American centre where the speciality is delving into the bio-chemical depths of nutrition that most regular doctors don't even know exist. As with most of these centres practising the new medicine, your transformation starts with an examination, but at the Berkeley Heart Lab – set up by Dr Robert Superko in conjunction with the University of California – tests of blood sugar and cholesterol are just the beginning.

You'll also have eight much newer, more specialised blood tests that combine to create a detailed snapshot of the workings of your metabolism. 'Over the past decade we have developed a much clearer picture of the factors leading to heart problems,' says Superko. 'The more precisely you can identify those putting you at risk, the more effectively we can treat you.' Just lowering cholesterol, he explains, can be worse than useless.

For instance, one of the tests, known as ALP (atherogenic lipoprotein profile), reveals what type of LDL cholesterol you have – something the standard cholesterol test can't. It detects if you have the gene for producing small dense LDLs (known as pattern B), which raises your risk of heart-disease risk by 300 per cent or more, even if your cholesterol level is low and you've no other risk factors.

'The gene responsible for pattern B is found in 30 per cent of the general population and 50 per cent of people with heart problems,' says Superko. 'Yet most people don't know about it because the best way to treat it is with diet and exercise, so the drug companies aren't interested.'

The treatment for pattern B shows just how sophisticated the Superko approach can be, and how it can turn conventional assumptions upside down. 'If you've got the gene but you remain a healthy weight, then nothing happens,' he explains. 'However, when you start putting on weight you get a rise of fatty acids in the blood and they trigger the gene to start producing the small dangerous LDLs. The way to turn it off is to exercise and lose weight.'

But there is more. 'If you have the gene but it's not causing any trouble and you go on a low-fat diet, that can also turn on the gene, sparking small LDL production. That's because the extra sugar which often goes with low-fat eating can raise those fatty acid levels. People who have been identified as having the gene with the ALP test do better on high-protein or Mediterranean type diets.'

And there are other twists and turns of individual metabolism that require different treatments. So Superko offers three different dietary packages, three levels of exercise and three supplement regimes. Depending on your personal 'cardiac fingerprint', as revealed by the new tests, you might be given any one of the nine different combinations, such as: supplements that focus on antioxidants, plus a diet that is low in carbohydrates and an intensive exercise programme. Drugs may also be used but they are just one option among many. The clinic also makes sure that the patients are followed up regularly to help them stick to their programme.

Putting it in the system

What we are talking about is diagnosing what kind of lifestyle, diet, supplement and exercise regime will move a person towards health, either from horizontal illness (secondary prevention) or from vertical illness (primary prevention).

The means for doing this are already available and being used by thousands of people every year. The vision of the Institute for Optimum Nutrition was to train a team of nutritional therapists who had that expertise to diagnose and motivate a person towards their perfect diet and lifestyle. Over a thousand such nutritional therapists have been trained by ION, and many more from other training colleges, treating an estimated 100,000 people a year. Few doctors work with or refer to nutritional therapists. (See Appendix 1 on page 392 to find one near you.)

As an illustration of how the ION vision might work, one company gave 25 directors and senior managers with highly stressful jobs a chance to have one-to-one consultations with a nutritional therapist, as well as encouragement to exercise on a regular basis with a personal trainer. Each person was asked to identify up to three health aims and tracked over six months. At the end of six months they reassessed their health aims. The results, shown below, show massive improvement in weight control, in lowering elevated cholesterol, in digestive health, energy, skin complaints, sleep and overall health.

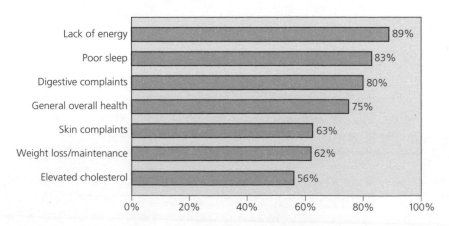

Percentage improvement in key health factors

Another way the new medicine could work would be for doctors to refer patients for educational courses that help teach people how to make the right nutritional and lifestyle changes. In the UK we've been testing exactly such a system, either as a weekend 100% Health workshop, or as 'Zest for Life', a series of 12 evening classes at Holford Diet and Nutrition Clubs.

The results are equally impressive. Thirty people attending a 100% Health weekend workshop had their overall health, diet and weight monitored before the weekend and three months later.

The group showed an improvement in their overall health (see figure below), and a big improvement in energy and hormonal issues (among the women); they also reported fewer food sensitivities, and better digestion and immunity. Their diets had also substantially improved. The higher their compliance with their personalised diet and supplement programmes, the better their improvement in health. The vast majority of those that were overweight also lost significant amounts of weight. These kinds of workshops run several times a year and would be the kind of thing a new-medicine doctor could easily refer patients to.

Our third pilot group was composed of 20 people whose main issue was losing weight. They attended eight evening sessions where they learnt about eating a low-GL diet, the importance of exercise, essential fats, supplements and food allergies, and had help and support in

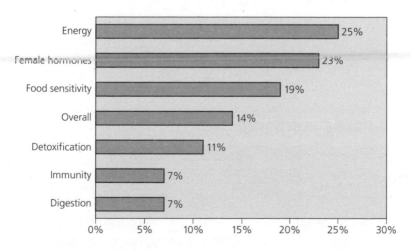

Percentage improvement in key health factors

developing a healthier low-GL diet, backed up with exercise and supplements. They lost, on average, 10lb (4.5kg) over the eight weeks.[38]

Savings plan

So the outlines of how the new medicine might work are already emerging. There would be some kind of testing, not to sell a particular product, but to highlight the strengths and weaknesses of your whole system. Depending on the findings, different sorts of diets would be recommended, backed up by appropriate supplementation, plus some doable lifestyle changes. As we've seen, giving patients the emotional and practical support they need to make the changes makes a big difference, and so do talks and information about what is going on in their bodies.

If nutritional medicine is allowed to develop fully, it will inevitably bring a significant reduction in the drugs bill, which could free up money to be spent in different ways. For instance, in the light of recent advice that psychotherapy was preferable to anti-depressants as a treatment for depression, researchers at the University of Bristol in the UK calculated that the money spent on anti-depressants between 1991 and 2002 could have employed 7,700 psychotherapists to give 1.54 million treatments of six sessions each year for depression.[39] How many health workshops, nutritional therapists, psychotherapists and fitness trainers might be paid for out of a significant cut in the budget for hypertension drugs? Ironically, the British NHS, faced with massive debts to which the ever-increasing drugs bill makes a big contribution, are making hundreds of psychotherapists redundant.

Mind–body medicine

But there is a bigger prize on offer from the nutritional non-drug approach than just making better use of health-care funding. Perhaps surprisingly, it holds out a greatly improved hope of treating psychological disorders by abolishing the mind–body split that has run through medicine for centuries. As we saw in Chapter 5, when you start treating unhealthy people as a complex adaptive network that is out of balance instead of a collection of faulty molecules to be targeted with drugs, the difference between a physical disorder and a psychological one disappears.

If your breathing is off kilter for any reason, your blood pressure rises and you feel anxious. Change your breathing, and your blood pressure drops and your mood lightens. The same multiple effects can be seen with food and supplements. Giving people antioxidants and omega-3 oils can change levels of cardiovascular risk factors in the blood, but it can also produce significant changes in behaviour. For instance, a carefully controlled study giving just the basic RDA of vitamins, minerals and essential fats to inmates at the maximum security Young Offenders Institution in Aylesbury in the UK resulted in a 35 per cent drop in reports of anti-social behaviour.[40]

A recognition of the interconnectedness of mind and body is a central feature of Patrick's Brain Bio Centre in London. A good example of how it works can be seen in the case of David.

> At the age of three, David was diagnosed as having a severe communication disorder. He had terrible tantrums, screamed at strangers, often avoided eye contact and was attending a special school. His parents were having serious difficulties controlling him.
>
> Within six months of attending the Brain Bio Centre he no longer had tantrums, he had been signed off at the special school – 'Something that almost never happens,' said his mother – and he was starting at a mainstream nursery school.

Although patients arrive at the Brain Bio Centre complaining of psychological symptoms, the team of experts, which includes a psychiatrist, psychologist and nutritional therapist, pay special attention to any physical problems. 'You rarely find psychological problems on their own,' said Lorraine Perretta, one of the clinical nutritionists. 'David presented with tantrums and delayed learning, but he was also not sleeping well, was constipated and had had several ear infections.'

So the first thing they do is run a series of tests. 'We run tests to see what levels of minerals and vitamins the person has,' says Perretta. 'Then we check out essential fatty acids because they are one of the basic building blocks of the brain and if you don't have enough or if they are being broken down too quickly, then you can be in trouble.'

The team also check the level of an amino acid called homocysteine, since higher than normal amounts in the blood are a good guide to the fact that the basic body chemistry isn't working very well. Most patients are also tested for allergies, using the latest pinprick blood test that has performed very well in a recent double-blind trial.[41]

'There is a pattern of physical symptoms we see quite often,' says Perretta, 'which is linked to sub-optimum nutrition. These patients have ear, nose and throat problems, with excess mucus and an above-average number of infections. That's combined with some kind of skin rash or allergy, like eczema, as well as a food intolerance of some sort. Finally, they suffer from chronic constipation or diarrhoea because their guts are disordered.'

This was very much the pattern that showed up with David. The tests showed that his zinc levels were low and he had raised levels of aluminium, which can be toxic. He also had high homocysteine levels and intolerance to dairy foods. But David's tests also showed something else. He had an excessive amount of what are called pyrroles in the urine. These act as oxidants and leach nutrients out of the body. The antidote is more nutrients, including B6, zinc and other antioxidants.

The key insight at the Brain Bio Centre is that when you sort out these imbalances, not only do the physical symptoms clear up but so do the psychological ones that came with them. This approach assumes that body and mind are seamlessly integrated. So high homocysteine is linked with heart disease but is also associated with depression. Food intolerances can show up as skin problems or ADHD. Perhaps the most interesting link in David's case comes with the high level of pyrroles, which has been linked with social phobia – a fearful reaction to strangers.

What's emerging here is the enormous flexibility of the new medicine. It can fit in with virtually any existing set-up. A doctor trained in nutrition might run his own clinic like Lindberg's, and form links with local sports centres and adult education classes so he could prescribe the relevant cookery and exercise classes needed. Or a regular doctor might work closely with a nutritional therapist, who in turn might liaise with a psychologist over cases involving depression or anxiety.

Cognitive behavioural therapy is likely to be far more effective for a patient who isn't feeling down because of high homocysteine levels or who has the kind of difficulty with focusing attention that can be helped with proper levels of fish oils. Professional athletes already pay a lot of attention to their nutrition. There's no reason why sports coaches in schools shouldn't be more involved in what their pupils are eating. And why stop at sport? The recent focus on school meals in the UK has led a number of teachers to make the link between academic performance and what children are eating.

A leading light in this field is the Food for the Brain Foundation, which is currently working with schools to develop an eating programme for children at school and at home that maximises their performance (for details, see www.foodforthebrain.org). Both parents and children take part in educational activities, which encourage the children to eat healthily. They are also given multivitamins and essential fat supplements every day.

Mainstream mantras

All of this sophistication is a far cry from the way mainstream medicine usually views the nutritional approach. While every doctor repeats the mantra about the importance of a healthy lifestyle, their hearts aren't really in it, which is part of the reason why they are generally so hopeless at helping patients through the necessary changes. What you can do about that is covered in the next chapter.

Reports in medical journals about lowering risk factors regularly make an obligatory nod in the direction of healthy living, but then remark that people aren't going to do that and get on to the latest drug study. Take, for example, a recent UK report that highlighted the real long-term crisis looming for the NHS: by 2031 the number of people over 65 is set to rise by over 50 per cent and the number of people with heart disease by 44 per cent, which will ratchet up the drug bill enormously. There could be fewer cases if people lead healthier lifestyles, the authors commented, but concluded limply: 'recent trends suggest this may not happen.'[42] Nothing doctors can do about that, then.

There is no serious disagreement with the fact that many people are eating themselves into an early grave. 'Diet-related diseases cost the NHS well over £15 billion a year,' according to Susan Fairweather-Tait of the

Nutrition Division, Institute of Food Research at Norwich Research Park. But the logical conclusion that actively discovering what aspects of patients' diets need improving, and helping them to do that, is largely ignored. 'Current medical practice places too great an emphasis on the use of drugs for disease prevention or control,' says Fairweather-Tait, 'because it is an easier alternative to implementing changes in diet and lifestyle. But the latter in fact can be far more effective and have obvious physiological and economic benefits.'[43]

However, the economic madness of putting huge numbers of people on costly preventative drugs for a few to benefit (see Chapter 2) may soon force a change. Take statins, on which the NHS spends more than on any other class of drug. The emerging evidence is that their role in preventing heart disease is minimal.

Many people may not be aware that deaths from heart disease have been dropping for some years – a decline of 54 per cent (68,000 fewer deaths) between 1991 and 2000.[44] Researchers from Liverpool University set out to find why. The biggest cause was the 35 per cent drop in smoking that saved nearly 30,000 lives, mostly in healthy people. Dietary changes resulted in 5,770 fewer deaths, while statin use lowered the rate by 2,135. But nearly 2,000 of those were people who had been given statins after a heart attack. The number of deaths prevented as a result of taking statins during that decade among people who had not actually had a heart attack was reckoned to be just 145! The authors of the research remarked with no further comment: 'this was less than the recently quoted UK government figure of 7,000 lives saved by statins in 2003'.[45]

So sticking with just the drug model doesn't seem a remotely sensible option. With the population ageing at a rapid rate and chronic diseases set to rise in step despite the increasing and increasingly expensive drug consumption, it must make sense for us to begin to demand a much more sophisticated approach to nutrition and other non-drug approaches to staying well and healthy. As we've seen, there is no shortage of examples of what is possible. How you can help to encourage your doctor, the medical charities and even the regulators to be more sympathetic to this new approach to medicine is covered in the final chapter.

21.

Bringing in the New Medicine

How to encourage your doctor to practise food medicine

IF YOU ARE LUCKY you will have a really sympathetic doctor who is interested in and knowledgeable about nutrition or regularly refers patients to nutritional therapists. If you are very lucky, you will have one who provides various forms of practical support if you need to change your eating habits or take more exercise. But most of us are most likely to have doctors who are more or less sceptical about the benefits of supplements and believe that you can get all the nutrients you need from a 'healthy balanced diet'. Faced with an overweight patient, they will recommend a low-fat/high-carbohydrate diet as the way to deal not just with that, but also with a raised risk of heart disease and possibly even type 2 diabetes. By now it should be clear why this is not the best option.

But don't despair. There is plenty you can do about it, although it may need a careful balance of determination and diplomacy. In theory it is now official government policy that patients should be more involved in their health, especially when suffering from chronic disease. A UK government report published very quietly in 2003 (*Securing Good Health for the Whole Population* by Derek Wanless[46]) estimated that involving patients in this way and concentrating on public health measures could save Britain's NHS £30 billion a year by 2022.

However, the gap between government policy and reality is infamously large and it's as well you know the worst before starting out. The simple fact is that when it comes to providing practical help on the best way to stay healthy, doctors have a pretty poor track record. One study, for instance, found that over 400 patients who got a brief 'obesity management training programme' from their doctor actually put on more weight after a year than the control group.[47] Another, an international study published nearly a year after the Wanless report, found that only 27 per cent of British patients felt their doctors had engaged them in making decisions about their health care, or offered them choices – compared with 41 per cent in New Zealand. 'And just 28 per cent reported receiving advice on weight, nutrition and exercise, compared with 52 per cent in the United States.'[48]

All this is set, of course, against a background of a really poor level of healthy living. Just three per cent of Americans are reckoned to follow even the most basic health rules of exercising, eating fruit and vegetables and so on,[49] and no one is suggesting the UK population is very much better. Only 20 per cent of children manage five portions of fruit and vegetables a day.[50]

Even once you become really ill – say, have a heart attack – the picture doesn't improve. For various reasons such as the influence of the drug companies on doctors' educations, and faulty studies about the benefits of certain supplements and the like, doctors are not all that focused on keeping you fit and healthy. But you might think at least heart-attack patients would get clear advice and support over healthy living once they left hospital; it's not as if there is any shortage of research showing this is very beneficial. In fact, the majority receive no information at all.

Based on a survey of 4,000 patients, researchers estimated that 63 per cent of heart patients treated in English NHS trusts had not had any formal rehabilitation and 37 per cent were not any regular programme to have their heart checked. Nearly half of all patients weren't given any advice on how to change their diet and over 33 per cent got no information about exercise.[51]

Handling any objections

So despite all the publicity about the importance of tackling obesity, encouraging people to exercise and the benefits of five to six servings of fruit and vegetables a day, you are dealing with a profession that still isn't entirely committed. But by now you should be aware of just how much evidence there is on the non-drug side, and it is certainly worth having a go at changing medical hearts and minds. As we saw in an earlier chapter there is no shortage of misinformation about the possible dangers of taking vitamins and supplements and 'natural cures' in general. So one place you might want to start – politely and diplomatically – is by countering some of the misinformation about the nutritional approach that your doctor may believe.

Here are the top five objections that doctors are likely to raise when you tell them about the low-GL diet and lifestyle changes you have taken on, or want to, and how to answer them.

Objection 1: *The diet seems reasonably sensible but you don't need supplements and you need to keep taking the drugs. Your improvement is really just a 'one-off' apparent success. It's probably got little to do with your new regime.*

Response: Ask your doctor what are his/her criteria for lowering or stopping medication? Is it being symptom-free, having a normal blood-sugar level or blood pressure? Make sure these are measured to objectively evaluate your new treatment. If this has been done already and you've got the measured proof of change, then insist firmly but not evangelically that this approach, diet, supplements or lifestyle change, has made a big difference and suggest they recommend it to others. Give them the details of the practitioner you saw or the book you read.

> Mary was diagnosed with systemic lupus erythematosis (SLE) and Sjögren's syndrome. Both of these conditions are auto-immune diseases, thought to be brought on by a virus. This means that Mary's body made antibodies that attacked her own body cells – auto-antibodies. Her symptoms included extreme fatigue, inflamed joints, leg haemorrhages, dry mouth and eyes. She came to see me (Patrick) for some nutritional advice.
>
> I put her on a healthier diet, cutting out all caffeine and limiting alcohol, and recommended a multivitamin and mineral formula containing plenty of B vitamins and additional vitamin C. Despite having had a very poor prognosis from her GP, she began to improve within three months.

After eight months her energy had returned to normal, her joints were no longer swollen or painful. In fact, her only remaining symptom was dry eyes. Even her auto-antibody count came down from 200 to 26.

Objection 2: *There is no evidence these treatments work.*
Response: This is a common one but, if you've looked at Part 3 of this book you'll see that it is just not true. Any properly trained nutritional therapist will be just as keen on basing treatment on the evidence as a doctor. In fact, you might argue that the diet and exercise approach is more firmly based in the evidence.

Not only have we seen that an average of 20 per cent of all drugs, and not just ones for children, are prescribed off-label – meaning that the trial evidence for the effectiveness is simply not there – but the evidence upon which doctors have based their prescribing often turns out to be faulty. Of course, they are not going to take kindly to this kind of comment from you, but you could show them this book, including the list of references, or even offer to lend it to them and ask for their opinion about the non-drug alternatives that you'd be interested in trying.

But it's still open to the sceptical doctor to ask for more evidence, and this is where you encounter one of the major blocks to getting nutritional medicine properly established. The amount of money available for testing non-drug therapies in tiny compared with the billions lavished on new pharmacological fixes and tracking down fresh genetic targets. One of the most striking conclusions of the government's Wanless report was that just getting good data on the effectiveness of such basic and obvious public-health issues as diet, drinking, smoking and exercise hasn't been done properly.

After setting out the possibility of saving billions of pounds by taking seriously the principle of encouraging patients to develop healthy lifestyles, Wanless admitted that there was a problem. 'At the moment,' he wrote, 'it's hard to know what the most effective interventions are' because nearly *all* the research money is tied up in the biomedical approach. But, he went on, 'the situation is too urgent to wait for the evidence. Promising initiatives should be evaluated as a series of natural experiments.'

The idea that we need some sort of funding for non-commercial treatments is a conclusion that a number of other experts and reports have reached. Writing about the way pharmaceutical companies dominate research, Richard Smith, ex-editor of the *British Medical Journal* and now Chief Executive of United Health Europe, comments: 'What we need is more public funding of trials, particularly of large head-to-head trials of all the treatments available for treating a condition.'[52] In other words, rather than just testing a new anti-inflammatory drug to treat arthritis against a placebo, try it out against omega-3 oil or even against a diet that reduces allergic reactions.

It's a radical idea that would certainly present challenges about how best to design the trials – the classic clinical trials now used to test drugs are based on comparing the effect of one molecule with another, rather than with the complex interactions of a diet or exercise. However, what patients actually want to know from research is what the best treatment is, not whether this drug is better than nothing. Positive results would also give the stamp of approval to non-drug treatments that would make doctors much more comfortable about using them.

Non-commercial testing was also one of the recommendations of the Parliamentary Health Committee's report, which proposed that: 'areas of research not of direct interest to the pharmaceutical industry, such as non-pharmacological treatments, but that may significantly benefit patients, should be funded by the government'.[53]

It's not just eminently sensible but also vital for developing a scientifically based system of medicine. Think about it. Suppose you were trying to plan a national transport policy but all the research was carried out by car manufacturers. Wouldn't be just a little difficult to get reliable evidence about the value of trains, buses and bikes? Unfortunately, in their response to the Parliamentary report, the government didn't even consider funding non-commercial research. We believe it should.

Objection 3: *Non-drug therapies are supposed to be very safe but supplements can have serious side effects. You should stop taking them except, perhaps, an RDA-type multivitamin.*
Response: A recent survey found that 29 per cent of people overall, and 37 per cent of people in the southeast of England take supplements –

and that the percentage of people taking supplements, and the amount of supplements that they take, is increasing.[54] So, despite all the negative hype, people are perceiving, and probably experiencing, benefits. Against this backdrop of almost 20 million people in Britain taking supplements, critics have a hard time coming up with any more examples of damage than maybe a few cases of diarrhoea as a result of taking high doses of vitamin C. That doesn't even begin to compare with over 2,000 people killed by gastrointestinal damage from aspirin-type drugs in the UK every year and over 10,000 people who die from prescription drugs.

Ask your doctor what their specific concern is in the context of your health problem. Is it the B vitamins, the vitamin A, E or C? Ask them how much they consider safe and on what evidence. Go armed with the evidence of the benefit of the supplements we recommend in this book, complete with the list of references. Too often doctors buy into an anti-supplement stance without ever having really examined the evidence. Ask them to come back to you with their opinion and of course show them Chapter 18 which details the bad science behind the main vitamin scares.

Objection 4: *Proper medicines go through stringent testing and so should any alternatives. I can't prescribe alternatives without this evidence.*
Response: It is hard to understand how anyone who knows anything about the way research trials are funded can say this with a straight face. Most non-drug practitioners would love to have a proper test of their treatment as compared with a drug. But drug companies pay for most of the trials and the higher the hoops (large-scale, randomised double-blind trials), the higher the cost and the higher the pharmaceutical companies' grip on the kind of research that gets done. The need for more robust research on new medicine approaches is obvious and we are campaigning for it. We would like to see it done in a way that does not conceal inconvenient data or downplay side effects. However, the fact is that there's a lot of positive research already and the downsides are minimal.

Ask your doctor if their concern is primarily about side effects. How confident are they that drug treatments are less likely to produce side effects than non-drug approaches? Ask them what you have to lose by exploring this option of your own free will, under their supervision.

Objection 5: *Health care involves wanting to get as near to the truth as possible but not giving vulnerable individuals false hope.*
Response: Absolutely. As the recent report by the parliamentary health committee found, doctors are being denied proper information about the drugs they are prescribing by drug companies' spinning of the data. A lot of false hope must have been generated as a result. Sleeping pills are still prescribed in their millions even though studies have shown they are not as effective as psychotherapy. What we need is doctors and patients working together with access to reliable information on both drug and non-drug medicine – and it starts with you giving this kind of information to your doctor.

How to 'train' your doctor

Once you have got the objections to the nutritional non-drug approach out of the way, you can then move on to establishing more of a two-way relationship with your doctor, so that you both decide on treatments together. Some useful hints about how you might go about it come from research done at the University of Michigan in the US, showing how important it was for patients and their doctors to agree on the basics, which is what are we trying to do here. The research team found that a key reason doctors weren't too successful at managing lifestyle treatments is that their goals weren't the same as the patients'.

The researchers asked 127 diabetes patients and their doctors to list their top three treatment goals and top three treatment strategies. Remarkably, only five per cent of the 'doctor patient pairs' agreed on all three goals and just ten per cent on all three treatment strategies.[55] The chances of successful and enduring lifestyle changes under those circumstances don't seem great.

Part of the problem the researchers identified was that the doctors were used to telling patients what to do 'often without giving very much information or being aware of the obstacles the patients may face'. It's not much use telling patients to eat fewer sweets, and more whole foods, fruit and vegetables without finding out about the complex psychological patterns that can often be associated with food – they may see it as a form of comfort, for instance – and helping them with buying and preparing the unfamiliar foods they may be recommended, as well as offering emotional and practical support as they make other lifestyle changes.

These problems remain not only because doctors aren't trained in the nutrition and lifestyle approach, but also because they believe the current system doesn't give them the time for it. They've got enough patients to see in a day without having to plan menus or map out exercise routines. All of which is perfectly true but, as we saw in the last chapter, they don't have to do all that themselves – they could collaborate with nurses, coaches and trainers, for instance. But the broad principles underpinning nutritional and non-drug medicine fit much better with the ideals that may well have originally prompted them to become a family doctor in the first place.

Doctors and nutrition – a marriage made in heaven

In conventional medicine, the doctors' main focus has been on treating people who are ill in order to reduce their risk of getting worse – secondary prevention. If you ask them why, they might reply that preventing people from getting ill in the first place, or primary prevention, isn't very effective. A major piece of evidence for this is a study by the respected Cochrane Collaboration that analysed ten primary care studies, involving counselling or education to lower cardiovascular risk, and found only a modest reduction and no change in the rate at which people died.[56]

Interestingly, though, the study concluded that the reason for the poor results could be that doctors are 'lacking the confidence or skills to influence complex behaviours like diet or smoking'. So a vicious circle develops: doctors don't concentrate on improving health because they find it doesn't work and the reason it doesn't work is because they aren't very good at it. Another reason given for skimping on primary care is a well-known estimate that you have to treat about five times as many people in primary prevention to prevent a heart-disease death as you do in secondary prevention.

But events are rapidly overtaking this establishment view. A recent analysis suggests that these figures are faulty.[57] Instead of being a waste of resources, preventing deaths with primary care turns out to be far more effective. The paper concludes: 'A death prevented or postponed in a patient with recognised coronary heart disease (secondary prevention) gained an additional 7.5 years of life vs. one prevented or postponed with primary prevention gained an additional 21 years.'

Now this may not be good news for ministers wrestling with pensions provision but from a health perspective the conclusion is obvious: 'The figures support the population prevention approach.' When you add that to the research mentioned in the last chapter, showing that the number of people over 65 is set to increase by over 50 per cent with a very high proportion of them expected to develop heart disease – let alone a range of other chronic disorders – it's obvious that there is going to have to be a switch of focus.

So on the one side you have mainstream physicians who in the past haven't been that hot on primary prevention but are going to have to get much better at it; and on the other side, practitioners of nutritional medicine whose whole expertise is in primary prevention and in keeping their patients healthy. Bringing them together would cover it all: a marriage made in heaven.

There are bonuses for doctors who adopt this approach too. Making the best use of cutting-edge modern medicine to analyse what is happening with a patient's metabolism and then working out what combination of non-drug treatments will bring it up to optimum performance is much more challenging and satisfying than simply prescribing the latest drug that, at best, will keep the symptoms at bay. It's a chance to claw back some of the clinical freedom that an exclusively drug-based model has taken away. Patients, too, are given more control and involvement (a well-documented stress reducer) rather than passively swallowing the prescribed drugs.

Once you've got your doctor on-side by dealing with the objections and pointing out the advantages, you've made a good start. But like all new relationships, there are plenty of things that can go wrong. One way is to improve co-operation is to make sure that you and your doctor have the same goals.

Keeping your doctor on-side

A major aim for you might be to manage your health problems over the long term without having to rely on drugs. So a good starting point would be to make sure you and your doctor are rowing in the same direction. Begin by letting them know what you want and ask what was expected of you. You also need to let them know when something isn't working for you.

Suppose that you are a diabetic and you are aware of all the research showing how effective diet and exercise are in treating diabetes. Ideally you would want your doctor to help you in that and you might assume that they would be aware of that research too. In fact, the Michigan study (see page 381) about the clash between doctors' and patients' goals, found that while most of the patients had 'avoiding insulin' and 'getting off all medications' at the top of their lists, the doctors' lists had 'lowering blood pressure or cholesterol levels' as first priority. Although three-quarters of the patients had high blood pressure, only 15 per cent thought it was a top priority to lower it. More evidence, if it was needed, that even when the research shows that non-drug treatments are effective, doctors still favour the pills.

So the first step to making sure that you and your doctor are working together is to let them know what your goals are and to check that the doctor agrees with them, so you can work together on your treatment. This is easy to say, but it can be hard to do, and can sometimes involve your having to take an independent line. What can be involved is illustrated by the case of Linda, who had to battle to get her doctor on-side but eventually managed it.

She was 43 when she was diagnosed with diabetes and prescribed medication. Her goal was to get her diabetes and her weight under control so she didn't have to be on medication for the rest of her life. However, she only got some rudimentary advice about diet and leaflets from her doctor, which weren't enough to catalyse the major change in her diet she knew she needed. She was still addicted to sweet foods and was actually gaining weight.

So Linda decided to take matters in her own hands. She bought *The Holford Low-GL Diet* book and attended Patrick Holford's 100 % Health weekend workshop, where she learnt about the benefits of a low-GL diet, how to prepare the meals and which supplements to take to stop her craving for sweet foods. This is how she described the experience:

'When I first started I thought it would be difficult. The thought of cooking three meals a day with all these new foods was daunting. But it's been so easy. My whole family used to be total chocaholics, eating sweets and chocolate every day. None of us have eaten any chocolate or sweets [since the course]. It's a miracle. We've had no cravings. I would never have believed this is possible. It's quite unbelievable.

My daughter, who loses weight very slowly, has lost between 11 and 13lb [5 and 6kg], I've lost 16lb [just over 7kg], my husband has lost 18lb [8kg], and my son, who is not so overweight, has lost 11lb [5kg] — all in the last six weeks.

The other thing is the energy. I was permanently tired. I could have spent the whole day in bed. Now my energy level is incredible. We are all feeling great.'

But then Linda encountered a problem, precisely the kind that a sympathetic doctor could have helped her with. From being too high, her blood-sugar levels went too low — the condition known as 'hypo' — when she took the sulfonylurea drug prescribed by her doctor. This was almost certainly because the new diet was doing its job, both stabilising her blood sugar and improving her sensitivity to insulin. At this point, in an ideal world, you might expect her doctor to have been jubilant — after all, Linda was better and was going to save the NHS lots of money. You might also have imagined he would want to investigate how she did it so he could recommend the method to other patients.

No one likes having their expertise challenged, however, especially by a system they have been taught to regard as inferior. The obvious solution to Linda's problem was to reduce her medication, but her doctor told her that there was no need for that. So once again she took matters into her own hands and started taking less of the drug anyway — something many people might not have had the confidence to do.

That reduced the hypos and at that point Linda might have abandoned her doctor. That's certainly what a lot of people do when they find a non-drug treatment that works for them. But instead she went back to him again. This time he was more sympathetic and stopped the drug completely, recognising that her new diet had made it redundant.

If you are committed to spreading the word about nutritional medicine and boosting support for it in the process, what Linda did was certainly the better option. The more people who continue to work with their doctors, the faster change is likely to happen. Of course, there are going to be times when you and your doctor going to be unable to work together. If that happens, see the 'Finding a "new-medicine" doctor' box below.

FINDING A 'NEW-MEDICINE' DOCTOR

If you are looking for a new doctor, here are a few questions worth asking:

- How do you feel about prescribing drugs for chronic conditions such as heart disease, diabetes and arthritis? Do you recommend specific diets?

- Do you actively encourage non-drug approaches? Do you refer to nutritional therapists, counsellors, osteopaths?

- How is your practice involved in primary prevention?

- What's your view on nutritional supplements?

If you draw a blank on any of these questions, this isn't the new doctor for you.

However, staying with a doctor who isn't particularly committed to 'new medicine' won't inevitably involve conflicts and challenging their judgement. As we saw in the last chapter, many of the most effective approaches used in clinics applying nutritional medicine don't need a doctor. You could suggest that your doctor refers patients like you to a nutritional therapist, or to a diet and nutrition club or to a weekend course (see Appendix 1, page 392). Meanwhile, if you've found 'outside help', make sure this practitioner contacts your doctor to explore ways of working together. There is no shortage of relatively simple changes that evidence and experience suggest can make a big difference.

You can also keep yourself informed. Although it is illegal to provide anything but the most general information about the action of any nutritional product in the place it is being sold, there are still plenty of other sources, such as books like this one, health newsletters, medical journals on the web and talking to your health-care practitioner, especially nutritionists.

You may only be interested in making nutritional medicine work for you, which is fine. But many people, once they find out what it can do for them, want to spread the word. If that's how you feel, then there is plenty more that you can do.

Encourage charities to help

Given the research showing that, where possible, many patients with chronic disorders would like to handle their condition without drugs, charities could do more to help them. Besides encouraging your doctor to become more aware of nutritional medicine, if you belong to one of the big medical charities you could check out just how much of their research funding is directed in finding yet more drug targets. Assuming you can get some like-minded supporters, you could start to campaign for maybe 50 per cent of funds to be devoted to non-drug approaches.

Of course a major reason why most charity research is dominated by the biomedical approach is because many of them receive considerable funding from the drug companies. Depression Alliance, for instance, is estimated to receive 80 per cent of its funding from drug companies. This level of drug-industry funding makes it increasingly difficult to remain impartial when evaluating the evidence for different treatments.

Often the role of drug-company funding is not made clear, as in the website funded by the UK Department of Health for the charity ADDISS (Attention Deficit Disorder Information and Support Service). This charity was also found to receive significant funding from several of the companies manufacturing variations on the Ritalin-type drugs prescribed to children with ADHD.[58] Recently, there have been moves to make charities more transparent about the source of their funding, but a shift in their research priorities would be even more valuable.

So, if you are a member of a charity, find out how much of their funding is from drug companies and, if they carry out research, how much is for non-drug approaches. If you don't like what you see, start a petition among like-minded members and propose to the board of governors to redress the balance. Also, let us know by emailing what you find to info@foodismedicine.co.uk.

Write to your MP or political representative

Now that you are aware of how vested interests and legal restrictions keep nutritional medicine on the fringes, you don't have to take that lying down. In most countries it won't become widely available to the millions who could benefit without changes to the law. That means getting involved with politics, campaign groups and contacting your political representative. So within the pages of this book there are 2 postcards for you to send to your MP and MEP or political representative to let them know your views. Hugely popular campaigns in the UK have already prevented legislation to outlaw certain supplements. So please take the time to complete these postcards and, in return, we'll send your MP a copy of this book if you let us know on our website www.foodismedicine.co.uk.

Better still, write them a letter arguing the case for:

- Legal recognition that food has a role to play in both prevention and treatment of disease

- A proper risk-assessment process to decide the upper limits of food supplements

- A proper risk-assessment system that will allow claims about benefit from nutrients

- Having food supplements excluded from current legislation affecting medicines.

If you live outside Britain many of the issues will be the same, but you'll need to write your own letter to your political representative making similar points. Also join your country's consumer health group to fight against any unnecessarily restrictive upper levels for nutrients or legislation that inhibits the truth being said about nutritional medicine. In Resources, page 405, you'll find the details of organisations campaigning for the freedom for people like you to access and be informed about nutritional medicine. They can advise you how best you can help.

A TEN-POINT PRESCRIPTION FOR GOOD MEDICINE

- Split the drug watchdogs – in the UK, Canada, the US and other countries the regulatory agency both licenses drugs and checks for dangerous side effects afterwards. This makes for an impossible conflict of interests and threatens our health.

- Experts on nutrition should sit on the drug regulatory committees to present the case for nutritional alternatives and explore ways in which nutritional medicine can be effectively used and claims made for it.

- Proper funding of national schemes for reporting adverse drug reactions (ADRs), such as the Yellow Card scheme in the UK.

- Campaign to encourage doctors and patients to report adverse side effects from treatments.

- Campaign to encourage doctors to take advantage of the health-boosting techniques developed by nutritional medicine and non-drug therapies.

- Establish a government-funded body to test nutritional and non-drug treatments against new drugs and against older ones too.

- Lobby health charities to spend at least a third if not half their research budget to investigate benefits of nutritional and non-drug therapies.

- Mandatory publishing of clinical trials so we can see which were successful and which were not. An independent body will need to maintain the register.

- A requirement for trials that actually relate to the people who are going to be taking the drugs. Subjects in clinical trials are often highly selected. They are frequently younger than the people who will actually be taking the drugs and they rarely have multiple disorders.

- Legal recognition that food has a role to play in both prevention and treatment of disease.

The way forward

You are part of a slow but irresistible change in the way medicine is practised. For years the medical establishment has dismissed all forms of treatment that didn't fit into the drugs and surgery model as unscientific. Some 26 years ago, the *British Medical Journal* published a paper about complementary/alternative medicine, 'The flight from science', which suggested that some aspects of it 'ought to be as extinct as divination of the future by examination of a bird's entrails'.[59]

It is a battle that still goes on today. In May 2006, a group of eminent British doctors headed by Professor Michael Baum wrote to all hospitals in the NHS urging them not to waste funds on unproven treatments, and that unless non-drug treatments had solid clinical trial evidence to back their use, they should not be available on the NHS.[60]

But Professor Baum's call is the last gasp of an era. As we have seen, drug-based medicine's claim to be firmly scientific is often shaky if not completely unfounded. During the last quarter century, mainstream medicine has been losing the battle to have exclusive control over how we heal ourselves. Despite constant warnings that going the non-drug route was irrational and most likely dangerous, patients have increasingly voted with their wallets to ignore this advice. In other businesses, the directors of a company that regularly blamed the customers for deserting them, rather than ordering an investigation into their own failings, would be fired.

As we said at the start of this book, medicine is changing because the Internet has made information about treatments that was once the professional preserve of doctors open to all; it is changing because patients have also become discerning consumers; it is changing because the nature of our diseases is shifting from acute to chronic. Most importantly, it is changing because we are all living longer, and no health service can support the cost of the drugs that the medical model suggests we use to treat the rise in chronic diseases. All these changes favour a major shift to the non-drug approach.

Imagine for a moment that medicine was delivering energy rather than health. Drugs are obviously the nuclear option – high-tech, expensive, top-down with the potential to cause considerable collateral damage. Your only responsibility as a consumer is to keep consuming; no need to address any of the issues driving energy demand unsustainably upwards. The nutritional and non-drug approach is the green option – combining high- and low-tech, decentralised, flexible and making use of existing natural systems. Every customer has the option of making a difference by the way they live.

We have emphasised the nutritional approach in this book and covered exercise, psychotherapy, breathing techniques, herbs and other avenues of complementary medicine in less depth, partly because the nutritional approach has the most evidence to support it, and partly because this is more our area of expertise. Eating healthily and taking the appropriate supplements is neither unduly difficult nor expensive, and it makes sense from the point of view of what doctors can recommend in response to the kinds of conditions you're likely to suffer from.

We believe this book can add years to your life – and life to your years. Let us know what works for you and what doesn't by sharing your experiences on our website, www.foodismedicine.co.uk.

Wishing you the best of health,

Patrick Holford and Jerome Burne

Appendix 1
100% Health – Creating Tomorrow's Medicine Today

YOU DON'T HAVE to wait for the new medicine of tomorrow. It's already here today. The first big shift is to stop thinking of curing disease and start thinking of promoting health. We call it '100% Health'.

What is 100% Health? You can define it for yourself. Ask yourself the question 'If you woke up 100% healthy how would you know?' You might find yourself listing things like boundless energy, radiant skin, great memory and mood or super-fitness. So why not make it happen – starting now? Rather than waiting for disease to strike, you can take a step in this direction. We've developed these ways of helping you get going.

1. Online 100% Health Profile. This online questionnaire, available at our www.foodismedicine.co.uk website, has been developed specifically to give you an in-depth report on how you are now (for example, the charts on Elaine, on page 104, were derived from her online profile) and exactly what you need to change in terms of diet, lifestyle and supplements to move towards 100% Health. Your goal is to get into the 'optimum' range for each of the key processes we've discussed – from blood-sugar balance to improved digestion.

2. One-to-one Nutrition Consultation. See a nutritional therapist trained in this form of medicine. We've been training just such

professionals since 1984 at the Institute for Optimum Nutrition. If you click 'consultations' at www.foodismedicine.co.uk and enter in your postcode we'll advise you who is best to see in your area.

3. 100% Health Workshop. This is a two-day event that provides a major transformation to your health. You'll learn exactly how to 'tune up' each of the six key factors (from balancing hormones to boosting immunity) necessary for 100% Health, learn how to prepare super-healthy foods, learn a 17-minute revitalising exercise system, and go away with your own action plan of diet, lifestyle changes and supplements. We then follow you up over three months. The workshop includes the online 100% Health Profile. These workshops are highly effective and are offered all over the world. See details on www.foodismedicine.co.uk. We hope interested doctors will start 'prescribing' workshops like these.

4. Fatburner workshops and seminars. If your goal is specifically to lose weight, there are also fatburner workshops and seminar series. You can sign up for a series of seminars and become part of a 'club' that supports you in achieving your goal, based on the low-GL (glycemic load) approach. See www.holforddiet.com for details.

5. 100% Health Newsletter and membership. By becoming a 100% Health member you will receive Patrick Holford's bi-monthly newsletter, with contributions from Jerome Burne, to keep you up to date on new health developments, and the advantages and disadvantages of different treatments including drugs. Our job is to give you the information you need to stay 100% healthy. Membership gives you instant access to all past issues, hundreds of special reports and a Q&A service. See www.patrickholford.com for details.

Appendix 2
Breathing Exercise

THIS BREATHING EXERCISE (reproduced with the kind permission of the Arica Institute, a school for self-knowledge), connects the *kath* point – the body's centre of equilibrium – with the diaphragm muscle so that deep breathing becomes natural and effortless. You can practise this exercise at any time, while sitting, standing or lying down, and for as long as you like. You can also do it unobtrusively during moments of stress. It is an excellent natural relaxant and energy booster, helping you to feel more connected and in tune.

The diaphragm is a dome-shaped muscle attached to the bottom of the rib cage. The *kath* is not an anatomical point like the navel, but is located in the lower belly, about three finger-widths below the navel. When you remember this point, you become aware of your entire body.

You can do this anywhere standing or sitting, but ideally find somewhere quiet first thing in the morning. As you inhale, you will expand your lower belly from the *kath* point and your diaphragm muscle. This allows the lungs to fill with air from the bottom to the top. As you exhale, the belly and the diaphragm muscle relax, allowing the lungs to empty from top to bottom. Inhale and exhale through your nose.

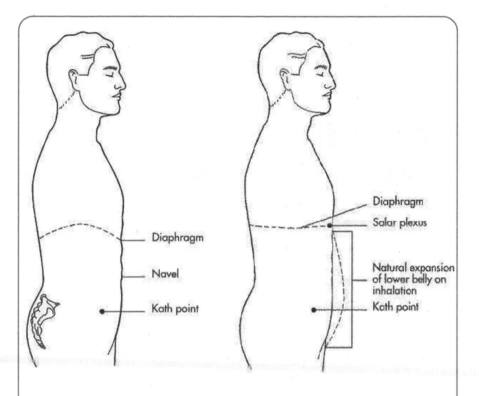

KATH POINT   BELLY EXPANDED

Diakath breathing

1. Sit comfortably, in a quiet place with your spine straight.

2. Focus your attention in your *kath* point.

3. Let your belly expand from the *kath* point as you inhale slowly, deeply and effortlessly. Feel your diaphragm being pulled down towards the *kath* point as your lungs fill with air from the bottom to the top. On the exhale, relax both your belly and your diaphragm, emptying your lungs from top to bottom.

4. Repeat at your own pace.

• Every morning, sit down in a quiet place before breakfast and practise Dia-Kath breathing for a few minutes.

- Whenever you are stressed throughout the day check your breathing. Practise Dia-Kath breathing for nine breaths. This is great to do before an important meeting, or when something has upset you.

© 2002 Oscar Ichazo. Diakath breathing is the service mark and Kath the trademark of Oscar Ichazo. Used by permission.

Measuring carbon dioxide levels in the blood

A capnometer is a device that measures the amount of carbon dioxide (CO_2) you are breathing out. This can be important because losing too much with each breath can destabilise your system. CO_2 is generally considered a waste product – the aim of breathing, we are told, is to get oxygen to the lungs – so you might think the more CO_2 breathed out, the better. In fact, CO_2 is an important regulator of the acid–alkaline balance in your blood. Too little of it and your body will shift in an acidic direction, which can cause many problems, including decreased blood flow to the brain and less oxygen reaching your neurons.

Chronic anxiety can lead to 'over-breathing' and an excessive loss of carbon dioxide. A capnometer can be used to check CO_2 loss. It also works as a biofeedback tool to show the patient how breathing correctly can bring CO_2 levels back to normal. It has been used to successfully help patients suffering from Post Traumatic Stress Disorder by a British medical doctor called David Beales. For further details see:

Mindful Physiology Institute
An organisation set up by David Beales to run educational programmes about breathing for health professionals and interested patients.
www.bp.edu/Index.htm

New Medicine Group (where David Beales works with other
practitioners in London)
144 Harley Street, W1G 7LE
0800 2888 682 (free phone)
www.newmedicinegroup.com

Physiotherapy for Hyperventilation
The organisation has practitioners around the UK who specialise in
breathing problems.
www.physiohypervent.org

Recommended Reading

For more on the nutritional approach

The books below give more details about the kind of diet, supplements and lifestyle changes that are outlined in Part 3 of this book.

General

Holford, Patrick, *The New Optimum Nutrition Bible*, Piatkus, 2005

Arresting diabetes

Haynes, Anthony, *The Insulin Factor*, Thorsons, 2004
Holford, Patrick, *The Holford Low-GL Diet*, Piatkus, 2004
Holford, Patrick and Fiona McDonald Joyce, *The Holford Low-GL Diet Cookbook*, Piatkus, 2005
Lindberg, Dr Fedon, *The Greek Doctor's Diet*, Rodale, 2006

Balancing hormones

Colgan, Dr Michael, *Hormonal Health – Nutritional and Hormonal Strategies for Emotional Well-being and Intellectual Longevity*, Apple Publishing, 1996
Holford, Patrick and Kate Neil, *Balance Hormones Naturally*, Piatkus, 1999
Lee, Dr John, with Hopkins, Virginia, *What Your Doctor May Not Tell You About the Menopause*, Warner Books, 1996

Solving attention and learning problems

Holford, Patrick and Deborah Colson, *Optimum Nutrition for Your Child's Mind*, Piatkus, 2006
Papalos, Demitri and Janice Papalos, *The Bipolar Child*, Broadway Books, 1999

Beating depression

Holford, Patrick, *Optimum Nutrition for the Mind*, Piatkus, 2003

Murray, Michael, *5-HTP, The Natural Way to Overcome Depression, Obesity and Insomnia*, Bantam, 1998

Noell McLeod, Malcolm, *Lifting Depression – The Chromium Connection*, Basic Health Publications, 2005

Puri, Basant K. and Hilary Boyd, *The Natural Way to Beat Depression*, Hodder and Stoughton, 2004

Ross, Julia, *The Mood Cure*, Viking, 2002

Servan-Schreiber, David, *Healing without Freud or Prozac*, Rodale, 2004

Improving your memory

Holford, Patrick, with Shane Heaton and Deborah Colson, *The Alzheimer's Prevention Plan*, Piatkus, 2005

Reducing pain

Darlington, Dr Gail and Linda Gamlin, *Diet and Arthritis*, Vermilion, 1996

Holford, Patrick, *Say No to Arthritis*, Piatkus, 2000

Eradicating asthma and eczema

Holford, Patrick and Natalie Savona, *Solve Your Skin Problems*, Piatkus, 2001

McKeown, Patrick, *Asthma-Free Naturally*, Harper Thorsons, 2003

Helping your heart

Cutting, Dr Derrick, *Stop that Heart Attack*, Class Publishing, 2001

Holford, Patrick, *Say No to Heart Disease*, Piatkus, 1998

For more on the pharmaceuticals industry and drugs

Abramson, John, *Overdosed America: The Broken Promise of American Medicine. How pharmaceutical companies distort medical knowledge, mislead doctors and compromise your health*, Harper Perennial, 2005

Angell, Marcia, *The Truth About Drug Companies: How They Deceive Us and What to Do about It*, Random House, 2004

Deyo, Richard and Donald Patrick, *Hope or Hype – The Obsession with Medical Advances and the High Cost of False Promises*, Amacom, 2005

Healy, David, *Let Them Eat Prozac*, New York University Press, 2004

Kassirer, Jerome P., *On the Take: How Medicine's Complicity with Big Business Can Endanger Your Health*, Oxford University Press, 2005

Law, Jacky, *Big Pharma: How the World's Biggest Drug Companies Market Illness*, Constable & Robinson, 2006

Medawar, C. and A. Hardon, *Medicines Out of Control? Antidepressants and the Conspiracy of Goodwill*, Askant, 2004. Available from www.socialaudit.org.uk/60403162.htm

Moynihan, Ray and Alan Cassels, *Selling Sickness: How Drug Companies Are Turning Us All into Patients*, Allen & Unwin, 2005

Servan-Schreiber, David, *Healing without Freud or Prozac: Natural Approaches to Curing Stress, Anxiety and Depression Without Drugs*, Rodale International Ltd, 2004

Walker, Martin J., *Dirty Medicine*, Slingshot Publications, 1993

Walker, Martin J., and Robert Schweizer, *HRT – Licensed to Kill and Maim: The Unheard Voices of Women Damaged by Hormone Replacement Therapy*, Slingshot Publications, 2006

Walker, Martin J., *The Brave New World of Zero Risk: Covert Strategies in British Science Policy*, downloadable from www.zero-risk.org

Resources

Useful websites

Australian Department of Health and Ageing
www.health.gov.au
Provides statistics, information on research and links to Australian and international health resources.

Center for Medical Consumers
www.medicalconsumers.org/
Information on drugs and treatment with an American focus.

The International Network of Cholesterol Skeptics
www.thincs.org/index.htm
As it says, campaigners who don't believe in the cholesterol and heart attack link. A lot of good material with links to articles from around the world.

Health Care Renewal
http://hcrenewal.blogspot.com/
A searchable blog with a range of postings on drug critiques.

Health Supreme
www.newmediaexplorer.org/sepp/index.htm
'News and perspectives you may not find in the media' site set up by Josef Hasslberger. Fairly eclectic but with a lot of useful links and a database with a number of news stories in this area.

Healthy Skepticism Inc
www.healthyskepticism.org/home.php?
'Countering misleading drug promotion'. A little difficult to find your way around, but a site with much drug company information. Provides links to recommended websites in the UK, Canada, USA, Australia, France, Pakistan and Malaysia.

Medical Research Council South Africa

www.mrc.ac.za

Provides information on research relating to South African medicine.

Medical Veritas

ww.vaccineveritas.com/pages/6/index.htm

'The Journal of Medical Truth', this is a heavyweight website focused on vaccines but covering other material as well.

Mindfully.org

www.mindfully.org/

Wide-ranging eco-aware site with health material, especially on pesticides, and other toxic materials. US based, but provides links to articles from all over the world.

New Zealand Ministry of Health

www.moh.govt.nz

Provides information, links to health-care resources in New Zealand and worldwide, data and statistics.

Public Citizen

www.citizen.org

The main American body campaigning for more rational and safety-aware attitudes to drugs.

Redflags daily

www.redflagsdaily.com/index.php

Very good site with daily postings on a range of health issues.

SA Health Info

www.sahealthinfo.org

Provides information on specific drugs (see www.sahealthinfo.org/admodule.sacendureport7.htm) and general information about health and nutrition.

South African Department of Health

www.doh.gov.za

Statistics, reports, links and resources for all aspects of health.

Therapeutic Initiative
www.ti.ubc.ca/
'Evidence based drug therapy' from the University of British Columbia in Vancouver, Canada. A source of carefully researched and independent reports.

UK Department of Health
www.dh.gov.uk
Provides statistics, health news and resources.

WorstPills.org
www.worstpills.org
A division of Public Citizen, this has detailed accounts of problem drugs but its nutritional information is basic. US based.

Useful addresses

Please help us campaign for change by writing to your MP or MEP using the postcards within the pages of this book.

General

The Brain Bio Centre is a London-based treatment centre founded by Patrick Holford that puts the optimum nutrition approach into practice for people with mental health problems, including learning difficulties, dyslexia, ADHD, autism, Alzheimer's, dementia, memory loss, depression, anxiety and schizophrenia.
For more information, visit www.brainbiocentre.com or call
+44 (0) 20 8871 9261.

British Association for Counselling and Psychotherapy is a leading professional body for counselling and psychotherapy and a useful and trustworthy reference point for anyone seeking information on counselling and psychotherapy in the United Kingdom. BACP also participates in the development of counselling and psychotherapy at an international level. For more information or to find a registered therapist near you: visit www.bacp.co.uk or call + 44 (0) 870 443 5252

The Institute for Optimum Nutrition (ION) offers a three-year foundation degree course in nutritional therapy that includes training in the optimum nutrition approach to mental health. There is a clinic, a list of nutrition practitioners across the UK and overseas, an information service and a quarterly journal – *Optimum Nutrition*.

Contact ION at Avalon House, 72 Lower Mortlake Road, Richmond TW9 2JY, UK, or call +44 (0) 870 979 1122 or visit www.ion.ac.uk

To find a nutritional therapist near you: visit www.patrickholford.com and click on consultations.

New Medicine Group runs a clinic that integrates the best from both mainstream and complementary medicine through a wide-ranging group of highly experienced practitioners.

Contact the NMG at 144 Harley Street, London W1G 7LE, UK, or call +44 (0) 20 7935 0023/+44 (0) 800 2888 682 (freephone in the UK), or email info@newmedicinegroup.com

Specific conditions

Food for the Brain is an educational charity to promote the link between optimum nutrition and mental health. The Food for the Brain Schools Campaign also gives schools and parents advice on how to make kids smarter by improving the quality of food in and outside school.

For more information, visit www.foodforthebrain.org

The Holford Diet Club provides advice and support for weight loss and health improvement through a series of weekly meetings.

For more information, visit www.holforddiet.com

The Hyperactive Children's Support Group is a registered charity that has been successfully helping ADHD/hyperactive children and their families for over 25 years. The HACSG is Britain's leading proponent of a dietary approach to the problem of hyperactivity.

For more information, visit www.hacsg.org.uk

The Natural Progesterone Information Service provides women and their doctors with details on how to obtain natural progesterone information packs for the general public and health practitioners, and books, tapes and videos relating to natural hormone health. For an order form and prescribing details (for doctors), please write, enclosing £1 in stamps and a large self-addressed envelope, to NPIS, PO Box 24, Buxton, SK17 9FB, UK.

The Sleep Assessment Advisory Service provides advice on overcoming insomnia.
For more information, call +44 (0) 28 9262 2266.

Campaigns

The Alliance for Natural Health is a UK-based, pan-European and international not-for-profit campaign organisation working to protect and promote natural health care through the use of good science and good law.
For more information, visit www.alliance-natural-health.org

Consumers for Health Choice is a successful lobbying and campaigning group on natural health matters. CHC is made up of dedicated individuals who actively promote the rights of consumers to have ready access to a wide range of natural health-care products, including vitamins and minerals, herbal remedies and other beneficial and safe supplements. Much of their work is in challenging adverse EU legislation.
For more information, visit www.healthchoice.org.uk

Products and techniques

Breathing tubes. Deviced by Frank Goddard, who suffered from asthma all his life, these tubes are intended to exercise the lungs.
For further information and ordering, see www.diyhealth.co.uk.

Buteyko (pronounced 'bu-tay-ko') is most commonly used as a treatment for those with asthma and other breathing disorders.
Visit www.buteykobreathing. org for a list of qualified teachers worldwide, and information on books and CDs; or you can read Patrick McKeown's *Asthma-Free Naturally* (Harper Thorsons, 2003).

Health Products for Life is an online shop for a range of health-promoting products including the relaxation CD *Silence of Peace*, which will bring you into an alpha state within four minutes; the Elanra range of ionisers to generate negative ions; full-spectrum lighting; and xylitol, the natural sugar alternative, plus a wide range of supplements.
Visit www.healthproductsforlife.com or call +44 (0) 20 8874 8038.

Psychocalisthenics

Psychocalisthenics is an exercise system that takes less than 20 minutes a day, and develops strength, suppleness and stamina and generates vital

energy. The best way to learn it is to do the Psychocalisthenics training. See
www.patrickholford.com (seminars) for details on this or call +44 (0) 20
8871 2949. Also available in the book *Master Level Exercise:
Psychocalisthenics* and on the Psychocalisthenics CD and DVD.
For further information, see www.pcals.com

Laboratory testing

Biolab carry out blood tests for essential fats, vitamin and mineral profiles,
chemical sensitivity panels, toxic element screens, and more. Only available
through qualified practitioners.
Contact Biolab at The Stone House, 9 Weymouth Street, London W1W
6DB, UK, or call +44 (0) 20 7636 5959, or visit www.biolab.co.uk

The European Laboratory of Nutrients (ELN) provide a wide range of
biochemical tests including platelet serotonin profiles, mineral profiles,
fatty acid profile, thyroid function test, hormone profiles and
neurotransmitter tests.
Contact ELN at Regulierenring 9, 3981 LA Bunnik, The Netherlands, or call
+31 (0) 30 287 1492 or visit www.europeanlaboratory.com

Food allergy (IgG ELISA) and homocysteine testing are available through
YorkTest Laboratories, using a home-test kit where you can take your own
pinprick blood sample and return it to the lab for analysis.
Contact FREEPOST NEA5 243 York YO19 5ZZ, UK, call freephone (in the
UK) +44 (0) 800 0746185 or visit www.yorktest.com

Hair mineral analyses are available from Trace Elements, Inc, a leading
laboratory for hair mineral analysis for health-care professionals
worldwide.
Visit www.traceelements.com for more details or contact the UK agent
Mineral Check at 62 Cross Keys, Bearsted, Maidstone, Kent ME14 4HR,
UK. Or call +44 (0) 1622 630044, or visit www.mineralcheck.com

The London Diabetes and Lipid Centre (14 Wimpole St, London W1G
9SX, UK, +44 (0) 207 636 9901) and **The Diagnostic Clinic** (50 New
Cavendish St, London W1G 8TL, UK, +44 (0) 870 789 7000) carry out
detailed metabolic testing.

References

Introduction

1. 'Fizzy drinks health risk', *The Daily Express*, 6 March 2006
2. 'The omega point', *The Economist*, 19 January 2006

Part 1

1. These developments are all well covered in James Lefanu's *The Rise and Fall of Modern Medicine*, Abacus, 2000
2. 'UK Vioxx Cases await Court Hearing', BBC News Online 11 April 2006, http://news.bbc.co.uk/1/hi/health/4901030.stm
3. A. Jack, 'Master or Servant: the US Drugs Regulator is put under Scrutiny', *Financial Times*, 7 January 2005
4. J. Lenzer, 'Secret US Report Surfaces on Antidepressants in Children', *British Medical Journal*, vol. 329, 2004, p.307
5. S. Boseley, 'Antidepressant Linked to Suicide Risk in Adults', *Guardian*, 13 May 2006
6. T. Lieberman, 'Bitter Pill', *Columbia Journalism Review*, July/August 2005
7. F. Hu *et al.*, 'Fish and Omega-3 Fatty Acid Intake and Risk of Coronary Heart Disease in Women', *Journal of the American Medical Association*, vol. 287 (14), 2002, pp. 1815–21
8. H. Tiemeier *et al.*, 'Plasma Fatty Acid Composition and Depression are Associated in the Elderly: The Rotterdam Study', *American Journal of Clinical Nutrition*, vol. 78 (1), 2003
9. W. C. Knowler *et al.*, 'Reduction in the Incidence of Type 2 Diabetes with Lifestyle Intervention or Metformin', *New England Journal of Medicine*, vol. 246, 2002, pp. 393–403
10. A. Trichopoulou *et al.*, 'Modified Mediterranean Diet and Survival: EPIC-elderly Prospective Cohort Study', *British Medical Journal*, vol. 30, 2005, p. 991
11. www.jr2.ox.ac.uk/bandolier/booth/painpag/nsae/nsae.html
12. M. Alexander, 'Vioxx – A Regulatory Timeline', *Andrews Special Report: Vioxx Litigation Issues and Perspectives*, Andrews Publications, 2005. Available from: http://west.thomson.com/product/40358501/product.asp
13. C. Bombardier *et al.*, 'Comparison of Upper Gastrointestinal Toxicity of Rofecoxib and Naproxen in Patients with Rheumatoid Arthritis', *New England Journal of Medicine*, vol. 343, 2000, pp. 150–2
14. D. Mukherjee *et al.*, 'Risk of Cardiovascular Events Associated With Selective COX-2 Inhibitors', *Journal of the American Medical Association*, vol. 286, 2001, pp. 954–9
15. E. Topol, 'Failing the Public Health – Rofecoxib, Merck and the FDA', *New England Journal of Medicine*, vol. 351, 2004, pp. 1707–9
16. E. Topol, 'Failing the Public Health – Rofecoxib, Merck and the FDA', *New England Journal of Medicine*, vol. 351, 2004, pp. 1707–9

17. M. Alexander, 'Vioxx – A Regulatory Timeline', *Andrews Special Report: Vioxx Litigation Issues and Perspectives*, Andrews Publications, 2005. Available from: http://west.thomson.com/product/40358501/product.asp

18. Available at www.pharmacist.com/warningletters/Yr2001/Merck0901.htm

19. J. Graham, 'FDA Knew in 2002 that Vioxx Posed Risk: Agency Chose Not to Warn Doctors', *Chicago Tribune*, 10 Feb 2005

20. J. Abramson, *Overdosed America: The Broken Promises of American Medicine*, Harper-Collins, 2004

21. M. Kaufman, 'FDA Is Criticized Over Drugs' Safety Problems; Response to Approved Medications Cited', *Washington Post*, 24 April 2006

22. A. Jack, 'Master or Servant: The US Drugs Regulator is Put under Scrutiny', *Financial Times*, 7 January 2005

23. K. Griffiths and D. Reece, 'The Pharmaceutical Industry Counts the Cost of the Drugs that Do Not Work', *Independent*, 23 August 2005

24. M. Angell, 'The truth about drug companies', *New York Review of Books*, 15 July 2004. Book published by Random House in 2004

25. M. Pirmohamed *et al.*, 'Adverse Drug Reactions as Cause of Admission to Hospital: Prospective Analysis of 18,820 Patients', *British Medical Journal*, vol. 329, 2004, pp. 15–19

26. M. Pirmohamed *et al.*, 'Adverse Drug Reactions as Cause of Admission to Hospital: Prospective Analysis of 18,820 Patients', *British Medical Journal*, vol. 329, 2004, pp. 15–19

27. Jason Lazarou *et al.*, 'Incidence of Adverse Drug Reactions in Hospitalized Patients: A Meta-analysis of Prospective Studies', *Journal of the American Medical Association*, vol. 279 (15), 1998, pp. 1200–5

28. J. R. Nebeker *et al.*, 'High Rates of Adverse Drug Events in a Highly Computerized Hospital', *Archives of Internal Medicine*, vol. 165 (10), 2005, pp. 1111–6. The number of cases may be even higher than that recorded in 1998. This paper studied admission to a new and highly computerised hospital for 20 weeks in 2000 and found that ADRs accounted for 41 per cent of all hospital admissions.

29. I. Heath, 'Who Needs Health Care – the Well or the Sick?', *British Medical Journal*, vol. 330, 2005, pp. 954–6

30. Common ones include 'daytime sedation, motor incoordination, cognitive impairments (anterograde amnesia), and related concerns about increases in the risk of motor vehicle accidents and injuries from falls' according to M. J. Sateia and P. D. Nowell, 'Insomnia', *The Lancet*, vol. 364 (9449), 2004, pp. 1959–73

31. Editorial, 'Treating Insomnia – Use of Drugs is Rising Despite Evidence of Harm and Little Meaningful Benefit', *British Medical Journal*, vol. 328, 2004, pp. 1198–9

32. M. J. Sateia and P. D. Nowell, 'Insomnia', *The Lancet*, vol. 364 (9449), 2004, pp. 1959–73

33. Professor Vaughn McCall, chairman of the Department of Psychiatry and Behavioral Medicine at Wake Forest University, Winston-Salem, North Carolina, giving evidence to the NIH State-of-the-Science Conference on Manifestations and Management of Chronic Insomnia in Adults, 9 June 2005. Press release from Newswise. McCall's research showed that the most widely used of these is one called trazodone , whose side effects, along with nausea, dizziness and agitation, include insomnia. However, there was one study showing that trazodone was better than a placebo in the first week of treatment, but no better in the second. www.newswise.com/

34. W. Miller, 'Insomnia: drug makers see huge numbers', *Providence Journal* (via Knight-Ridder/*Tribune Business News*), 30 January 2005

35. C. Nathan, 'Antibiotics at the Crossroads' *Nature*, vol. 43, 21 October 2004, pp. 899–902

36. C. Nathan, 'Antibiotics at the Crossroads' *Nature*, vol. 43, 21 October 2004, pp. 899–902

37. R. Moynihan, 'The Marketing of a Disease: Female Sexual Dysfunction', *British Medical Journal*, vol. 330, 22 January 2005, pp. 192–4

38. 'Coroner's drug inquiry call', *BBC News*, 11 March 2003. Available at http://news.bbc.co.uk/1/hi/wales/2841171.stm

39. S. Boseley, 'Four People Dead is Four Too Many', *Guardian*, 9 August 2001

40. J. Law, *Big Pharma: How the World's Biggest Drug Companies Market Illness*, Constable and Robinson, 2006, p. 58

41. D. Graham *et al.*, 'Risk of acute myocardial infarction and sudden cardiac death in patients treated with cyclo-oxygenase 2 selective and non-selective non-steroidal anti-inflammatory drugs: nested case-control study, *The Lancet*, vol. 365 (9458), 2005, pp. 475–81

42. G. Harris, 'New Drugs Hit the Market but Promised Trials go Undone', *New York Times*, 4 March 2006

43. See website www.pharmalive.com – The Pulse of the Pharmaceutical Industry. Summary of a report entitled 'Top 500 Prescription Drugs' contains a chart on this page: http://www.pharmalive.com/special_reports/sample.cfm?reportID=191 Med Ad News May 2005: 'Top 500 prescription drugs'

44. G. Hodge, 'Happiness . . . Is a Pill that Makes You Lose Weight, Sorts Out PMT, and Really Cheers You Up. Its name? Prozac', *Independent on Sunday*, 17 February 2002

45. M. H. Teicher *et al.*, 'Emergence of Intense Suicidal Preoccupation during Fluoxetine Treatment', *American Journal of Psychiatry*, vol. 147, 1990, pp. 207–10

46. H. Melander *et al.*, 'Evidence B(i)ased Medicine – Selective Reporting from Studies Sponsored by Pharmaceutical Industry: Review of Studies in New Drug Applications', *British Medical Journal*, vol. 326, 2003, pp. 1171–3. The research revealed that out of 42 placebo-controlled trials only half had shown a benefit from the drug. But while 19 of those papers had been published, sometimes several times, only six of the unfavourable ones had been published alone, while four others had never been published at all. 'Any attempt to recommend a specific SSRI from publicly available data is likely to be based on biased evidence' the paper concluded.

47. Personal communication with Dr David Healy, reader in psychological medicine at the North Wales Department of Psychological Medicine, Cardiff University, and the leading campaigner on the links between SSRIs and suicide. His main concern was that doctors should be warned of the possibility of suicide among a small section of patients so they could take appropriate action. Among his evidence for this risk was the fact that even before the drug was licensed in the UK, precisely such a warning had been insisted on by the German licensing authorities in 1988. It read: 'Patients must be sufficiently observed until the effects of the anti-depressive effect sets in. Taking an additional sedative may also be necessary.'

48. Personal communication to Jerome Burne from Dr David Healy. He told how in 2000 the American paper, the *Boston Globe*, alerted to the fact that the patent on Prozac was about to expire, conducted a search of the US patent office to discover if there was a replacement in the pipeline. A new form of Prozac, known as R-fluoxetine, had been patented in 1993 (US patent no. 5,708,035). Now a patent application requires that you say why your new version is an improvement. So what were the benefits of R-fluoxetine? 'It will not produce several existing side effects, including akathisia, suicidal thoughts and self-mutilation . . . one of its [Prozac's] more significant side effects.' Precisely the side effects the company had been denying for a decade. The quote is taken from the *Boston Globe* story which in turn is quoting the patent application. L. Garnett, 'Debate about Effects of Prozac Continues As Drug Patent Nears Expiration', *Boston Globe* (Knight-Ridder/*Tribune Business News*), 7 May 2000.

49. A. Khan *et al.*, 'Symptom Reduction and Suicide Risk in Patients Treated with Placebo in Antidepressant Clinical Trials: An Analysis of the Food and Drug Administration Database', *Archives of General Psychiatry*, vol. 57 (4), 2000, pp. 311–7. The total of 5,200 pages of documents examined revealed that not only were the SSRIs no better than the older tricyclic anti-depressants, but they were not even 10 per cent more effective than placebos, which produced an average of a 30.9 per cent improvement in depression.

50. I. C. K. Wong *et al.*, 'Increased Prescribing Trends of Paediatric Psychotropic Medications, *Archive of Disease in Childhood*, vol. 89, 2004, pp. 1131–2

51. M. Frith, 'Dramatic Increase in Overdoses Linked to Antidepressants', *Independent*, 25 February 2005

52. J. Dowards and R. McKie, 'Dark Secrets Lurking in the Drugs Cabinet', *Observer*, 7 November 2004

53. From the official record of the proceedings of the British House of Commons, known as Hansard. In a speech on 23 February 2004, Paul Flynn, the MP for Newport West, stated that in October 1998 the manufacturers of Seroxat had prepared a report headed 'confidential: for internal use only' giving details of studies conducted in 1993 and 1996 on children with Seroxat vs. a placebo that showed an increase in suicides on the drug. However, this data was only made available to the regulators in 2003

54. E. Marshall, 'Antidepressants and Children: Buried Data Can Be Hazardous to a Company's Health', *Science*, vol. 304 (5677), 2004, pp. 1576–7

55. J. Couzin, 'Volatile Chemistry: Children and Antidepressants', *Science*, vol. 305 (5683), 2004, pp. 468–70

56. An internal memorandum of the company involved (GlaxoSmithKline) dated 1998 – five years earlier – discussed these unfavourable results and concluded that their target should be 'effectively to manage the dissemination of these data in order to minimise any potential negative commercial impact'. C. Medawar and A. Hardon, *Medicines out of Control? – Antidepressants and the Conspiracy of Goodwill*, Askant Academic Publishers, 2004, p. 202

57. E. Marshall, 'Antidepressants and Children: Buried Data Can Be Hazardous to a Company's Health', *Science*, vol. 304 (5677), 2004, pp. 1576–7

58. S. Mayor, 'Psychological Therapy Must Accompany Antidepressants in Young People', *British Medical Journal*, vol. 331, 2005, p. 714

59. J. Moncrieff and I. Kirsch, 'Efficacy of Antidepressants in Adults', *British Medical Journal*, vol. 331, 2005, pp. 155–7

60. J. Lenzer, 'FDA Warns that Antidepressants may Increase Suicidality in Adults', *British Medical Journal*, vol. 331, 2005, p. 70

61. S. Mayor, 'NICE Calls for Wider Use of Statins', *British Medical Journal*, vol. 332, 2006, p. 256

62. Confusingly, the UK and the US measure the amount of cholesterol you have in your blood in different ways. In the UK we use 'millimoles per litre' abbreviated mmol/l, while the American use 'milligrams per decilitre' abbreviated mg/dl.

63. This is because statins are recommended if you have a mild to moderate risk of having a heart attack; a risk of between 1/7 and 1/10. It's not hard to show up as having a moderate risk – factors include simply being male and 55 or over; being 45 and male and having one risk factor like smoking, or being female and over 55 and having one risk factor.

64. M. A. Silver *et al.*, 'Effect of Atorvastatin on Left Ventricular Diastolic Function and Ability of Coenzyme Q10 to Reverse that Dysfunction', *American Journal of Cardiology*, vol. 94, 2004, pp. 1306–10

65. J. Abramson, *Overdosed America: The Broken Promises of American Medicine*, Harper-Perennial, 2005

66. Editorial, *British Medical Journal*, vol. 305, 1992, pp. 15–19

67. U. Ravnskov, 'High Cholesterol May Protect Against Infections and Atherosclerosis', *Quarterly Journal of Medicine*, vol. 96, 2003, pp. 927–34. Dr Uffe Ravnskov is a Danish physician and long-time sceptic about the links between cholesterol and heart disease. This commentary shows that in people over 65 higher cholesterol is linked with living longer, possibly because of the role cholesterol plays in the immune system.

68. From an interview by Jerome Burne, *The Times*, 24 January 2004. R. Superko, a fellow of the American College of Cardiology who has developed a treatment plan for heart patients that combines drugs, food, vitamins and exercise asserts: 'My key message is that cholesterol is not the most common cause of heart disease. We've known for 20 years that 50 per cent of people with heart problems have the same cholesterol levels as those who don't.

    'Of course, very high levels are dangerous and should be brought down,' he continues, 'but within the normal range, cholesterol level is a poor predictor of risk.' So lowering it isn't that effective at reducing risk either. 'Statin-type drugs reduce risk by about 25 per cent, which is not good enough. What's worse is drug company publicity has persuaded people that low cholesterol equals low risk. That is deceptive and unfair.' See also his fascinating book: R. Superko, *Before the Heart Attacks: A Revolutionary Approach to Detecting, Preventing and even Reversing Heart Disease*, Rodale, 2004

69. http://www.cbc.ca/story/science/national/2005/04/11/statins050411.html CBC news, 'Improve cholesterol drug prescribing habits, medical team advises', 11 April 2005. Between 1988 and 1992, Toronto's Institute for Clinical Evaluative Sciences (ICES) looked at Canadians aged 18 to 74 who were considered at low risk for heart disease but who qualified for statin therapy, to estimate how many such people would need to take the drugs to save one life.

70. Petition to the US National Institutes of Health seeking an independent review panel to re-evaluate the National Cholesterol Education Program guidelines, 23 September 2004. Available from www.cspinet.org/new/pdf/finalnihltr.pdf This is from the website of the Integrity in Science Project, Center for Science in the Public Interest, 1875 Connecticut Ave. NW #300, Washington DC 20009, US. tel: (202) 777–8374 www.cspinet.org

71. Testimony from Graham Vidler, Head of Policy at *Which?*, before the Parliamentary health committee hearings into the influence of the pharmaceutical industry, 14 October 2004: 'We know that the drug (Zocor) works at a particular dose for high-risk patients. To speed up the reclassification process, it is being allowed to be sold over the counter at a lower dose and to patients at lower risk. We simply do not know if it will be effective for that group, but what that group is being asked to do is spend £13 a month to participate in a clinical trial, to see if the product works in those conditions.'

72. E. W. Gregg *et al.*, 'Relationship of Walking to Mortality Among US Adults with Diabetes', *Archives of Internal Medicine*, vol. 163, 2003, pp. 1440–7

73. J. Shepherd *et al.*, 'Prevention of Coronary Heart Disease with Pravastatin in Men with Hypercholesterolemia', *New England Journal of Medicine*, vol. 333 (20), 1995, pp. 1301–8

74. J. R. Downs *et al.*, 'Primary Prevention of Acute Coronary Events With Lovastatin in Men and Women With Average Cholesterol Levels: Results of AFCAPS/TexCAPS', *Journal of the American Medical Association*, vol. 279 (20), 1998, pp. 1615–22

75. L. Getz *et al.*, 'Estimating the High Risk Group for Cardiovascular Disease in the Norwegian HUNT 2 Population according to the 2003 European Guidelines: Modelling Study', *British Medical Journal*, vol. 331, 2005, p. 551

76. U. Ravnskov *et al.*, 'Controversy: Should we Lower Cholesterol as Much as Possible?' *British Medical Journal*, vol. 332, 2006, pp. 1330–32

77. S. Kelleher and D. Wilson, 'The Hidden Big Business behind Your Doctor's Diagnosis', *Seattle Times*, 26–30 June 2005

78. I. Heath, 'Who Needs Health Care – The Well or the Sick?', *British Medical Journal*, vol. 330, 2005, pp. 954–6

79. Petition to the US National Institutes of Health seeking an independent review panel to re-evaluate the National Cholesterol Education Program guidelines, 23 September 2004. Available from www.cspinet.org/new/pdf/finalnihltr.pdf This is from the website of the Integrity in Science Project, Center for Science in the Public Interest, 1875 Connecticut Ave. NW #300, Washington DC 20009, US. tel: (202) 777–8374 www.cspinet.org See also: Third Report of the Expert Panel on Detection, Evaluation, and Treatment of High Blood Cholesterol in Adults (Adult Treatment Panel III). Details of the financial links between those members of the panel and manufacturers of statins can be found at: www.nhlbi.nih.gov/guidelines/cholesterol/atp3upd04_disclose.htm For a sceptical overview of the value of cholesterol-lowering advice see www.cholesterol-and-health.com/index.html

80. The old UK high level of 5mmol/l before the guideline change in 2001 was equal to 200mg/dl. It's estimated that 70 per cent of people in UK have cholesterol above 5mmol/l, so the number achieving the new target of 3mmol/l is tiny.

81. Petition to the US National Institutes of Health seeking an independent review panel to re-evaluate the National Cholesterol Education Program guidelines, 23 September 2004. Available from Integrity in Science Project, Center for Science in the Public Interest, 1875 Connecticut Ave. NW #300, Washington DC 20009, US. tel: (202) 777–8374 www.cspinet.org 'On July 12, 2004, the National Cholesterol Education Program of the National Heart, Lung and Blood Institute, issued revised guidelines for cholesterol levels advising that people at moderately high risk of developing, but no previous history of heart disease ("primary prevention") and LDL-cholesterol levels between 100 and 129mg/dl be offered the "therapeutic option" of cholesterol-lowering therapy with a statin.'

82. J. Abramson, *Overdosed America: The Broken Promises of American Medicine*, Harper Perennial, 2005. In this book Abramson analyses a study known as ALLHAT ('Major Outcomes in Moderately Hypercholesterolemic, Hypertensive Patients Randomized to Pravastatin vs. Usual Care: the Antihypertensive and Lipid-Lowering Treatment to Prevent Heart Attack Trial (ALLHAT-LLT)', *Journal of the American Medical Association*, vol. 288, 2002, pp. 2998–3007), which started in 1994 and involved over 10,000 people with a high risk of heart disease. There were an equal number of men and women, some in their fifties, some older, some who'd had heart attacks and some who hadn't, some with cholesterol above 130 and some below it. At the beginning of the study patients either got a statin or 'usual care'. By the end of the study, 26 per cent of the 'usual care' patients had also been put on statins. So at the end of the study you had one group of whom just over a quarter had got statins and another group of whom over three-quarters had statins – some had stopped taking them. Now if tripling the number of people taking statins, as the 2001 guidelines had done, was going to bring big benefits, you'd expect much better survival rates in the group most of whom had statins. In fact there was no difference between the two groups. The medical establishment largely ignored these results. As an editorial in the *Journal of the American Medical Association* declared: 'Physicians might be tempted to conclude that this large study demonstrates that statins do not work: however, it is well known that they do.' Abramson comments: 'So much for science-based medicine.'

83. D. Wilson, 'New Blood-Pressure Guidelines Pay Off – for Drug Companies', *Seattle Times*, 26–30 June 2005

84. ALLHAT Collaborative Research Group, 'Major Cardiovascular Events in Hypertensive Patients Randomized to Doxazosin vs Chlorthalidone: The Antihypertensive and Lipid-lowering Treatment to Prevent Heart Attack Trial (ALLHAT)', *Journal of the American Medical Association*, vol. 283 (15), 2000, pp. 1967–75

85. ALLHAT Collaborative Research Group, 'Major Outcomes in High-risk Hypertensive Patients Randomized to Angiotensin-converting Enzyme Inhibitor or Calcium Channel Blocker vs Diuretic: The Antihypertensive and Lipid-lowering Treatment to Prevent Heart Attack Trial (ALLHAT)', *Journal of the American Medical Association*, vol. 288 (23), 2002, pp. 2981–97

86. D. Wilson, 'New Blood-pressure Guidelines Pay Off – for Drug Companies', *Seattle Times*, 26–30 June, 2005. See http://seattletimes.nwsource.com/html/health/sick1.html

87. J. Abramson, *Overdosed America: The Broken Promises of American Medicine*, Harper Perennial, 2005, pp. 107–09

88. B. Dahlof *et al.*, 'Prevention of Cardiovascular Events with an Antihypertensive Regimen of Amlodipine adding Perindopril as required versus Atenolol adding Bendro-flumethiazide as required, in the Anglo-Scandinavian Cardiac Outcomes Trial-Blood Pressure Lowering Arm (ASCOT-BPLA): a Multicentre Randomised Controlled Trial', *The Lancet*, vol. 366 (9489), 2005, pp. 895–906

89. Editorial: 'Behavioural Medicine: Changing Our Behaviour', *British Medical Journal*, vol. 332, 2006, pp. 437–8

90. K. Dunder *et al.*, 'Increase in Blood Glucose Concentration During Anti-hypertensive Treatment as a Predictor of Myocardial Infarction: Population Cohort Based Study', *British Medical Journal*, vol. 326, 2003, p. 681

91. R. E. Ferner, 'Is Concordance the Primrose Path to Health?', *British Medical Journal*, vol. 327, 2003, pp. 821–2

92. G. Harris and E. Koli, 'Lucrative Drug, Danger Signals and the FDA', *New York Times*, 10 June 2005

93. J. Doward, '$90 Million Payout over Child Abuse Drug', *Observer*, 8 February 2004

94. J. Law, *Big Pharma: How the World's Biggest Drug Companies Market Illness*, Constable and Robinson, 2006, p. 76

95. 'Consumers Sue Pharmaceutical AstraZeneca Over Misleading Nexium Campaign: AFL–CIO Joins Suit Alleging Scheme to Deceive Consumers, Increase Profits', 18 October 2004. The case is continuing – see www.communitycatalyst.org/index.php?doc_id=571

96. 'Spin Doctored: How Drug Companies Keep Tabs on Physicians', online journal *Slate*, 31 May 2005

97. R. E. Ferner, 'The Influence of Big Pharma', *British Medical Journal*, vol. 330, 2005, pp. 855–6

98. L. Reich, 'Are GPs In Thrall to Drug Companies?' *Daily Telegraph*, 2 March 2005

99. J. Lexchin *et al.*, 'Pharmaceutical Industry Sponsorship and Research Outcome and Quality', *British Medical Journal*, vol. 326, 2003, pp. 1167–70

100. K. Niteesh *et al.*, 'Relationships Between Authors of Clinical Practice Guidelines and the Pharmaceutical Industry', *Journal of the American Medical Association*, vol. 287, 2002, pp. 612–17

101. R. Taylor and J. Giles, 'Cash Interests Taint Drug Advice', *Nature*, vol. 437, 2005, p. 1070. An investigation by *Nature* found that a third of the academics involved in writing clinical guidelines and who declared a conflict of interest had financial links with the companies who made the drugs they were recommending. Around 70 per cent of the committees (panels) who drew up the recommendations were affected. The report pointed out that less than half of the 200 guidelines studied had any information about

conflict of interests at all and noted that in those ones 'the problem could be even worse'. All the members of one of the committees had financial links with the drug – for the treatment of anaemia in AIDS – that the committee recommended. These guidelines are specifically intended to affect doctors' prescribing habits. 'The practice stinks,' said the deputy editor of the *Journal of the American Medical Association*.

102. L. Wayne and M. Petersen, 'A Muscular Lobby Rolls Up Its Sleeves', *New York Times*, 11 November 2001

103. 'Big Pharmaceuticals Buy More Influence than Ever', *New Scientist*, 16 July 2005. A news item reports that drug firms have spent $800 million since 1998 buying influence, including $675 million on direct lobbying of Congress. During that period, according to the Center for Public Integrity 'federal oversight of the pharmaceutical industry was weakened' and protection for patents was strengthened. The companies spend $87 million on campaign donations. In 2004 alone they spent $128 million on 1,300 lobbyists.

104. For instance, Wyeth, the fifth largest supplier of drugs to the NHS, funds a lobby group – Networking for Industry – which has set up four other groups, the most active of which is the Associate Parliamentary Group for Health (APGH) whose members include MPs, ministers and executives from at least eight drug companies. APGH arranges a range of talks and seminars to advise MPs and staff from NHS and other government departments and to introduce them to drug company executives. Wyeth also provides primary care training programmes for nurses and practices managers. Wyeth has a trust fund worth $3.7 billion to meet claims from patients who say they were damaged by their slimming drugs Pondimin and Redux, which caused valvular heart disease. M. Walker, *Brave New World of Zero Risk: Covert Strategy in British Science Policy*, Slingshot Publications, 2005. Downloadable free from: www.zero-risk.org

105. 'Drug industry: Human Testing Masks Death, Injury; Compliant FDA', 2 November 2005, available at http://www.bloomberg.com/apps/news?pid=specialreport&sid=aspHJ_sFen1s&refer=news

106. M. Petersen, 'Madison Avenue Plays Growing Role in Drug Research', *New York Times*, 22 November 2002

107. R. Smith, 'Medical Journals Are an Extension of the Marketing Arm of Pharmaceutical Companies', *Public Library of Science – Medicine*, vol. 2 (5), 2005, e138

108. P. A. Rochon *et al.*, 'A Study of Manufacturer-supported Trials of Nonsteroidal Anti-inflammatory Drugs in the Treatment of Arthritis', *Archives of Internal Medicine*, vol. 154, 1994, pp. 157–63

109. J. Lexchin *et al.*, 'Pharmaceutical Industry Sponsorship and Research Outcome and Quality', *British Medical Journal*, vol. 326, 2003, pp. 1167–70

110. T. Finucane and C. Boult, 'Commercial Support and Bias in Pharmaceutical Research' *American Journal of Medicine*, vol. 117, 2004, pp. 842–5. This article explores the association of funding and findings of pharmaceutical research at a meeting of a medical professional society. 'What commercially supported research can be trusted?' asked the authors. 'To make it worse, physicians do not reliably detect bias in the information presented to them' and there is 'no evidence that bias in individual studies is reliably detected and discounted'.

111. L. Eaton, News roundup: 'Editor Claims Drugs Companies have a "Parasitic" Relationship with Journals', *British Medical Journal*, vol. 330, 2005, p. 9

112. J. N. Jureidini *et al.*, 'Efficacy and Safety of Antidepressants for Children and Adolescents', *British Medical Journal*, vol. 328, 2004, pp. 879–83

113. D. William, 'The National Institutes of Health: Public Servant or Private Marketer?' *Los Angeles Times*, 22 December 2004

114. M. Petersen, 'Madison Avenue Plays Growing Role in Drug Research', *New York Times*, 22 November 2002

115. S. Boseley, 'Junket Time in Munich for the Medical Profession – and it's All on the Drug Firms', *Guardian*, 5 October 2004

116. S. Frederick *et al.*, 'Medical Students' Exposure to and Attitudes About Drug Company Interactions: A National Survey', *Journal of the American Medical Association*, vol. 294, 2005, pp. 1034–42

117. R. E. Ferner, 'The Influence of Big Pharma', *British Medical Journal*, vol. 330, 2005, pp. 855–6

118. Parliamentary health committee report, *The Influence of the Pharmaceutical Industry*, April 2005

119. S. Hulley *et al.*, 'Randomized Trial of Estrogen Plus Progestin for Secondary Prevention of Coronary Heart Disease in Postmenopausal Women', *Journal of the American Medical Association*, vol. 280, 1998, pp. 605–13

120. K. McPherson and E. Hemminki, 'Synthesising Data to Assess Drug Safety', *British Medical Journal*, vol. 328, 2004, pp. 518–20. How two researchers, simply by analysing existing trials, found a raised risk for heart disease from HRT back in 1997. At the time the paper was ridiculed but it turned out to be just about right.

121. J. E. Rossouw *et al.*, 'Risks and Benefits of Estrogen Plus Progestin in Healthy Post-menopausal Women: Principal Results from the Women's Health Initiative Randomized Controlled Trial', *Journal of the American Medical Association*, vol. 288 (3), 2002, pp. 321–33

122. S. Frederick *et al.*, 'Medical Students' Exposure to and Attitudes About Drug Company Interactions: A National Survey', *Journal of the American Medical Association*, vol. 294, 2005, pp. 1034–42

123. P. Vallance, 'Developing an Open Relationship with the Drug Industry', *The Lancet*, vol. 366, 2005, pp. 1062–4

124. S. Schneeweiss *et al.*, 'A Medicare Database Review found that Physician Preferences Increasingly Outweighed Patient Characteristics as Determinants of First-time Prescriptions for COX-2 Inhibitors', *Journal of Clinical Epidemiology*, vol. 58, 2005, pp. 98–102

125. S. Morgan *et al.*, '"Breakthrough" Drugs and Growth in Expenditure on Prescription Drugs in Canada', *British Medical Journal*, vol. 331, 2005, pp. 815–16

126. J. Law, *Big Pharma: How the World's Biggest Drug Companies Market Illness*, Constable and Robinson, 2006, p. 127

127. R. Ferner, 'The Influence of Big Pharma', *British Medical Journal*, vol. 330, 2005, pp. 855–6

128. An example of the MHRA's culture of secrecy and intimacy with the drug companies they were supposed to be regulating emerged when an 'intensive review' was set up to look into SSRIs in the wake of the British *Panorama* TV programme aired on 13 October 2003 (see http://news.bbc.co.uk/1/hi/programmes/panorama/2321545.stm) on with-drawal problems with Seroxat. It turned out that the chairman of the review committee had already sat on an early committee that concluded that withdrawal problems with SSRIs were rare, while two of the other four members had financial links with the manu-facturers of Seroxat. (C. Medawar, A. Hardon, *Medicines Out of Control? Antidepressants and the Conspiracy of Goodwill*, Aksant Academic Publishers, 2004, p. 16). Officially the US Federal Drugs Adminstration bans such links, but between 1998 and 2000 it waived this ban on no fewer than 800 occasions. (D. Cauchon, 'FDA advisors tied to industry', *USA Today*, 24 September 2000)

129. R. Evans and S. Boseley, 'The Drugs Industry and its Watchdog: a Relationship Too Close for Comfort', *Guardian*, 4 October 2004

130. R. Brook, 'Upset and Angry at Lack of Action', BBC News online (http://news.bbc.co.uk/1/hi/programmes/panorama/3710380.stm), 3 October 2004

131. Drug companies actively push off-label prescribing, sometimes with little or no evidence or fabricated evidence. One of the most shocking examples was revealed in a court case involving a drug called Neurontin, licensed to treat epileptic seizures. However the drug company had aggressively pushed for it to be prescribed off-label for at least 11 other neurological conditions, such as ADHD in children, neurological pain and bipolar disorder. A *New York Times* article ('Whistle-Blower Says Marketers Broke the Rules to Push a Drug', 14 March 2002) reported that most of the evidence for the safety and effectiveness of the drug for these uses appears to have been fabrications by the corporation. In 2004 Neurontin was the 16th bestselling drug in the world, with sales worth $2.73 billion.

132. X. Bosch, 'Europe follows US in testing drugs for children', *Science*, vol. 309, 2005, p. 799

133. D. C. Radley *et al.* 'Off-label Prescribing Among Office-Based Physicians', *Archive of Internal Medicine*, vol. 166, 2006, pp. 1021–6. See also S. Boodman, 'Off Label, Off Base? Many Drug Uses Don't Rest on Strong Science', *Washington Post*, 23 May 2006

134. For a fuller account of this see R. Shepherd, 'Death of the Magic Bullet', *Sunday Times Magazine*, 31 July 2005

135. One of the few researchers to have actually looked at the workings of the Yellow Card scheme is Charles Medawar, whose website Social Audit (www.socialaudit.org.uk) played a major role in getting the Seroxat withdrawal problems officially recognised. In his thorough and shocking book with A. Hardon, *Medicines Out of Control? Antidepressants and the Conspiracy of Goodwill* (Aksant Academic Publishers, 2004, pp. 183–94), he describes just how uninformative the Yellow Cards were when he looked at the scheme for the British TV programme *Panorama*. 'Three in four said nothing about past medical history, one in four recorded the outcome of the reported reaction as "unknown". There was no evidence of regulatory follow-up of any reports of suicidal behaviour and injury/poisonings.'

   Medawar and Hardon describe how an average doctor could expect to see about 50 'significant' adverse drug reactions or ADRs in a year, and yet it's estimated that they would report only about 1 per cent of them. Doctors send in about half of the total 19,000 or so Yellow Card reports every year. But poor as their response is, it is positively thorough compared with the performance of hospital doctors, who send in most of the rest, even though it is estimated that out of 6 million UK hospital admissions a year, about 5 per cent involve ADRs. And this is the system that the Committee for the Safety of Medicines (a division of the MHRA, the main drug regulatory body) has described as being 'of the utmost importance for monitoring drug safety'. What's more, the information collected is regarded as secret and has never been subject to any independent review or evaluation. Medawar and Hardon concluded that the reason five investigations into problems of suicide and dependency with SSRIs had found nothing was due to the 'generally low standards of reporting, miscoding and flawed analyses of Yellow Cards [which] had led to substantial under-estimation of risks'. See also: R. Shepherd, 'Death of the Magic Bullet', *Sunday Times Magazine*, 31 July 2005

136. The Parliamentary health committee was clearly unimpressed with the whole post-marketing system. After a drug has been licensed for use by the MHRA the agency is also required to monitor it and watch for signs that it may be causing unexpected side effects and problems. The main method used by the agency for this is the criticised Yellow Card system. In its report, *The Influence of the Pharmaceutical Industry*, 2005, the committee said it didn't believe that the MHRA had 'sufficient resources for effective post-marketing

surveillance', commenting that the 'current process seems to be extremely passive' So it recommended that 'the MHRA employ sufficient numbers of staff to monitor effectively drugs which have been recently licensed' and that it should 'investigate options for the development of more effective post-marketing surveillance systems'.

137. B. Kermode-Scott, 'Agencies "Failed Miserably" over COX-2 Inhibitor', *British Medical Journal*, vol. 330, 2005, p. 113. This was a news item about an editorial in a leading Canadian journal about the post-marketing system in that country which made recommendations that were almost identical to the ones contained in the Parliamentary health committee report, *The Influence of the Pharmaceutical Industry*, 2005. It said that if an active system of surveillance had been used, the problems with Vioxx would have been picked up much sooner. It went on to describe the existing post-marketing system as: 'a fragmentary and under-funded mechanism for post-approval surveillance based on physician reporting of isolated adverse events' and concluded: 'New national agencies are needed to monitor drug safety independently from the approval process . . . only then can doctors and patients be assured an unbiased safety assessment of the drugs they are prescribing and taking.'

138. S. Gottlieb, 'Journal Calls for New System to Monitor Post-marketing Drug Safety', *British Medical Journal*, vol. 329, 2004, p. 1258. This was a report of an article in the *Journal of the American Medical Association* only a few months earlier which recommended something similar in the US. The editors of *JAMA* have called for a 'major restructuring' of the way that US drug regulators respond to concerns over the safety of drugs after they go on the market. The call comes after a group of doctors uncovered delays in issuing warnings about the cholesterol-lowering drug Cerivastatin despite the fact that the manufacturer, Bayer, had evidence of its adverse effects for more than 18 months. The editors propose a new system that uncouples drug approval from post-marketing safety surveillance and adds new oversight requirements.'

139. R. Rabin, 'Lawsuit Questions Drugs Need,' www.newsday.com 9 October 2005. This article is available for free, along with further comment and links, from: www.healthyskepticism.org/library/ref.php?id=3062

140. www.jr2.ox.ac.uk/bandolier/band50/b50-8.html

141. R. Lenzner and M. Maiello, 'The $22 Billion Gold Rush', *Forbes*, 10 April 2006. This article also raises questions about the extent to which the claims are driven by the sufferings of the patients or by lawyers in search of fees.

142. K. Griffiths and D. Reece, 'The Pharmaceutical Industry Counts the Cost of the Drugs that Do Not Work', *Independent*, 23 August 2005

143. K. Griffiths and D. Reece, 'The Pharmaceutical Industry Counts the Cost of the Drugs that Do Not Work', *Independent*, 23 August 2005

144. N. Shute, 'Pills Don't Come with a Seal of Approval', *US News and World Report*, 29 September 1997

Part 2

1. K. Powell, 'Stem-cell Niches: It's the Ecology Stupid!' *Nature*, vol. 435 (7040), 19 May 2005, pp. 268–70

2. S. Frantz, 'Drug Discovery: Playing Dirty', *Nature*, vol. 437 (7061), 13 October 2005, pp. 942–3

3. The UK gets more bang for its bucks than Israel, Finland, Iceland and Germany, whose spend ranges from $1,402 to $2,365; we don't stay healthy for so long as they do in France

(73.1) but then they do spend nearly twice as much, while Australians get 73.2 years for $500 more than the UK. Data taken from the World Health Organization in 2000 and analysed in C. Medawar and A. Hardon, *Medicines Out of Control? Antidepressants and the Conspiracy of Goodwill*, Askant Academic Publishers, 2004, p. 217

4. A. Oswald, 'Will Hiring More Doctors make you Live Longer?' *The Times*, 24 April 2002. See also A. Oswald's website www2.warwick.ac.uk/fac/soc/economics/staff/faculty/oswald/

5. S. Lister, 'Recovery of NHS Under Way at Cost of £90 Billion', *The Times*, 13 July 2004

6. I. Heath, 'Who Needs Health Care – The Well or the Sick?', *British Medical Journal*, vol. 330, 2005, pp. 954–6

7. L. E. Dahners *et al.*, 'Effects of Nonsteroidal Anti-Inflammatory Drugs on Bone formation and Soft-Tissue Healing', *Journal of the American Academy of Orthopaedic Surgeons*, vol. 12 (3), 2004, pp. 139–43

8. C. Paton and I. N. Ferrier, 'SSRIs and Gastrointestinal Bleeding', *British Medical Journal*, vol. 331, 2005, pp. 529–30

9. M. Nelson *et al.*, 'Epidemiologial Modelling of Routine Use of Low Dose Aspirin for the Primary Prevention of Coronary Heart Disease and Stroke in Those Aged >70', *British Medical Journal*, vol. 330, 2005, p. 1306

10. D. Phizackerley, 'Statins: Customers Will Need to Make Informed Choices', *Pharmaceutical Journal*, vol. 272, 2004, p. 706

11. 'Do Statins have a Role in Primary Prevention?' *Therapeutics Letter 48*, April/June 2003

12. P. Breggin, 'Recent US, Canadian and British Regulatory Agency Actions concerning Antidepressant-induced Harm to Self and Others: A review and analysis', *International Journal of Risk & Safety in Medicine*, vol. 16 (4), 2004, pp. 247–59

13. D. Healy *et al.*, 'Lifetime Suicide Rates in Treated Schizophrenia: 1875–1924 and 1994–98 Cohorts Compared', *British Journal of Psychiatry*, vol. 188, 2006, pp. 223–8

14. Much of the work on this has been done by Gloucestershire GP Dr David Beales, who is also a research associate at Buckingham and Chilterns University College and an expert on stress and the direct effects it can have on physiology. Also see J. G. Laffey and B. P. Kavanagh, 'Hypocapnia – A review', *New England Journal of Medicine*, vol. 347, 2002, pp. 43–53

15. A. H. Mokdad *et al.*, 'Actual Causes of Death in the United States 2000', *Journal of the American Medical Association*, vol. 291 (10), 2004, pp. 1238–45. This states: 'The leading causes of death in 2000 were tobacco (435,000 deaths; 18.1 per cent of total US deaths), poor diet and physical inactivity (365,000 deaths; 15.2 per cent), and alcohol consumption (85,000 deaths; 3.5 per cent). Other actual causes of death were microbial agents (75,000), toxic agents (55,000), motor vehicle crashes (43,000), incidents involving firearms (29,000), sexual behaviors (20,000), and illicit use of drugs (17,000). However, poor diet and physical inactivity may soon overtake tobacco as the leading cause of death. The need to establish a more preventive orientation in the US health care and public health systems has become more urgent.'

16. Institute of Medicine, 'The Future of the Public's Health in the 21st Century', November 2002, www.iom.edu/Object.File/Master/4/165/0.pdf

17. R. Molteni, 'Exercise Reverses the Harmful Effects of Consumption of a High-fat Diet on Synaptic and Behavioral Plasticity Associated to the Action of Brain-derived Neurotrophic Factor', *Neuroscience*, vol. 123 (2), 2004, pp. 429–40

18. H. Phillips, 'How Life Shapes the Brainscape: From Meditation to Diet, Life Experiences Profoundly Change the Structure and Connectivity of the Brain', *New Scientist*, 26 November 2005

19. E. M. Friedman *et al.*, 'Social Relationships, Sleep Quality, and Interleukin-6 in Aging Women', *Proceedings of the National Academy of Sciences of the United States of America*, vol. 102 (51), 2005, pp. 18757–62

20. C. P. Fischer *et al.*, 'Supplementation with Vitamins C and E Inhibits the Release of Interleukin-6 from Contracting Human Skeletal Muscle', *Journal of Physiology*, vol. 558 (2), 2004, pp. 633–45

21. J. H. Christensen *et al.*, 'Heart Rate Variability and n-3 Polyunsaturated Fatty Acids in Patients with Diabetes Mellitus', *Journal of Internal Medicine*, vol. 249, 2001, pp. 545–52

22. L. Bernardi *et al.*, 'Effect of Rosary Prayer and Yoga Mantras on Autonomic Cardiovascular Rhythms: Comparative Study', *British Medical Journal*, vol. 323, 2001, pp. 1446–9

23. P. Poirier *et al.*, 'Impact of Diet-Induced Weight Loss on the Cardiac Autonomic Nervous System in Severe Obesity', *Obesity Research*, vol. 11 (9), 2003, pp. 1040–7

24. H. Hemingway and M. Marmot, 'Psychosocial Factors in the Aetiology and Prognosis of Coronary Heart Disease: Systematic Review of Prospective Cohort Studies', *British Medical Journal*, vol. 318, 1999, pp. 1460–7; M. Marmot and R. Wilkinson, 'Psychosocial and Material Pathways in the Relation between Income and Health: a Response to Lynch *et al.*', *British Medical Journal*, vol. 322, 2001, pp. 1233–6

25. P. Lichtenstein *et al.*, 'Environmental and Heritable Factors in the Causation of Cancer – Analyses of Cohorts of Twins from Sweden, Denmark, and Finland', *New England Journal of Medicine*, vol. 343 (2), 2000, pp. 78–85

26. R. A. Waterland and R. L. Jirtle, 'Transposable Elements: Targets for Early Nutritional Effects on Epigenetic Gene Regulation', *Molecular and Cellular Biology*, vol. 23 (15), 2003, pp. 5293–5300

27. A. Motluk, 'The Food You Eat may Change your Genes for Life', *New Scientist*, 17 November 2005. Another more detailed account of this work can be found at the *Science Daily* website in 'Epigenetics Means What we Eat, How we Live and Love, Alters How our Genes Behave', www.sciencedaily.com/releases/2005/10/051026090636.htm

28. J. Bland, *Genetic Nutritioneering*, McGraw-Hill, 1999

29. R. Girling, 'Poison: A Day at Home Exposes us to Ferocious Chemical Bombardment from what we Breathe, Wear and Eat. Even Organic Food Produces Pesticides that Kill Rats. So How can we Stay Safe?' *Sunday Times*, 4 July 2004. Published on the Scientific Alliance Website, http://www.scientific-alliance.org/news_archives/chemicals/poison.htm

30. C. Courtney, 'Long-term Donepezil Treatment in 565 Patients with Alzheimer's Disease (AD2000): Randomized Double-blind Trial', *The Lancet*, vol. 363 (9427), 2004, pp. 2105–15

31. W. H. Herman *et al.*, 'The Cost-Effectiveness of Lifestyle Modification or Metformin in Preventing Type 2 Diabetes in Adults with Impaired Glucose Tolerance', *Annals of Internal Medicine*, vol. 142 (5), 2005, pp. 323–33

32. T. Jones *et al.*, 'Enhanced Adrenomedullary Response and Increased Susceptibility to Neuroglycopenia: Mechanisms Underlying the Adverse Effects of Sugar Ingestion in Healthy Children', *Journal of Pediatrics*, vol. 126 (2), 1995, pp. 171–7

33. G.R. Heninger, 'Serotonin, Sex, Psychiatric Illness', *Proceedings of the National Academy of Sciences of the United States of America*, vol. 94 (4), 1997, pp. 823–4

34. X. Protopopescu *et al.*, 'Orbitofrontal Cortex Activity Related to Emotional Processing Changes Across the Menstrual Cycle', *Proceedings of the National Academy of Sciences of the United States of America*, vol. 102 (44), 2005, pp. 16060–5

35. Press release from American College of Rheumatology, 17 October 2004. Available from: www.rheumatology.org/press/2004/fedutes_nsaidp.pdf This is for the year 2002–2003

36. M. Wolfe and D. Lichtenstein, 'Gastrointestinal Toxicity of Nonsteroidal Anti-inflammatory Drugs', *New England Journal of Medicine*, vol. 340, 1999, pp. 1888–99. This

is for the years 1997 and 1998 and estimates 103,000 hospitalisations and 16,500 deaths each year.

37. F. Shanahan and P. J. Whorwell, 'IgG-Mediated Food Intolerance in Irritable Bowel Syndrome: A Real Phenomenon or an Epiphenomenom?', *American Journal of Gastro-enterology*, vol. 100 (7), 2005, p. 1558

38. W. Atkinson *et al.*, 'Food Elimination Based on IgG Antibodies in Irritable Bowel Syndrome: a Randomised Controlled Trial', *Gut*, vol. 53, 2004, pp. 1459–64

Part 3

1. 'Diabetes spreads to 275 a day', *The Australian*. See www.news.com.au/story/0,10117,19136554-2,00.html?from=rss

2. See www.health24.com/dietnfood/General/15-742-775,29907.asp

3. J. Marx, 'Unravelling the Cause of Diabetes', *Science*, vol. 296 (5568), 2002, pp. 686–9

4. M. Lazar, 'How Obesity causes Diabetes: Not a tall tale', *Science*, vol. 307 (5708), 2005, pp. 373–5

5. L. Hermann *et al.*, 'Vitamin B12 Status of Patients Treated with Metformin: A Cross-sectional Cohort Study', *British Journal of Diabetes and Vascular Disease*, vol. 4 (6), 2004, pp. 401–6. D. Buvat, Letter: 'Use of metformin is cause of vitamin B12 deficiency', *American Family Physician*, 15 June 2004

6. L. D. May *et al.*, 'Mixed Hepatocellular-cholestatic Liver Injury After Pioglitazone Therapy', *Annals of Internal Medicine*, vol. 136 (6), 2002, pp. 449–52

7. A. Garg, 'Thiazolidinedione-Associated Congestive Heart Failure and Pulmonary Edema', *Mayo Clinic Proceedings*, vol. 78, 2003, p. 1088

8. US Food and Drug Administration Medical Officer Review of Rosiglitazone (Avandia), 16 April 1999, p. 40

9. S.E. Nissen, K.Wolski and E.J. Topol, 'Effect of Muraglitazar on Death and Major Adverse Cardiovascular Events in Patients with Type 2 Diabetes Mellitus', *Journal of the American Medical Association*, vol. 294 (20), 2005, pp. 2581–6

10. S. L. Norris *et al.* 'Pharmacotherapy for Weight Loss in Adults with Type 2 Diabetes', The Cochrane Database of Systematic Reviews 2005, issue 1, article no.: CD004096

11. J. S Torgerson *et al.*, 'Xenical in the Prevention of Diabetes in Obese Subjects (XENDOS) Study: A Randomized Study of Orlistat as an Adjunct to Lifestyle Changes for the Prevention of Type 2 Diabetes in Obese Patients', *Diabetes Care*, vol. 27 (1), 2004, pp. 155–61

12. In April 2006 the health research group Public Citizen called for its withdrawal on these grounds. The full text of the petition can be found at www.citizen.org/publications/release.cfm?ID=7423

13. 'FDA drug testimony sets off alarms', *The Sacramento Bee*, 20 November 2004

14. T. Gura, 'Obesity Drug Pipeline Not So Fat', *Science*, vol. 299, 2003, p. 849. Health research group Public Citizen petitioned for the withdrawal of Reductil in 2002

15. K. Dunder, 'Increase in Blood Glucose Concentration During Anti-hypertensive Treat-ment as a Predictor of Myocardial Infarction: Population Cohort Based Study', *British Medical Journal*, vol. 326, 2003, p. 681

16. D. Bell *et al.*, 'Do sulfonylurea drugs increase the risk of cardiac events?', *Canadian Medical Association Journal*, vol. 174, 2006, pp. 185–6

17. T. Orchard *et al.*, 'The Effect of Metformin and Intensive Lifestyle Intervention on the Metabolic Syndrome: the Diabetes Prevention Program randomized trial', *Annals of Internal Medicine*, vol. 142 (8), 2005, pp. 61–19

18. J. Wylie-Rosett *et al.*, 'Lifestyle Intervention to Prevent Diabetes: Intensive AND Cost Effective', *Current Opinion in Lipidology*, vol. 17 (1), 2006, pp. 37–44
19. W.C. Knowler *et al.*, 'Reduction in the Incidence of Type 2 Diabetes with Lifestyle Intervention or Metformin', *New England Journal of Medicine*, vol. 346, 2002, pp. 393–403
20. K. Christian *et al.*, 'Effect of a Short-Term Diet and Exercise Intervention on Oxidative Stress, Inflammation, MMP-9 and Monocyte Chemotactic Activity in Men with Metabolic Syndrome Factors', *Journal of Applied Physiology*, vol. 100, 2006, pp. 1657–65.
21. G. Boden, 'Short-term Effects of Low-carbohydrate Diet Compared with the Usual Diet in Obese Patients with Type 2 Diabetes', *Annals of Internal Medicine*, vol. 142 (6), 2005, pp. 1–44
22. M. C. Gannon, 'Effect of a High-protein, Low Carbohydrate Diet on Blood Glucose Control in People with Type 2 Diabetes', *Diabetes*, vol. 53 (9), 2004, pp. 2375–82
23. A. Khan *et al.*, 'Cinnamon Improves Glucose and Lipids of people with Type 2 Diabetes', *Diabetes Care*, vol. 26, 2003, pp. 3215–18
24. P. Wursch and F. X. Pi-Sunyer, 'The Role of Viscous Soluble Fiber in the Metabolic Control of Diabetes: A Review with Special Emphasis on Cereals Rich in Beta-glucan', *Diabetes Care*, vol. 20 (11), 1997, pp. 1774–80
25. L. Tappy *et al.*, 'Polyclinique Medicale Universitaire, Lausanne, Switzerland. Effects of Breakfast Cereals Containing Various Amounts of Beta-glucan Fibers on Plasma Glucose and Insulin Responses in Non-insulin-dependent Diabetes Mellitus subjects', *Diabetes Care*, vol. 19 (8), 1996 pp. 831–4
26. M. Bernstein, www.eurekalert.org/pub_releases/2005-11/acs-sfa111705.php, American Chemical Society via Eurekalert, public release date: 17 November 2005
27. R. A. Anderson, 'Nutritional Factors Influencing the Glucose/insulin system: Chromium', *Journal of the American College of Nutrition*, vol. 16, 1997, pp. 404–410
28. See National Institute of Health summary on chromium's role in health and disease at http://dietary-supplements.info.nih.gov/factsheets/chromium.asp
29. M. Pereira *et al.*, 'Effects of a Low-Glycemic Load Diet on Resting Energy Expenditure and Heart Disease Risk Factors During Weight Loss', *Journal of the American Medical Association*, vol. 292, 2004, pp. 2482–90
30. S. A. La Haye *et al.*, 'Comparison Between a Low Glycemic Load Diet and a Canada Food Guide Diet in Cardiac Rehabilitation Patients in Ontario', *Canadian Journal of Cardiology*, vol. 21 (6), 2005, pp. 489–94
31. D.B. Pawlak *et al.*, 'Effects of Dietary Glycaemic Index on Adiposity, Glucose Homeostasis and Plasma Lipids in Animals', *The Lancet*, vol. 364 (9436), 2004, pp. 778–85
32. J. Salmeron *et al.*, 'Dietary Fiber, Glycemic Load, and Risk of Non-insulin-dependent Diabetes Mellitus in Women', *Journal of the American Medical Association*, vol. 277 (6), 1997, pp. 472–7
33. J. Salmeron *et al.*, 'Dietary Fiber, Glycemic Load, and Risk of Non-insulin-dependent Diabetes Mellitus in Men,' *Diabetes Care*, vol. 20 (4), 1997, pp. 545–550
34. C. B. Ebbeling *et al.*, 'A Reduced-Glycemic Load Diet in the Treatment of Adolescent Obesity', *Archives of Pediatrics and Adolescent Medicine*, vol. 157, 2003, pp. 773–9
35. Holford P. *et al.* 'The Effects of a Low Glycemic Load Diet on Weight Loss and Key Health Risk Indicators', *Journal of Orthomolecular Medicine*, vol. 21 (2), 2006, pp. 71–8
36. W. T. Cefalu *et al.*, 'Role of Chromium in Human Health and in Diabetes', *Diabetes Care*, vol. 27, 2004, pp. 2741–51
37. N. Cheng *et al.*, 'Follow-up Survey of People in China with Type 2 Diabetes Mellitus Consuming Supplemental Chromium', *Journal of Trace Elements in Experimental Medicine*, vol. 12, 1999, pp. 55–60

38. M. F. McCarty, 'High-dose Biotin, an Inducer of Glucokinase Expression, May Synergize with Chromium Picolinate to Enable a Definitive Nutritional Therapy for Type II Diabetes', *Medical Hypotheses*, vol. 52 (5), 1999, pp. 401–6. Review.

39. M. F. McCarty. 'High-dose Biotin, an Inducer of Glucokinase Expression, May Synergize with Chromium Picolinate to Enable a Definitive Nutritional Therapy for Type II Diabetes', *Medical Hypotheses*, vol. 52 (5), 1999, pp. 401–6. Review.

40. W. C. Knowler *et al.*, 'Reduction in the Incidence of Type 2 Diabetes with Lifestyle Intervention or Metformin', *New England Journal of Medicine*, vol. 246, 2002, pp. 393–403

41. W. T. Cefalu *et al.*, 'Effect of Chromium Picolinate on Insulin Sensitivity in Vivo', *Journal of Trace Elements in Experimental Medicine*, vol. 12, 1999, pp. 71–83

42. J.A. Janus and E.I. Krajnc, 'Integrated Criteria Document Chromium: Effects', National Institute of Public Health and Environmental Protection, Report No. 710401002, Bilthoven, The Netherlands, 1990, p. 89

43. Institute of Medicine (IOM), 'Chromium picolinate: prototype monograph', in *Dietary Supplements: A Framework for Evaluating Safety*, Institute of Medicine, 2004, pp. B1–B80

44. J. Marx, 'Unravelling the Cause of Diabetes', *Science*, vol. 296 (5568), 2002, pp. 686–9

45. A. McIntosh *et al.*, 'Clinical Guidelines and Evidence Review for Type 2 Diabetes: Management for Blood Glucose', available at www.nice.org.uk/page.aspx?o=guidelines

46. *Physician's Desk Reference*, 49th edition, Montvale NJ: Medical Economics, 1995

47. C. M. F. Antune *et al.*, 'Endometrial Cancer and Oestrogen Use: Report of a Large Case Control Study', *New England Journal of Medicine*, vol. 300, 1979, pp. 9–13. R. R. Paganini-Hill and B. E. Henderson, 'Endometrial Cancer and Patterns of Use of Oestrogen Replacement Therapy: a Cohort Study', *British Journal of Cancer*, vol. 59, 1989, pp. 445–7. P. K. Green *et al.*, 'Risk of Endometrial Cancer Following Cessation of Menopausal Hormone Use', *Cancer Causes Control*, vol. 7, 1996, pp. 575–80

48. J. Beresford *et al.*, 'Risk of Endometrial Cancer in Relation to Use of Oestrogen Combined with Cyclic Progestogen Therapy in Postmenopausal Women', *The Lancet*, vol. 349, 1997, pp. 458–61. E. Weiderpass *et al.* 'Risk of Endometrial Cancer Following Oestrogen Replacement with and without Progestins', *Journal of the National Cancer Institute*, vol. 91, 1999, pp. 1131–7

49. L. Bergkvist *et al.*, 'The Risk of Breast Cancer After Estrogen and Estrogen-progestin Replacement', *New England Journal of Medicine*, vol. 321 (5), 1989, pp. 293–7

50. G. A. Colditz *et al.*, 'The Use of Estrogens and Progestins and the Risk of Breast Cancer in Postmenopausal Women', *New England Journal of Medicine*, vol. 332 (24), 1995, pp. 1589–93

51. G. A. Colditz *et al.*, 'The Use of Estrogens and Progestins and the Risk of Breast Cancer in Postmenopausal Women', *New England Journal of Medicine*, vol. 332 (24), 1995, pp. 1589–93

52. V. Beral *et al.*, 'Breast Cancer and Hormone-replacement Therapy in the Million Women Study', *The Lancet*, vol. 362 (9382), 2003, pp. 419–27

53. S. Batt, Kaiser-permanent Medical Centre study, *Patients No More: The Politics of Breast Cancer*, Scarlet Press, 1997

54. J. Robbins, *Reclaiming Our health: Exploring the Medical Myth and Embracing the Source of True Healing*, H. J. Kramer, 1996

55. T. W. McDonald *et al.*, 'Exogenous Estrogen and Endometrial Carcinoma: Case-control and Incidence Study', *American Journal of Obstetrics and Gynecology*, vol. 127 (6), 1997, pp. 572–80

56. S. A. A. Beresford *et al.*, 'Risk of Endometrial Cancer in Relation to Use of Oestrogen Combined with Cyclic Progestogen Therapy in Postmenopausal Women', *The Lancet*, vol. 349, 1977, pp. 458–61; A. Cerin *et al.*, 'Adverse Endometrial Effects of Long-cycle Oestrogen and Progestogen Replacement Therapy, *New England Journal of Medicine*, vol. 334, 1996, pp. 668–9; G. A. Colditz *et al.*, 'The Use of Oestrogens and Progestins and the Risk of Breast Cancer in Postmenopausal Women', *New England Journal of Medicine*, vol. 332, 1995, pp. 1589–93; E. Dale *et al.*, 'Risk of Venous Thromboembolism in Users of Hormone Replacement Therapy', *The Lancet*, vol. 348, 1996, pp. 977–80; F. Grodstein *et al.*, 'Post-menopausal Oestrogen and Progestin Use and the Risk of Cardiovascular Disease', *New England Journal of Medicine*, vol. 335, 1996, pp. 453–61; F. Grodstein *et al.*, 'Prospective Study of Exogenous Hormones and Risk of Pulmonary Embolism in Women', *The Lancet*, vol. 348, 1996, pp. 983–7; E. Hemminki and K. McPherson, 'Impact of Postmenopausal Hormone Therapy on Cardiovascular Events and Cancer: Pooled Data from Clinical Trials', *British Medical Journal*, vol. 315, 1997, pp. 149–55; M. V. Pike *et al.*, 'Oestrogen-progestin Replacement Therapy and Endometrial Cancer', *Journal of the National Cancer Institute*, vol. 89, 1997, pp. 1110–16

57. www.cancer.gov/cancertopics/mothers-prescribed-des. The study detected a modest association between DES exposure and breast cancer risk, with a relative risk of about 1.3. In other words, 16 per cent of women prescribed DES during pregnancy developed breast cancer, in comparison with 13 per cent of women not prescribed DES. Therefore, it is estimated that one in six women who were prescribed DES will develop breast cancer, whereas one in eight women in the general population will develop the disease.

58. K. Hunt *et al.*, 'Long-term Surveillance of Mortality and Cancer Incidence in Women Receiving Hormone Replacement Therapy', *British Journal of Obstetrics and Gynaecology*, vol. 94, 1987, pp. 620–35; K. Hunt *et al.* 'Mortality in a Cohort of Long Term Users of Hormone Replacement Therapy: An Updated Analysis,' *British Journal of Obstetrics and Gynaecology*, vol. 97, 1990, pp. 1080–6

59. L. Bergkvist *et al.*, 'The Risk of Breast Cancer After Estrogen and Estrogen-progestin Replacement', *New England Journal of Medicine*, vol. 321 (5), 1989, pp. 293–7

60. Mary Cushman *et al.*, 'Oestrogen Plus Progestin and Risk of Venous Thrombosis', *Journal of the American Medical Association*, vol. 292, 2004, pp. 1573–80

61. J. E. Rossouw *et al.*, 'Risks and Benefits of Oestrogen Plus Progestin in Healthy Post-menopausal Women: Principal Results from the Women's Health Initiative Randomized Controlled Trial', *Journal of the American Medical Association*, vol. 288, 2002, pp. 321–33

62. A. H. MacLennan *et al.*, 'Oral Oestrogen and Combined Oestrogen/progestogen Therapy Versus Placebo for Hot Flushes', The Cochrane Database of Systematic Reviews 2004, issue 4, article no.: CD002978

63. J. E. Rossouw *et al.*, 'Risks and Benefits of Oestrogen Plus Progestin in Healthy Post-menopausal Women: Principal Results from the Women's Health Initiative Randomized Controlled Trial', *Journal of the American Medical Association*, vol. 288, 2002, pp. 321–33

64. D. T. Felson *et al.*, 'The Effect of Postmenopausal Oestrogen Therapy on Bone Density in Elderly Women', *New England Journal of Medicine*. vol. 329, 1993, pp. 1141–6; J. E. Rossouw *et al.*, 'Risks and Benefits of Oestrogen plus Progestin in Healthy Post-menopausal Women: Principal Results from the Women's Health Initiative Randomized Controlled Trial', *Journal of the American Medical Association*, vol. 288, 2002, pp. 321–33

65. D. T. Felson *et al.*, 'The Effect of Postmenopausal Oestrogen Therapy on Bone Density in Elderly Women', *New England Journal of Medicine*, vol. 329, 1993, pp. 1141–6

66. C. Minelli *et al.* 'Benefits and Harms Associated with Hormone Replacement Therapy: Clinical Decision Analysis', *British Medical Journal*, vol. 328, 2004, p. 371

67. P. A. Komesaroff *et al.*, 'Effects of Wild Yam Extract on Menopausal Symptoms, Lipids and Sex Hormones in Healthy Menopausal Women', *Climacteric*, vol. 4, 2001, pp. 144–50

68. J. Lee *et al.*, *What Your Doctor May Not Tell You About Breast Cancer*, Thorsons, 2002

69. H. B. Leonetti *et al.*, 'Transdermal Progesterone Cream for Vasomotor Symptoms and Postmenopausal Bone Loss', *Obstetrics and Gynecology*, vol. 94, 1999, pp. 225–8

70. G. Holzer *et al.*, 'Effects and Side Effects of 2% Progesterone Cream on the Skin of Peri- and Postmenopausal Women: Results from a Double-blind, Vehicle-controlled, Randomized Study', *British Journal of Dermatology*, vol. 153 (3), 2005, pp. 626–34

71. J. T. Hargrove *et al.*, 'Menopausal Hormone Replacement Therapy with Continuous Daily Oral Micronized Estradiol and Progesterone', *Obstetrics and Gynecology*, vol. 73 (4), 1989, pp. 606–12. Also see http://www.project-aware.org/Resource/Studies/warner.html

72. J. A. Tice *et al.*, 'Phytooestrogen Supplements for the Treatment of Hot Flashes: The Isoflavone Clover Extract (ICE) Study: A Randomized Controlled Trial', *Journal of the American Medical Association*, vol. 290 (2), 2003, pp. 207–14

73. 'Treatment of Menopause-associated Vasomotor Symptoms: Position Statement of the North American Menopause Society', *Menopause*, vol. 11 (1), 2004, pp. 11–33

74. FSA Committee on Toxicology (COT) report on Phytooestrogens and Health, May 2003, available from www.food.gov.uk/science/ouradvisors/toxicity/reports/phytooestrogens andhealthcot

75. B. K. Jacobsen *et al.*, 'Does High Soy Milk Intake Reduce Prostate Cancer Incidence? The Adventist Health Study (United States)', *Cancer Causes Control*, vol. 9 (6), 1998, pp. 553–7

76. S. L. Dormire and N. K. Reame, 'Menopausal Hot Flash Frequency Changes in Response to Experimental Manipulation of Blood Glucose', *Nursing Research*, vol. 52 (5), 2003, pp. 338–43

77. P. T. McSorley *et al.*, 'Vitamin C Improves Endothelial Function in Healthy Oestrogen-deficient Postmenopausal Women', *Climacteric*, vol. 6 (3), 2003, pp. 238–47

78. R. R. McLeanet *et al.*, 'Homocysteine as a Predictive Factor for Hip Fracture in Older Persons', *New England Journal of Medicine*, vol. 350 (20), 2004, pp. 2042–9

79. J. B. van Meurs *et al.*, 'Homocysteine Levels and the Risk of Osteoporotic Fracture', *New England Journal of Medicine*, vol. 350 (20), 2004, pp. 2033–41

80. J. Homik *et al.*, The Cochrane Database of Systematic Reviews 2000, issue 2, article no.: CD000952

81. J. Porthouse *et al.*, 'Randomised Controlled Trial of Calcium and Supplementation with Cholecalciferol (Vitamin D3) for Prevention of Fractures in Primary Care', *British Medical Journal*, vol. 330, 2005, p. 1003

82. R. Jackson, 'Calcium Plus Vitamin D Supplementation and the Risk of Fractures', *New England Journal of Medicine,* vol. 354 (7), 2006, pp. 669–83

83. W. Wuttke *et al.*, 'The Cimicifuga Preparation BNO 1055 vs Conjugated Estrogens in a Double-blind Placebo-controlled Study: Effects on Menopause Symptoms and Bone Markers', *Mauritas*, vol. 44 (suppl 1), 2003, pp. S67–S77; Jacobsen J. *et al.*, 'Randomised Trial of Black Cohosh for the Treatment of Hot Flashes Among Women with a History of Breast Cancer', *Journal of Clinical Oncolgy*, vol. 19, 2001, pp. 2739–45; W. Stoll, 'Cimifuga vz Estrogenis Substances' *Mediziische Welt*, vol. 36, 1985, pp. 871–4

84. R. Lupu *et al.*, 'Black cohosh, A Menopausal Remedy, Does Not Have Oestrogenic Activity and Does Not Promote Breast Cancer Cell Growth', *International Journal of Oncology*, vol. 23 (5), 2003, pp. 1407–12

85. C. Kupfersztain *et al.*, 'The Immediate Effect of Natural Plant Extract, *Angelica Sinensis* and *Matricaria Chamomilla* (Climex) For the Treatment of Hot Flushes During

Menopause: A Preliminary Report', *Clinical and Experimental Obstetrics and Gynecology*, vol. 30 (4), 2003, pp. 203–6

86. J. D. Hirata *et al.*, 'Does Don Quai Have Oestrogenic Effects in Postmenopausal Women?', *Fertility and Sterility*, vol. 68, 1997, pp. 981–6

87. B. Grube *et al.*, 'St. John's Wort Extract: Efficacy for Menopausal Symptoms of Psychological Origin', *Advances in Therapy*, vol. 16 (4), 1999, pp. 177–86

88. R. Uebelhack *et al.*, 'Black Cohosh and St John's Wort for Climacteric Complaints: A Randomized Trial', *Obstetrics and Gynecology*, vol. 107 (2 Pt 1), 2006, pp. 247–55

89. B. Roemheld-Hamm, 'Chasteberry', *American Family Physician*, vol. 72(5), 2005, pp. 821–4

90. C. Li *et al.*, 'Menopause-related Symptoms: What Are the Background Factors? A Prospective Population-based Cohort Study of Swedish Women (The Women's Health in Lund Area Study)', *American Journal of Obstetrics and Gynecology*, vol. 189 (6), 2003, pp. 1646–53

91. L. Germaine *et al.*, 'Behavioural Treatment of Menopausal Hot Flushes', *American Journal of Obstetrics and Gynecology*, vol. 167, 1992, pp. 436–9; R. Freedman *et al.*, 'Behavioural Treatment of Menopausal Hot Flushes: Evaluation by Ambulatory Monitoring', *American Journal of Obstetrics and Gynecologytrics and Gynecology*, vol. 167, 1992, pp. 436–9; R. Freedman *et al.*, 'Biochemical and Thermoregulatory Effects of Behavioural Treatment for Menopausal Hot Flashes', *Menopause*, vol. 2, 1995, pp. 211–18

92. D. Fobbester *et al.*, 'Optimum Nutrition UK survey', October 2004. Available from www.ion.ac.uk

93. S. Weich *et al.*, 'Rural/non-rural Differences in Rates of Common Mental Disorders in Britain: Prospective Multilevel Cohort Study', *British Journal of Psychiatry*, vol. 188, 2006 pp. 51–7

94. Ian B. Hickie, 'Preventing Depression: A Challenge for the Australian Community', *Medical Journal of Australia*, vol. 177 (7), 2002, pp. 85–6

95. A. Tylee and P. Ghandhi, 'The Importance of Somatic Symptoms in Depression in Primary Care', *Journal of Clinical Psychology*, vol. 7 (4), 2005, pp. 167–76. Also see NICE Guideline for Depression www.nice.org <http://www.nice.org>

96. Daniel Chisholm quoted in 'Depression: social and economic timebomb: strategies for quality care' by A. Dawson in *The Economic Consequences of Depression* edited by A. Tylee, BMJ Books for WHO Regional Office for Europe, 2001, ISBN 0-727-91573-8

97. P. Farley, 'The anatomy of despair', *New Scientist*, 1 May 2004

98. R. A. Hansen *et al.*, 'Efficacy and Safety of Second-generation Anti-depressants in the Treatment of Major Depressive Disorder', *Annals of Internal Medicine*, vol. 143 (6), 2005, pp. 415–26, Review

99. Anti-Depressant, Heart Risk Association Needs Further Study: In a surprise finding, patients with coronary artery disease who take commonly used anti-depressant drugs may be at a significantly higher risk of death. See http://dukemednews.duke.edu/news/article.php?id=9535

100. NICE report on anti-depressants. See www.nice.org.uk/page.aspx?o=cg023

101. J. R. Geddes *et al.*, 'Selective Serotonin Reuptake Inhibitors (SSRIs) for Depression', The Cochrane Database of Systematic Reviews, issue 4, 1999, article no: CD001851

102. R. A. Hansen *et al.*, 'Efficacy and Safety of Second-generation Anti-depressants in the Treatment of Major Depressive Disorder', *Annals of Internal Medicine*, vol. 143 (6), 2005, pp. 415–26, Review

103. A. Khan *et al.*, 'Symptom Reduction and Suicide Risk in Patients Treated with Placebo in Antidepressant Clinical Trials', *Archives of General Psychiatry*, vol. 57, 2000, pp. 311–24

104. J. Moncrieff and I. Kirsch, 'Efficacy of Anti-depressants in Adults', *British Medical Journal*, vol. 331, 2005, pp. 155–7

105. J. Moncrieff *et al.*, 'Active Placebos Versus Anti-depressants for Depression', The Cochrane Database of Systematic Reviews 2004, issue 1, article. no.: CD003012

106. J. Davidson *et al.*, 'Effect of Hypericum Perforatum (St John's Wort) in Major Depressive Disorder: A Randomized Controlled Trial', *Journal of the American Medical Association*, vol. 287, 2002, pp. 1807–14

107. D. Fergusson *et al.*, 'Association Between Suicide Attempts and Selective Serotonin Re-uptake Inhibitors: Systematic Review of Randomised Controlled Trials', *British Medical Journal*, vol. 330, 2005, p. 396

108. C. R. Sharpe, *et al.*, 'The Effects of Tricyclic Anti-depressants on Breast Cancer Risk', *British Journal of Cancer*, vol. 86 (1), 2002, pp. 92–7

109. M. Cotterchia, *et al.*, 'Antidepressant Medication Use and Breast Cancer Risk', *American Journal of Epidemiology*, vol. 151 (10), 2002, pp. 951–7

110. J. Swiatek, 'Antidepressant Maker GlaxoSmithKline Held Liable in Wrongful-Death Case" copyright (c) 2001 KRTBN Knight-Ridder Tribune Business News; Source: World Reporter (TM) 7 June 2001. http://www.baumhedlundlaw.com/SSRIs/Paxil-Schell.htm

111. D. Williams, 'Bitter Pills: They're Prescribed to Millions, But Do the New Anti-depressants Work? And Are They Worth the Risk?', *Time International* (South Pacific Edition), 21 November 2005

112. See S. Boseley, 'Murder, Suicide. A Bitter Aftertaste for the "Wonder" Depression Drug' at www.guardian.co.uk/Archive/Article/0,4273,4201752,00.html

113. D. G. Perahia *et al.*, 'Symptoms Following Abrupt Discontinuation of Duloxetine Treatment in Patients with Major Depressive Disorder', *Journal of Affective Disorders*, vol. 89 (1–3), 2005, pp. 207–12

114. F. Bogetto *et al.*, 'Discontinuation Syndrome in Dysthymic Patients Treated with Selective Serotonin Reuptake Inhibitors: A Clinical Investigation', *CNS Drugs*, vol. 16 (4), 2002, pp. 273–83

115. T. Audhya, 'Advances in Measurement of Platelet Catecholamines at Sub-picomole Level for Diagnosis of Depression and Anxiety', *Clinical Chemistry*, Abstract no. 128 published in the 2005 Annual Meeting, p. A248.

116. T. Audhya, 'Advances in Measurement of Platelet Catecholamines at Sub-picomole Level for Diagnosis of Depression and Anxiety', *Clinical Chemistry*, Abstract no. 128 published in the 2005 Annual Meeting, p. A248.

117. T. Audhya, *Journal of Nutritional Medicine* (accepted for publication).

118. K. A. Smith *et al.*, 'Relapse of Depression After Rapid Depletion of Tryptophan', *The Lancet*, vol. 349, 1997, pp. 915–19

119. E. H. Turner *et al.*, 'Serotonin a la Carte: Supplementation with the Serotonin Precursor 5-hydroxytryptophan', *Pharmacology and Therapeutics*, vol. 109 (3), 2006, pp. 325–38

120. W. Poldinger *et al.*, 'A Functional-dimensional Approach to Depression: Serotonin Deficiency and Target Syndrome in a Comparison of 5-hydroxytryptophan and Fluvoxamine', *Psychopathology*, vol. 24 (2), 1991, pp. 53–81

121. E. H. Turner *et al.*, 'Serotonin a la Carte: Supplementation with the Serotonin Precursor 5-hydroxytryptophan', *Pharmacology and Therapeutics*, vol. 109 (3), 2006, pp. 325–38

122. I. Bjelland *et al.*, 'Folate, Vitamin B12, Homocysteine, and the MTHFR 677CT Polymorphism in Anxiety and Depression: The Hordaland Homocysteine Study', *Archives of General Psychiatry*, vol. 60, 2003, pp. 618–26

123. A. Coppen and J. Bailey, 'Enhancement of the Antidepressant Action of Fluoxetine by Folic Acid: A Randomized, Placebo-controlled Trial', *Journal of Affective Disorders*, vol. 60 (2), 2000, pp. 121–30

124. M. J. Taylor *et al.*, 'Folate for Depressive Disorders', The Cochrane Database of Systematic Reviews 2003, issue 2, article no.: CD003390

125. J. R. Hibbeln, 'Fish Consumption and Major Depression', *The Lancet*, vol. 351 (9110), 1998, p. 1213

126. M. Peet and R. Stokes, 'Omega-3 Fatty Acids in the Treatment of Psychiatric Disorders', *Drugs*, vol. 65 (8), 2005, pp. 1051–9

127. S. Frangou *et al.*, 'Efficacy of Ethyl-eicosapentaenoic Acid in Bipolar Depression: Randomised Double-blind Placebo-controlled Study', *British Journal of Psychiatry*, vol. 188, 2006, pp. 46–50

128. A. Stoll *et al.*, 'Omega-3 Fatty Acids in Bipolar Disorder: A Preliminary Double-blind, Placebo-controlled Trial', *Archives of General Psychiatry*, vol. 56 (5), 1999, pp. 407–12

129. B. Nemets *et al.*, 'Addition of Omega-3 Fatty Acid to Maintenance Medication Treatment for Recurrent Unipolar Depressive Disorder,' *American Journal of Psychiatry*, vol. 159, 2002, pp. 477–9

130. S. Frangou *et al.*, 'Efficacy of Ethyl-eicosapentaenoic Acid in Bipolar Depression: Randomised Double-blind Placebo-controlled Study', *British Journal of Psychiatry*, vol. 188, 2006, pp. 46–50

131. D. Benton *et al.*, 'Mild Hypoglycaemia and Questionnaire Measures of Aggression', *Biological Psychology*, vol. 14 (1–2), 1982, pp. 129–35

132. A. Roy *et al.*, 'Monoamines, Glucose Metabolism, Aggression Toward Self and Others', *International Journal of Neuroscience*, vol. 41 (3–4), 1988, pp. 261–4

133. A. G. Schauss, *Diet, Crime and Delinquency*, Parker House, 1980

134. M. Virkkunen, 'Reactive Hypoglycaemic Tendency Among Arsonists', *ACTA Psychiatrica Scandinavica*, vol. 69 (5), 1984, pp. 445–52

135. M. Virkkunen and S. Narvanen, 'Tryptophan and Serotonin Levels During the Glucose Tolerance Test Among Habitually Violent and Impulsive Offenders', *Neuropsychobiology*, vol. 17 (1–2), 1987, pp. 19–23

136. J. Yaryura-Tobias and F. Neziroglu, 'Violent Behaviour, Brain Dysrythmia and Glucose Dysfunction. A New Syndrome', *Journal of Orthomolecular Psychiatry*, vol. 4, 1975, pp. 182–5

137. M. Bruce and M. Lader, 'Caffeine Abstention and the Management of Anxiety Disorders', *Psychological Medicine*, vol. 19, 1989, pp. 211–14

138. O. W. Wendel and W. E. Beebe, 'Glycolytic Activity in Schizophrenia', in D. Hawkins & L. Pauling, *Orthomolecular Psychiatry: Treatment of Schizophrenia*. San Francisco, W. H. Freeman, 1973 ISBN: 0716708981

139. L. Christensen, 'Psychological Distress and Diet – Effects of Sucrose and Caffeine', *Journal of Applied Nutrition*, vol. 40 (1), 1988, pp. 44–50

140. L. Christensen, 'Psychological Distress and Diet – Effects of Sucrose and Caffeine', *Journal of Applied Nutrition*, vol. 40 (1), 1988, pp. 44–50

141. M. McLeod, 'Lifting Depression – The Chromium Connection', Basic Health Publications, 2005

142. J. R. Davidson *et al.*, 'Effectiveness of Chromium in Atypical Depression: A Placebo-controlled Trial, *Biological Psychiatry*, vol. 53 (3), 2003, pp. 261–4

143. J. Docherty *et al.*, 'A Double-Blind, Placebo-Controlled, Exploratory Trial of Chromium Picolinate in Atypical Depression', *Journal of Psychiatric Practice*, vol. 11 (5), 2005, pp. 302–14

144. L. Craft and F. Perna, 'The Benefits of Exercise for the Clinically Depressed', *Journal of Clinical Psychiatry*, vol. 6 (3), 2004, pp. 104–11

145. N. A. Singh, 'A Randomized Controlled Trial of High versus Low Intensity Weight Training versus General Practitioner Care for Clinical Depression in Older Adults', *Journals of Gerontology, Series A, Biological Sciences and Medical Sciences*, vol. 60 (6), 2005, pp. 768–76

146. S. Leppamaki *et al.*, 'Drop-out and Mood Improvement: A Randomised Controlled Trial with Light Exposure and Physical Exercise', *BMC Psychiatry*, vol 4 (1), 2004, p. 22

147. K. Martiny *et al.*, 'Adjunctive Bright Light in Non-seasonal Major Depression: Results from Clinician-rated Depression Scales', *ACTA Psychiatrica Scandinavica*, vol. 112 (2), 2005, pp. 117–25

148. L. Swiecicki *et al.*, 'Platelet Serotonin Transport in the Group of Outpatients with Seasonal Affective Disorder Before and After Light Treatment, and in Remission (in the Summer)', *Psychiatria Polska*, vol. 39 (3), 2005, pp. 459–68

149. N. Goel *et al.*, 'Controlled Trial of Bright Light and Negative Air Ions for Chronic Depression', *Psychological Medicine*, vol. 35 (7), 2005, pp. 945–55

150. G. Brown *et al.*, 'Social Support, Self-esteem and Depression', *Psychological Medicine*, vol. 16 (4), 1986, pp. 813–31

151. See www.alzheimers.org.au/index.cfm

152. C. Courtney *et al.*, 'Long-term Donepezil Treatment in 565 Patients with Alzheimer's Disease (AD2000): Randomised Double-blind Trial', *The Lancet*, vol. 363 (9427), 2004, pp. 2105–15

153. A. Areosa Sastre *et al.*, 'Memantine for dementia', The Cochrane Database of Systematic Reviews 2006, issue 2, article no.: CD003154

154. National Institute for Health and Clinical Excellence, 'Appraisal Consultation Document: Alzheimer's disease – Donepezil, Rivastigmine, Galantamine and Memantine (review)'. See www.nice.org.uk/page.aspx?o=245908

155. K. A. Jost *et al.*, 'Rapidly Progressing Atrophy of Medial Temporal Lobe in Alzheimer's Disease', *The Lancet*, vol. 343 (8901), pp. 829–30

156. S. Seshadri *et al.*, 'Plasma Homocysteine as a Risk Factor for Dementia and AD', *New England Journal of Medicine*, vol. 346 (7), 2002, pp. 476–83

157. P. S. Sachdev *et al.*, 'Relationship Between Plasma Homocysteine Levels and Brain Atrophy in Healthy Elderly Individuals', *Neurology*, vol. 58, 2002, pp. 1539–41

158. S. J. Duthie, *et al.*, 'Homocysteine, B Vitamin Status, and Cognitive Function in the Elderly', *American Journal of Clinical Nutrition*, vol. 75 (5), 2002, pp. 908–13

159. M. Corrada, *Alzheimer's & Dementia*, vol. 1, 2005, pp. 11–18

160. T. Bottiglieri *et al.*, 'Plasma Total Homocysteine Levels and the C677T Mutation in the Methylenetetrahydrofolate Reductase (MTHFR) Gene: A Study in an Italian Population with Dementia', *Mechanical Ageing Development*, vol. 122 (16), 2001, pp. 2013–23

161. J. Durga, 'Effect of Folic Acid Supplementation on Cognitive Function', *5th International Conference on Homocysteine Metabolism*, 25–30 June 2005, Milan, Italy

162. S. J. Eussen *et al.*, 'Oral Cyanocobalamin Supplementation in Older People with Vitamin B12 Deficiency: A Dose-finding trial', *Archives of Internal Medicine*, vol. 165 (10), 2005, pp. 1167–72

163. M. Morris, *et al.*, 'Consumption of Fish and N-3 Fatty Acids and Risk of Incident Alzheimer's Disease', *Archives of Neurology*, vol. 60, 2003, pp. 940–6

164. M. Morris *et al.*, 'Dietary Intake of Antioxidant Nutrients and the Risk of Incident Alzheimer's Disease in a Biracial Community Study', *Journal of the American Medical Association*, vol. 284 (24), 2002, pp. 3230–7

165. M. Sano, *et al.*, 'A Controlled Trial of Selegiline, Alpha Tocopherol or Both as Treatment of AD', *New England Journal of Medicine*, vol. 336, 1997, pp. 1216–22

166. S. J. Colcombe *et al.*, 'Neurocognitive Aging and Cardiovascular Fitness: Recent Findings and Future Directions', *Journal of Molecular Neuroscience*, vol. 24, 2004, pp. 9–14

167. P. Callaghan, 'Exercise: A Neglected Intervention in Mental Health Care?', *Journal of Psychiatric & Mental Health Nursing*, vol. 11, 2004, pp. 476–83

168. M. E. Lytle *et al.*, 'Exercise Level and Cognitive Decline: The MoVIES Project', *Alzheimer's Disease and Associated Disorders*, vol. 18, 2004, pp. 57–64

169. B. P. Sobel, 'Bingo vs. Physical Intervention in Stimulating Short-term Cognition in Alzheimer's Disease Patients', *American Journal of Alzheimer's Disease and Other Dementias*, vol. 16, 2001, pp. 115–20

170. D. Laurin *et al.*, 'Physical Activity and Risk of Cognitive Impairment and Dementia in Elderly Persons', *Archives of Neurology*, vol. 58 (2–1), pp. 498–504

171. R. S. Wilson *et al.*, 'Cognitive Activity and Incident AD in a Population-based Sample of Older Persons', *Neurology*, vol. 59, 2002, pp. 1910–14

172. J. Verghese *et al.*, 'Leisure Activities and the Risk of Dementia in the Elderly', *New England Journal of Medicine*, vol. 348 (2–3), pp. 2508–16

173. R. S. Wilson *et al.*, 'Participation in Cognitively Stimulating Activities and Risk of Incident Alzheimer Disease', *Journal of the American Medical Association*, vol. 287, 2002, pp. 742–8

174. J. G. Crawford, 'Alzheimer's Disease Risk Factors as Related to Cerebral Blood Flow', *Medical Hypotheses*, vol. 46, 1996, pp. 367–77

175. A. Osawa *et al.*, 'Relationship Between Cognitive Function and Regional Cerebral Blood Flow in Different Types of Dementia', *Disability and Rehabilitation*, vol. 26, 2004, pp. 739–45

176. D. Laurin *et al.*, 'Physical Activity and Risk of Cognitive Impairment and Dementia in Elderly Persons', *Archives of Neurology*, vol. 58, 2001, pp. 498–504

177. T. Satoh *et al.*, 'Walking Exercise and Improved Neuropsychological Functioning In Elderly Patients with Cardiac Disease', *Journal of Internal Medicine*, vol. 238, 1995, pp. 423–8

178. E. Larson *et al.*, 'Exercise is Associated with Reduced Risk for Incident Dementia Among Persons 65 years and Older', *Annals of Internal Medicine*, vol. 144, 2006, pp. 73–81

179. S. J. Colcombe *et al.*, 'Aerobic Fitness Reduces Brain Tissue Loss in Aging Humans', *Journals of Gerontology, Series A, Biological Sciences and Medical Sciences*, vol. 58, 2003, pp. 176–80

180. L. Teri *et al.*, 'Exercise Plus Behavioral Management in Patients with Alzheimer Disease: A Randomized Controlled Trial', *Journal of the American Medical Association*, vol. 290, 2003, pp. 2015–22

181. D. Fobbester *et al.*, 'Optimum Nutrition UK survey', October 2004. Available from www.ion.ac.uk

182. M. J. Sateia and P. D. Nowell, 'Insomnia', *The Lancet*, vol. 364 (9449), 2004, pp. 1959–73

183. Clinical Guideline: Anxiety, 22 December 2004, National Institute for Health and Clinical Excellence, NHS Management of anxiety (panic disorder, with or without agoraphobia, and generalised anxiety disorder) in adults in primary, secondary and community care

184. Editorial: 'Treating Insomnia', *British Medical Journal*, vol. 29, 2004, pp. 1198–9

185. C. Nystrom, 'Effects of Long-term Benzodiazepine Medication. A Prospective Cohort Study: Methodological and Clinical Aspects', *Nordic Journal of Psychiatry*, vol. 59 (6), 2005, pp. 492–7

186. A. Hirst and R. Sloan, 'Benzodiazepines and Related Drugs for Insomnia in Palliative Care', The Cochrane Database of Systematic Reviews 2001, issue 4, article no.: CD003346

187. National Institute for Health and Clinical Excellence, 'Insomnia: Newer Hypnotic Drugs' (no. 77) – see http://www.nice.org.uk/page.aspx?o=ta077

188. See www.netdoctor.co.uk/medicines/100002841.html

189. G. D. Jacobs *et al.*, 'Cognitive Behavior Therapy and Pharmacotherapy for Insomnia: A Randomized Controlled Trial and Direct Comparison', *Archives of Internal Medicine*, vol. 164 (17), 2004, pp. 1888–96

190. M. J. Sateia and P. D. Nowell, 'Insomnia', *The Lancet*, vol. 364 (9449), 2004, pp. 1959–73

191. P. Montgomery and J. Dennis, 'Physical Exercise for Sleep Problems in Adults aged 60+', The Cochrane Database of Systematic Reviews 2002, issue 4, article no.: CD003404

192. L. Yai, '"Brain music" in the Treatment of Patients with Insomnia', *Neuroscience and Behavioral Physiology*, vol. 28, 1998, pp. 330–5

193. I. Olszewska and M. Zarow, 'Does Music During Dental Treatment Make a Difference?' See www.silenceofmusic.com/pdf/dentists.pdf

194. L. Shilo, 'The Effects of Coffee Consumption on Sleep and Melatonin Secretion', *Sleep Medicine*, vol 3 (3), 2002, pp. 271–3

195. I. S. Shiah and N. Yatham, 'GABA Functions in Mood Disorders: An Update and Critical Review', *Life Sciences*, vol. 63 (15), 1998, pp. 1289–303

196. G. R. Heninger, 'Serotonin, Sex, Psychiatric Illness', *Proceedings of the National Academy of Sciences*, vol. 94 (4), 1997, pp. 823–4

197. G. R. Heninger, 'Serotonin, Sex, Psychiatric Illness', *Proceedings of the National Academy of Sciences*, vol. 94 (4), 1997, pp. 823–4

198. A. Brzezinski *et al.*, 'Effects of Exogenous Melatonin on Sleep: A Meta-analysis', *Sleep Medicine Reviews*, vol. 9 (1), 2005, pp. 41–50

199. S. Esteban, 'Effect of Orally Administered L-tryptophan on Serotonin, Melatonin, and the Innate Immune Response in the Rat', *Molecular and Cellular Biochemistry*, vol. 267 (1–2), 2004, pp. 39–46

200. T. C. Birdsall, '5-Hydroxytryptophan: A Clinically-effective Serotonin Precursor', *Alternative Medicine Review*, vol. 3 (4), 1998, pp. 271–80

201. O. Bruni *et al.*, 'L-5-Hydroxytryptophan Treatment of Sleep Terrors in Children', *European Journal of Pediatrics*, vol. 163 (7), 2004, pp. 402–7

202. S. Young, 'The Clinical Psychopharmacology of Tryptophan', pp. 49–88 in *Nutrition and the Brain* (vol. 7), ed. J. and R. Wurtman, Raven Press, New York, 1996

203. M. Hornyak, 'Magnesium Therapy for Periodic Leg Movements-related Insomnia and Restless Legs Syndrome: An Open Pilot Study', *Sleep*, vol. 21 (5), 1998, pp. 501–5

204. D. Wheatley, 'Medicinal Plants for Insomnia: A Review of their Pharmacology, Efficacy and Tolerability', *Journal of Psychopharmacology*, vol. 19 (4), 2005, pp. 414–21

205. M. Spinella, *The Psychopharmacology of Herbal Medicine*, MIT Press, 2001

206. M. Dorn, 'Valerian Versus Oxazepam: Efficacy and Tolerability in Nonorganic and Nonpsychiatric Insomniacs – a Randomized, Double-blind Clinical Comparative Study', *Forschende Komplementärmedizin und Klassische naturheilkunde*, vol. 7, 2000, pp. 79–81.

207. E. U. Vorbach *et al.*, 'Treatment of Insomnia: Effectiveness and Tolerance of a Valerian Extract', *Psychopharmakotherapie*, vol. 3, 1996, pp. 109–15.

208. C. Stevinson, E. Ernst, 'Valerian for Insomnia: A Systematic Review of Randomized Clinical Trials', *Sleep Medicine*, vol. 1, 2000, pp. 91–9.

209. *The Big Picture*, published by the Arthritis Research Campaign. See www.arc.org.uk/about_arth/bidoctoric.htm

210. See www.arthritisvic.org.au/downloads/Bottom%20Line.pdf

211. R. D. Rudic *et al.*, 'COX-2-derived Prostacyclin Modulates Vascular Remodelling', *Circulation Research*, vol. 96 (12), 2005, pp. 1240–7

212. X. Liang *et al.*, 'Prostaglandin D2 Mediates Neuronal Protection via the DP1 Receptor', *Journal of Neurochemistry*, vol. 92 (3), 2005, pp. 477–8. This essentially found that one of the

effects of the prostglandins blocked by COX-2 inhibitors was to protect brain cells after a stroke, so cutting down their production with the drug could increase stroke damage.

213. C. Dai *et al.*, 'National Trends in Cyclooxygenase-2 Inhibitor Use Since Market Release: Nonselective Diffusion of a Selectively Cost-effective Innovation', *Archives of Internal Medicine*, vol. 165, 2005, pp. 171–7

214. S. Chaplin, 'Volume and Cost of Prescribing in England, 2004', *Prescriber*, vol. 16, (5), 5 August 2005. To print hard copy go to http://www.escriber.com/Prescriber/Features.asp?ID=989&GroupID=40&Action=View

215. J. Hippisley-Cox and C. Coupland, 'Risk of Myocardial Infarction in Patients Taking Cyclo-oxygenase-2 Inhibitors or Conventional Non-steroidal Anti-inflammatory Drugs: Population Based Nested Case-control Analysis', *British Medical Journal*, vol. 330, 2005, pp. 1366–9

216. P. Elwood *et al.*, 'For and Against: Aspirin for Everyone Older than 50?': FOR, *British Medical Journal*, vol. 330, 2005, pp. 1440–1 and C. Baigent, 'For and against: Aspirin for everyone older than 50?': AGAINST, *British Medical Journal*, vol. 330, 2005, pp. 1442–3

217. See www.jr2.ox.ac.uk/bandolier/booth/painpag/nsae/nsae.html#Heading10

218. D. Y. Graham *et al.*, 'Visible Small-intestinal Mucosal Injury in Chronic NSAID Users', *Clinical Gastroenterology and Hepatology*, vol. 3 (1), 2005, pp. 55–9

219. P. M. Brooks *et al.*, 'NSAIDs and Osteoarthritis – Help or Hindrance?', *Journal of Rheumatology*, vol. 9, 1982, pp. 3–5

222. Raffa *et al.*, 'Discovery of "Self-Synergistic" Spinal/Supraspinal Antinociception Produced by Acetaminophen (Paracetamol)', *Journal of Pharmacology and Experimental Therapeutics*, vol. 295, 2000, pp. 291–4

221. Dr Anthony Temple, 'Max daily OTC dose of Acetaminophen Shows Efficacy Comparable to Rx Doses of Naproxen for OA Pain', 2nd Joint Scientific Meeting of the American Pain Society and the Canadian Pain Society, 7 May 2004

222. I. E. Towheed *et al.*, 'Acetaminophen for Osteoarthritis', The Cochrane Database of Systematic Reviews 2006 , issue 4, article no.: CD004257

223. T. Wienecke and P. C. Gøtzsche, 'Paracetamol Versus Nonsteroidal Anti-inflammatory Drugs for Rheumatoid Arthritis', The Cochrane Database of Systematic Reviews 2004, issue 1, article no.: CD003789

224. K. Hawton, 'UK legislation on Analgesic Packs: Before and After Study of Long Term Effect on Poisonings', *British Medical Journal*, vol. 329 (7474), 2004, p. 1076

225. L. Hunt, 'Ban Pain Drug, Says Leading Surgeon', *Independent*, 1 October 1996

226. Arthritis Society, see www.arthritis.ca/types%20of%20arthritis/osteoarthritis/default.asp?s=1

227. J. Magnus Bjordal, 'Primary Care Non-steroidal Anti-inflammatory Drugs, Including Cyclo-oxygenase-2 Inhibitors, in Osteoarthritic Knee Pain: Meta-analysis of Randomised Placebo Controlled Trials', *British Medical Journal*, vol. 329, 2004, p. 1317

228. A. Wilde Mathews and B. Martinez, 'Warning Signs: Emails Suggest Merck Knew Vioxx's Dangers at Early Stage – As Heart-risk Evidence Rose, Officials Played Hardball; Internal Message: Dodge! – Company says "Out of Context"', the *Wall Street Journal*, 1 November 2004

229. G. D. Curfman *et al.*, 'Expression of Concern', *New England Journal of Medicine*, vol. 353, 2005, pp. 2813–14; Bombardier *et al.*, 'Comparison of Upper Gastrointestinal Toxicity of RofeCoxib and Naproxen in Patients with Rheumatoid Arthritis', *New England Journal of Medicine*, vol. 343, 2000, pp. 1520–8

230. M. Herper and R. Langreth, 'Merck Study May Have Hidden Vioxx Data', *Forbes*, 8 December 2005. Go to http://www.forbes.com/2005/12/08/merck-vioxx-study-1208 markets14.html

231. G. Fitzgerald, 'Effect of Ibuprofen on Cardioprotective Effect of Aspirin', *The Lancet*, vol. 361 (9368), 2003, p. 1561

232. J. Reginster *et al.*, 'Long-term Effects of Glucosamine Sulphate on Osteoarthritis Progression: A Randomised, Placebo-controlled Clinical Trial', *The Lancet*, vol. 357 (9252), 2001, pp. 251–6

233. Results presented at the American College of Rheumatology Annual Scientific Meeting, 2005. Available at http://arthritis.about.com/od/glucosamine/a/glucosaminesulf.htm

234. T. Towheed *et al.*, 'Glucosamine Therapy for Treating Osteoarthritis', The Cochrane Database of Systematic Reviews 2005, issue 2, article no.: CD002946

235. D. Clegg *et al.*, 'Glucosamine, Chondroitin Sulfate, and the Two in Combination for Painful Knee Osteoarthritis', *New England Journal of Medicine*, vol. 354 (8), 2006, pp. 795–808

236. D. Clegg *et al.*, 'Glucosamine, Chondroitin Sulfate, and the Two in Combination for Painful Knee Osteoarthritis', *New England Journal of Medicine*, vol. 354 (8), 2006, pp. 795–808

237. B. Mazieres *et al.*, 'Chondroitin Sulfate in Osteoarthritis of the Knee: a Prospective, Double Blind, Placebo Controlled Multicenter Clinical Study', *Journal of Rheumatology*, vol. 28 (1), 2001, pp. 173–81

238. F. Richy *et al.*, 'Structural and Symptomatic Efficacy of Glucosamine and Chondroitin in Knee Osteoarthritis: A Comprehensive Meta-analysis', *Archives of Internal Medicine*, vol. 163 (13), 2003, pp. 1514–22

239. 'Methylsulfonylmethane (MSM) Monograph', *Alternative Medicine Review*, vol. 8 (4), 2003, pp. 442–50

240. P. R. Usha and M. Naidu, 'Randomised, Double-blind, Parallel, Placebo-controlled Study of Oral Glucosamine, Methylsulfonylmethane and their Combination in Osteoarthritis', *Clinical Drug Investigation*, vol. 24 (6), 2004, pp. 353–63

241. S. W. Jacob and J. Appleton, *MSM: The Definitive Guide. A Comprehensive Review of the Science and Therapeutics of Methylsulfonylmethane*, Freedom Press, 2003, pp. 107–21

242. S. W. Jacob and J. Appleton, *MSM: The Definitive Guide. A Comprehensive Review of the Science and Therapeutics of Methylsulfonylmethane*, Freedom Press, 2003, pp. 107–21

243. L. Clare *et al.*, 'Pathologic Indicators of Degradation and Inflammation in Human Osteoarthritic Cartilage Are Abrogated by Exposure to N-3 Fatty Acids', *Arthritis & Rheumatism*, vol. 46 (6), 2002, pp. 1544 –53

244. W. J. Kraemer *et al.*, 'Effect of a Cetylated Fatty Acid Topical Cream on Functional Mobility and Quality of Life of Patients with OA' , *Journal of Rheumatology*, vol. 3 (4), 2004, pp. 767–74

245. R. Hesslink *et al.*, 'Cetylated Fatty Acids Improve Knee Function in Patients with Osteoarthritis', *Journal of Rheumatology*, vol. 29 (8), 2002, pp. 1708–12

246. N. Chainani-Wu, 'Safety and Anti-Inflammatory Activity of Curcumin: A Component of Turmeric (Curcuma longa)', *Journal of Alternative and Complementary Medicine*, vol. 9 (1), 2003, pp. 161–8

247. A. Y. Fan *et al.*, 'Effects of an Acetone Extract of Boswellia Carterii Birdw. (Burseraceae) Gum Resin on Rats with Persistent Inflammation', *Journal of Alternative and Complementary Medicine*, vol. 11 (2), 2005, pp. 323–31; A. Y. Fan *et al.*, 'Effects of an Acetone Extract of Boswellia Carterii Birdw. (Burseraceae) Gum Resin on Adjuvant-induced Arthritis in Lewis Rats', *Journal of Ethnopharmacology*, vol. 101 (1–3), 2005, pp. 104–9

248. N. Kimmatkar *et al.*, 'Efficacy and Tolerability of Boswellia Serrata Extract in Treatment of Osteoarthritis of Knee: A Randomized Double Blind Placebo Controlled Trial', *Phytomedicine*, vol. 10 (1), 2003, pp. 3–7.

249. R. Kulkarni *et al.*, 'Treatment of Oesteoarthritis with a Herbal Formulation: A Double-blind, Placebo Controlled, Crossover Study', *Journal of Ethnopharmaceuticals*, vol. 33, 1991, pp. 91–5

250. M. Lemay *et al.*, 'In Vitro and Ex Vivo Cyclooxygenase Inhibition by a Hops Extract', *Asia Pacific Journal of Clinical Nutrition*, vol. 13 (suppl.), 2004, p. S110

251. D. J. Pattison *et al.*, 'Dietary Beta-cryptoxanthin and Inflammatory Polyarthritis: Results from a Population-based Prospective Study', *American Journal of Clinical Nutrition*, vol. 82 (2), 2005, pp. 451–5

252. G. Beauchamp *et al.*, 'Ibuprofen-like Activity in Extra-virgin Olive Oil', *Nature*, vol. 437, 1 September 2005

253. C. Bitler *et al.*, 'Hydrolyzed Olive Vegetation Water in Mice has Anti-inflammatory Activity', *Journal of Nutrition*, vol. 135 (6), 2005, pp. 1475–9.

254. M. A. van der Laar and J. K. van der Korst, 'Food Intolerance in Rheumatoid Arthritis I: A Double Blind Controlled Trial of the Clinical Effects of Elimination of Milk Allergens and Azo Dyes', *Annals of the Rheumatic Diseases*, vol. 51, 1992, pp. 298–302; M. A. van der Laar, and J. K. van der Korst, 'Food Intolerance in Rheumatoid Arthritis II: Clinical and Histological Aspects, *Annals of the Rheumatic Diseases*, vol. 51, 1992, pp. 303–6

255. National Asthma Campaign, 'Out in the Open: A True Picture of Asthma in the United Kingdom Today, National Asthma Campaign Audit 2001', *Asthma Journal*, vol. 6 (suppl. 1–14), 2001; also see H. C. Williams, 'Is the Prevalence of Atopic Dermatitis Increasing?', *Clinical and Experimental Dermatology*, vol. 17, 1992, pp. 385–91

256. J. Kay *et al.*, 'The Prevalence of Childhood Atopic Eczema in a General Population', *Journal of the American Academy of Dermatology*, vol. 30, 1994, pp. 35–9

257. See www.mydr.com.au/default.asp?article=3783

258. M. Masoli *et al.*, 'Dose-response Relationship of Inhaled Budesonide in Adult Asthma: A Meta-analysis', *European Respiratory Journal*, vol. 23 (4), 2004, pp. 552–8

259. A. Cranney *et al.*, 'Corticosteroid-induced Osteoporosis: A Guide to Optimum Management', *Treatments in Endocrinology*, vol. 1 (5), 2002, pp. 271–9

260. D. W. McGraw *et al.*, 'Antithetic Regulation by ß-adrenergic Receptors of Gq Receptor Signaling via Phospholipase C Underlies the Airway ß-agonist Paradox, *Journal of Clinical Investigation*, vol. 112, 2003, pp. 619–26

261. See www.aaaai.org/aadmc/ate/betaagonists.html

262. D. H. Au *et al.*, 'Risk of Mortality and Heart Failure Exacerbations Associated with Inhaled ß-Adrenoceptor Agonists Among Patients with Known Left Ventricular Systolic Dysfunction', *Chest*, vol. 123, 2003, pp. 1964–9

263. H. Boushey *et al.*, 'Daily Versus As-needed Corticosteroids for Mild Persistent Asthma', *New England Journal of Medicine*, vol. 352, 2005, pp. 1589–91

264. H. Boushey, 'Daily versus As-needed Corticosteroids for Mild Persistant Asthma', *New England Journal of Medicine*, vol. 352 (15), 2005, pp. 1519–28

265. 'Topical Steroids for Atopic Dermatitis in Primary Care', *Drug and Therapeutics Bulletin*, vol. 41, 2003, pp. 5–8

266. M. A. Firer *et al.*, 'Cow's Milk Allergy and Eczema: Patterns of the Antibody Response to Cow's Milk in Allergic Skin Disease', *Clinical Allergy*, vol. 12, 1982, pp. 385–90

267. F. Shakib *et al.*, 'Relevance of Milk- and egg-specific IgG4 in Atopic Eczema', *International Archives of Allergy and Applied Immunology*, vol. 75, 1984, pp. 107–12; F. Shakib *et al.*, 'Study of IgG Sub-class Antibodies in Patients with Milk Intolerance', *Clinical Allergy*, vol. 16, 1986, pp. 451–8

268. S. Husby *et al.*, 'IgG Subclass Antibodies to Dietary Antigens in Atopic Dermatitis', *ACTA Dermato-Venereologica*, vol. 144, 1989, pp. 88–92

269. Y. Iikura *et al.*, 'How to Prevent Allergic Disease Study of Specific IgE, IgG, and IgG4 Antibodies in Serum of Pregnant Mothers, Cord Blood, and Infants', *International Archives of Allergy and Applied Immunology*, vol. 88, 1989, pp. 250–2

270. S. Lucarelli *et al.*, 'Specific IgG and IgA Antibodies and Related Subclasses in the Diagnosis of Gastrointestinal Disorders or Atopic Dermatitis due to Cow's Milk and Egg', *International Journal of Immunopathology and Pharmacology*, vol. 11, 1998, pp. 77–85

271. B. Niggemann *et al.*, 'Outcome of Double-blind, Placebo-controlled Food Challenge Tests in 107 Children with Atopic Dermatitis', *Clinical and Experimental Allergy*, vol. 29, 1999, pp. 91–96

272. D. Panagiotakos *et al*,. 'The Association Between Coffee Consumption and Plasma Total Homocysteine Levels: The ATTICA Study', *Heart Vessels*, vol. 19 (6), 2004, pp. 280–6

273. A. Zampelas *et al.*, 'Associations Between Coffee Consumption and Inflammatory Markers in Healthy Persons: The ATTICA Study', *American Journal of Clinical Nutrition*, vol. 80 (4), 2004, pp. 862–7

274. M. Kulig *et al.*, 'Long-lasting Sensitization to Food During the First Two Years Precedes Allergic Airway Disease [asthma and rhinitis]', *Pediatric Allergy and Immunology*, vol. 9 (2), 1998, pp. 61–7

275. D. Gustafsson, 'Development of Allergies and Asthma in Infants and Young Children with Atopic Dermatitis a Prospective Followup to 7 Years of Age', *Allergy*, vol. 55, 2000, pp. 240–5

276. N. L. Misso *et al.*, 'Plasma Concentrations of Dietary and Nondietary Antioxidants are Low in Severe Asthma', *European Respiratory Journal*, vol. 26 (2), 2005, pp. 257–64

277. G. Riccioni and N. D'Orazio, 'The Role of Selenium, Zinc and Antioxidant Vitamin Supplementation in the Treatment of Bronchial Asthma: Adjuvant Therapy or Not?', *Expert Opinion on Investigational Drugs*, vol. 14 (9), 2005, pp. 1145–55.

278. V. Garcia *et al.*, 'Dietary Intake of Flavonoids and Asthma in Adults', *European Respiratory Journal*, vol. 26 (3), 2005, pp. 449–52

279. A. Soutar, 'Bronchial Reactivity and Dietary Antioxidants', *Thorax*, vol. 52, 1997, pp. 166–70

280. A. Fogarty *et al.*, 'Corticosteroid Sparing Effects of Vitamin C and Magnesium in Asthma: A Randomised Trial', *Respiratory Medicine* , vol. 100(1), 2006, pp. 174–9

281. A. Fogarty *et al.*, 'Dietary Vitamin E, IgE Concentrations, and Atopy', *The Lancet*, vol. 356, (9241), 2000, pp. 1573–4

282. G. Panin *et al.*, 'Topical Alpha-tocopherol Acetate in the Bulk Phase: Eight Years of Experience in Skin Treatment', *Annals of the New York Academy of Sciences*, vol. 1031, 2004, pp. 443–7 Review

283. See www.uclm.es/inabis2000/posters/files/070/index.htm – *The treatment of skin atopy with vitamin A and antioxidant vitamins*

284. E. Tanabe, 'Treatment of Intractable Facial Lesions of Adult Atpoic Dermatitis with Environ Mild Night Cream', *Aesthetic Dermatology*, vol. 5, 1995, pp. 1119–22

285. L. Hodge *et al.*, 'Consumption of Oily Fish and Childhood Asthma', *Medical Journal of Australia*, vol. 164, 1996, pp. 137–40

286. D. A. de Luis *et al.*, 'Dietary Intake in Patients with Asthma: A Case Control Study', *Nutrition*, vol. 21 (3), 2005, pp. 320–4

287. T. D. Mickleborough and R. W. Rundell, 'Dietary Polyunsaturated Fatty Acids in Asthma- and Exercise-induced Bronchoconstriction', *European Journal of Clinical Nutrition*, vol. 59 (12), 2005, pp. 1335–46

288. P. Kankaanpää *et al.*, 'Dietary Fatty Acids and Allergy', *Annals of Medicine*, vol. 31, 1999, pp. 282–7

289. K. W. Wong, 'Clinical of N-3 Fatty Acid Supplementation in Patients with Asthma', *Journal of the American Dietetic Association*, vol. 105 (1), 2005, pp. 98–105 Review

290. J. K. Peat *et al.*, 'Three-year Outcomes of Dietary Fatty Acid Modification and House Dust Mite Reduction in the Childhood Asthma Prevention Study', *Journal of Allergy and Clinical Immunology*, vol. 114 (4), 2004, pp. 807–13

291. T. Mickleborough *et al.*, 'Protective Effect of Fish Oil Supplementation on Exercise-Induced Bronchoconstriction in Asthma', *Chest*, vol. 129, 2006, pp. 39–49

292. E. Grandjean *et al.*, 'Efficacy of Oral Long-term N-acetylcysteine in Chronic Broncho-pulmonary Disease: A Meta-analysis of Published Double-blind Placebo-controlled Clinical Trials', *Clinical Therapuetics*, vol. 22 (2), 2000, pp. 209–21

293. E. Mindell, *The MSM Miracle*, Keats Publishing Inc, New Canaan, Connecticut, 1997, p. 25

294. H. A. Klein *et al.*, 'Dimethylsulfoxide in Adult Respiratory Stress Syndrome', *Annals of the New York Academy of Sciences*, 1983

295. E. Middleton and G. Drzewiecki, 'Effects of Flavanoids and Transitional Metal Cations on Antigern-induced Histamine Relase from Human Basiphils', *Biochemical Pharmacology*, vol. 31 (7), 1982, pp. 1449–53; E. Middleton and G. Drzewicki, 'Flavinoid inhibition of Human Basophil Histamine Release Stimulated by Various Agents', *Biochemical Pharma cology*, vol. 33 (21), 1984, pp. 3333–8

296. S. Claverie-Benureau, 'Magnesium Deficiency Allergy-like Crisis in Hairless Rats: A Suggested Model for Inflammation Studies', *Journal de Physiologie* (Paris), vol. 76 (2), 1980, pp. 173–5

297. D. K. Cheuk *et al.*, 'A Meta-analysis on Intravenous Magnesium Sulphate for Treating Acute Asthma', *Archives of Disease in Childhood*, vol. 90 (1), 2005, pp. 74–7 Review

298. B. H. Rowe and C. A. Camargo Jr, 'The Use of Magnesium Sulfate in Acute Asthma: Rapid Uptake of Evidence in North American Emergency Departments', *Journal of Allergy and Clinical Immunology*, vol. 117 (1), 2006, pp. 53–8

299. M. Blitz *et al.*, 'Inhaled Magnesium Sulfate in the Treatment of Acute Asthma', The Cochrane Database of Systematic Reviews 2005, issue 4, art. no.:CD003898

300. J. E. Sprietsma, 'Modern Diets and Diseases: NO-zinc Balance. Zinc and Nitrogen Monoxide (NO) Collectively Protect Against Viruses, AIDS, Autoimmunity, Diabetes, Allergies, Asthma, Infectious diseases, Atherosclerosis and Cancer', *Medical Hypotheses*, vol. 53, 1999, pp. 6–16

301. M. Richter *et al.*, 'Zinc Status Modulates Bronchopulmonary Eosinophil Infiltration in a Murine Model of Allergic Inflammation', *Chest*, vol. 123 (3 suppl.), 2003, p. 446S

302. Y. N. Clement *et al.*, 'Medicinal Herb Use Among Asthmatic Patients Attending a Specialty Care Facility in Trinidad', *BMC Complementary and Alternative Medicine*, vol. 5 (1), 2005, p. 3

303. B. B. Aggarwal and S. Shishodia, 'Suppression of the Nuclear Factor-kappaB Activation Pathway by Spice-derived Phytochemicals: Reasoning for Seasoning', *Annals of the New York Academy of Sciences*, vol. 1030, 2004, pp. 434–41 Review

304. A. Ram *et al.*, 'Curcumin Attenuates Allergen-induced Airway Hyperresponsiveness in Sensitized Guinea Pigs', *Biological and Pharmaceutical Bulletin*, vol. 26 (7), 2003, pp. 1021–4

305. P. McHugh *et al.*, 'Buteyko Breathing Technique for Asthma: An Effective Intervention', *New Zealand Medical Journal*, vol. 116 (1187), 2003, p. U710

306. A. Bruton and G. T. Lewith, 'The Buteyko Breathing Technique for Asthma: A Review', *Complementary Therapies in Medicine*, vol. 13 (1), 2005, pp. 41–6

307. British Heart Foundation report in reference to Office for National Statistics 2005, www.bhf.org.uk/news/index.asp?secID=16&secondlevel=241&thirdlevel=1875&artID=8198

308. S. Chaplin, 'Volume and Cost of Prescribing in England', *Prescriber*, 5 August 2005, pp. 36–8

309. *Prescriber*, 5 August 2005; see www.escriber.com N. P. Stocks *et al.*, 'Statin Prescribing in Australia: Socioeconomic and Sex Differences', *Medical Journal of Australia*, vol. 180 (5), 2004, pp. 229–31

310. T. Pickering, 'Tension and hypertension', *Journal of the American Medical Association*, vol. 370, 1993, p. 2494

311. D. Wald *et al.*, 'Homocysteine and Cardiovascular Disease: Evidence on Causality from a Meta-analysis', *British Medical Journal*, vol. 325, 2002, p. 202

312. A. G. Bostom *et al.*, 'Nonfasting Plasma Total Homocysteine Levels and Stroke Incidence in Elderly Persons: The Framingham Study, *Annals of Internal Medicine*, 7 September 1999, vol. 131 (5), pp. 352–5 and P. K. Sarkar and L. A. Lambert, 'Aetiology and treatment of hyperhomocysteinaemia causing ischaemic stroke', *International Journal of Clinical Practice*, vol. 55 (4), May 2001, pp. 262–8

313. M. R. Law *et al.*, 'Quantifying Effect of Statins on Low Density Lipoprotein Cholesterol, Ischaemic Heart Disease, and Stroke: Systematic Review and Meta-analysis', *British Medical Journal*, vol. 326, 2003, p. 1423

314. See P. Langsjoen, 'Introduction to coenzyme Q10', at http://faculty.washington.edu/~ely/coenzq10.html

315. P. Langsjoen, 'Statin-induced cardiomyopathy', Redflagsweekly.com 8 July 2002

316. D. Graveline, *Lipitor: Thief of Memory, Statin Drugs and the Misguided War on Cholesterol*, Infinity Publishing, 2004

317. R. H. Grimm Jr, 'Hypertension Management in the Multiple Risk Factor Intervention Trial (MRFIT). Six-year Intervention Results for Men in Special Intervention and Usual Care Groups', *Archives of Internal Medicine*, vol. 145 (7), 1985, pp. 1191–9

318. C. D. Furberg *et al.*, 'ALLHAT Officers and Coordinators for the ALLHAT Collaborative Research Group. Major Outcomes in Moderately Hypercholesterolemic, Hypertensive Patients Randomized to Pravastatin vs Usual Care: The Antihypertensive and Lipid-Lowering Treatment to Prevent Heart Attack Trial (ALLHAT-LLT)', *Journal of the American Medical Association*, vol. 288 (23), 2002, pp. 2998–3007

319. Multiple Risk Factor Intervention Trial Research Group, 'Baseline Rest Electrocardiographic Abnormalities, Antihypertensive Treatment, and Mortality in the Multiple Risk Factor Intervention Trial', *American Journal of Cardiology*, vol. 55 (1), 1985, pp. 1–15; J.A. Cutler *et al.*, 'Coronary Heart Disease and All-causes Mortality in the Multiple Risk Factor Intervention Trial: Subgroup Findings and Comparisons with Other Trials', *Preventive Medicine*, vol. 14 (3), 1985, pp. 293–311; R. H. Grimm *et al.*, 'Hypertension Management in the Multiple Risk Factor Intervention Trial (MRFIT), Six-year Intervention Results for Men in Special Intervention and Usual Care Groups', *Archives of Internal Medicine*, vol. 145 (7), 1985, pp. 1191–9; 'Mortality after 10? years for Hypertensive Participants in the Multiple Risk Factor Intervention Trial', *Circulation*, vol. 82 (5), 1990, pp. 1616–28

320. R. Burton, 'Withdrawing Antihypertensive Treatment', *British Medical Journal*, vol. 303, 1991, pp. 324– 5

321. C. D. Furberg *et al.*, 'Nifedipine. Dose-related increase in Mortality in Patients with Coronary Heart Disease', *Circulation*, vol. 92 (5), 1995, pp. 1326–30

322. 'Medical Error May Have Caused Sharon's Stroke', Associated Press in Jerusalem, *Guardian*, 21 April 2006

323. British National Formulary (published by British Medical Association and the Royal Pharmaceutical Society of Great Britain) March, 2004, see www.bnf.org

324. D. Jenkins, 'A Dietary Portfolio Approach to Cholesterol Reduction,' *Metabolism*, vol. 51 (12), 2002, pp. 1596–604

325. D. Jenkins, 'Direct Comparison of a Dietary Portfolio of Cholesterol-lowering Foods with a Statin in Hypercholesterolemic Participants', *American Journal of Clinical Nutrition*, vol. 81, 2005, pp. 380–7; D. Jenkins, 'Assessment of the Longer-term Effects of a Dietary Portfolio of Cholesterol-lowering Foods in Hypercholesterolemia,' *American Journal of Clinical Nutrition*, vol. 83 (3), 2006, pp. 582–91.

326. G. Yang *et al.*, 'Longitudinal Study of Soy Food Intake and Blood Pressure Among Middle-aged and Elderly Chinese Women', *American Journal of Clinical Nutrition*, vol. 81 (5), 2005, pp. 1012–17

327. M. D. Ashen and R. S. Blumenthal, 'Low HDL Cholesterol Levels', *New England Journal of Medicine*, 2005, vol. 353, pp. 1252–60

328. See www.nlm.nih.gov/medlineplus/druginfo/natural/patient-niacin.html

329. S. M. Grundy *et al.*, 'Efficacy, Safety, and Tolerability of Once-daily Niacin for the Treatment of Dyslipidemia Associated with Type 2 Diabetes: Results of the Assessment of Diabetes Control and Evaluation of the Efficacy of Niaspan Trial', *Archives of Internal Medicine*, vol. 162 (14), 2002, pp. 1568–76

330. W. J. Mroczek *et al.*, ' Effect of Magnesium Sulfate on Cardiovascular Hemodynamics', *Angiology*, vol. 28, 1977, pp. 720–4

331. B. T. Altura and B. M. Altura, 'Magnesium in Cardiovascular Biology', *Scientific American*, May/June 1995, pp. 28–36

332. J. Geleijnse *et al.*, 'Reduction of Blood Pressure with a Low Sodium, High Potassium, High Magnesium Salt in Older Subjects with Mild to Moderate Hypertension', *British Medical Journal*, vol. 309, 1994, pp. 436–40

333. Lyn Steffen, 'Eat Your Fruit and Vegetables, *The Lancet*, vol. 367, 2006, pp. 278–9

334. N. Stephens *et al.*, 'Randomised Controlled Trial of Vitamin E in Patients with Coronary Disease: Cambridge Heart Antioxidant Study (CHAOS)', *The Lancet*, vol. 347, 1996, pp. 781–6

335. M. J. Stampfe *et al.*, 'Vitamin E Consumption and the Risk of Coronary Disease in Women', *New England Journal of Medicine*, vol. 328, 1993, pp. 1444–9.

336. E. B. Rimm *et al.*, 'Vitamin E Consumption and the Risk of Coronary Heart Disease in Men', *New England Journal of Medicine*, vol. 328, 1993, pp.1450–6

337. K. G. Losonczy, T. B. Harris, R. J. Havlik, 'Vitamin E and Vitamin C Supplement Use and Risk of All-Cause and Coronary Heart Disease Mortality in Older Persons: The Established Populations for Epidemiologic Studies of the Elderly', *American Journal of Clinical Nutrition*, vol. 64 (2), 1996, pp. 190–6.

338. A. M. Heck *et al.*, 'Potential Interactions Between Alternative Therapies and Warfarin', *American Journal of Health-System Pharmacy*, vol. 57, 2000, pp. 1221–30

339. K. Jones, K. Hughes, L. Mischley, D. J. McKenna, 'Coenzyme Q-10 and Cardiovascular Health', *Alternative Therapies in Health and Medicine*, vol. 10 (1), 2004, pp. 22–30; also M. Dhanasekaran, J. Ren, 'The Emerging Role of Coenzyme Q-10 in Aging, Neuro-degeneration, Cardiovascular Disease, Cancer and Diabetes Mellitus', *Current Neurovascular Research*, vol. 2 (5), 2005, pp. 447–59

340. K. Folkers and Y. Yamamura eds., *Biomedical and Clinical Aspects of Coexzyme Q*, Elsevier Science Publishers, Amsterdam 1986

341. K. Folkers and Y. Yamamura eds., *Biomedical and Clinical Aspects of Coexzyme Q*, Elsevier Science Publishers, Amsterdam 1986

342. F. Rosenfeldt, F. Miller, P. Nagley *et al.*, 'Response of the Senescent Heart to Stress: Clinical Therapeutic Strategies and Quest for Mitochondrial Predictors of Biological Age', *Annals of the New York Academy of Sciences*, vol. 1019, 2004, pp. 78–84; also see F. Rosenfeldt, S. Marasco, W. Lyon *et al.*, 'CoEnzyme Q10 Therapy

Before Cardiac Surgery Improves Mitochondrial Function and In Vitro Contractility of Myocardial Tissue', *Journal of Thoracic and Cardiovascular Surgery*, vol. 129 (1), 2005, pp. 25–32

343. K. Folkers and Y. Yamamura eds., B*iomedical and Clinical Aspects of Coexzyme Q*, Elsevier Science Publishers, Amsterdam 1986

344. B. Burke, 'Randomized, Double Blind, Placebo-controlled Trial of COQ10 in Isolated Systolic Hypertension', *Southern Medical Journal*, vol. 94 (11), 2001, pp. 1112–17

345. J. M. Hodgson *et al.*, 'Coenzyme Q10 Improves Blood Pressure and Glycaemic Control: A Controlled Trial in Subjects with Type 2 Diabetes', *European Journal of Clinical Nutrition*, vol. 56 (11), 2002, pp. 1137–42

346. P. Langsjoen and A. Langsjoen, 'Overview of the Use of CoQ10 in Cardiovascular Disease', *Biofactors*, vol. 9 (2–4), 1999, pp. 273–84

347. O. Osilesi *et al.*, 'Blood Pressure and Plasma Lipids During Ascorbic Acid Supplementation in Borderline Hypertensive and Normotensive Adults', *Nutrition Research*, vol. 11, 1991, pp. 405–12

348. P. Jacques, 'Effects of Vitamin C on High Density Lipoprotein Cholesterol and Blood Pressure', *Journal of the American College of Nutrition*, vol. 11 (2), 1992, pp. 139–44; S. J. Duffy *et al.*, 'Treatment of Hypertension with Ascorbic Acid', *The Lancet*, vol. 354 (9195), 1999, pp. 2048–9

349. P. Knekt *et al.*, 'Antioxidant Vitamins and Coronary Heart Disease Risk: A Pooled Analysis of 9 Cohorts', *American Journal of Clinical Nutrition*, vol. 80 (6), 2004, pp. 1508–20

350. K. G. Losonczy *et al.*, 'Vitamin E and Vitamin C Supplement Use and Risk of All-cause and Coronary Heart Disease Mortality in Older Persons: The Established Populations for Epidemiologic Studies of the Elderly', *American Journal of Clinical Nutrition*, vol. 64 (2), 1996 pp. 190–6; K. G. Losonczy, T. B. Harris, R. J. Havlik, 'Vitamin E and Vitamin C Supplement Use and Risk of All-cause and Coronary Heart Disease Mortality in Older Persons: The Established Populations for Epidemiologic Studies of the Elderly', *American Journal of Clinical Nutrition*, vol. 64 (2), 1996, pp. 190–6.

351. R. Clarke, 'Homocysteine-lowering Trials for Prevention of Heart Disease and Stroke', *Seminars in Vascular Medicine*, vol. 5 (2), 2005, pp. 215–22.

352. J. Spence *et al.*, 'Vitamin Intervention for Stroke Prevention', *Stroke*, vol. 36 (11), 2005, pp. 2404–9

353. Q. Yang, 'Improvement in Stroke Mortality in Canada and the United States, 1990 to 2002', *Circulation*, vol. 113 (10), 2006, pp. 1335–43

354. HOPE 2 Investigators, 'Homocysteine Lowering with Folic acid and B Vitamins in Vascular Disease', *New England Journal of Medicine*, vol. 354, 2006, pp. 1567–77

355. K. Bonaa, *et al.*, 'Homocysteine Lowering and Cardiovascular Events after Acute Myocardial Infarction', *New England Journal of Medicine*, vol. 354, 2006, pp. 1578–88

356. A. Lewis *et al.*, 'Treatment of Hypertriglyceridemia with Omega-3 fatty Acids: A Systemic Review', *Journal of the American Acadamy of Nurse Practitioners*, vol. 16 (9), 2004, pp. 384–95

357. British Nutrition Foundation, 'N-3 Fatty Acids and Health', briefing paper, 1999

358. Gruppo Italiano per lo Studio della Sopravvivenza nell'Infarto miocardico (GISSI), 'Dietary Supplementation with N-3 Polyunsaturated Fatty Acids and Vitamin E after Myocardial Infarction: Results of the GISSI-Prevenzione Trial', *The Lancet*, vol. 354 (9177), 1999, pp. 447–55

359. J. N. Din *et al.*, 'Omega-3 Fatty Acids and Cardiovascular Disease – Fishing for a Natural Treatment', *British Medical Journal*, vol. 328, 2004, pp. 30–35

360. M.Yokoyama, 'Effects of Eicosapentaenoic Acid (EPA) on Major Cardiovascular Events in Hypercholesterolemic Patients: The Japan EPA Lipid Intervention Study (JELIS)', American Heart Association Scientific Sessions, 13–16 November 2005, Dallas, Texas

361. M. S. Buckley *et al.*, 'Fish Oil Interaction with Warfarin', *Annals of Pharmacotherapy*, vol. 38 (1), 2004, pp. 50–2

362. L. Hooper *et al.* 'Risks and Benefits of Omega-3 Fats for Mortality, Cardiovascular Disease, and Cancer: Systematic Review', *British Medical Journal*, vol. 332, 2006, pp. 752–60

363. S. Warshafsky, 'Effect of Garlic on Total Serum Cholesterol. A meta-analysis', *Annals of Internal Medicine*, vol. 119 (7.1), 1993, pp. 599–605

364. C. Silagy, 'Garlic as a Lipid Lowering Agent – A Meta-analysis', *Journal of the Royal College of Physicians*, vol. 28 (1), 1994, pp. 39–45

365. A. Adler and B. Holub, 'Effect of Garlic and Fish Oil Supplementation on Serum Lipid and Lipoprotein Concentrations in Hypercholesterolemic Men', *American Journal of Clinical Nutritionists*, vol. 65 (2), 1997, pp. 445–50

366. H. Goto *et al.*, 'Effect of Curcuma Herbs on Vasomotion and Hemorheology in Spontaneously Hypertensive Rats', *American Journal of Chinese Medicine*, vol. 33 (3), 2005, pp. 449–57

367. M. Zahid Ashraf *et al.*, 'Antiatherosclerotic Effects of Dietary Supplementations of Garlic and Turmeric: Restoration of Endothelial Function in Rats', *Life Sciences*, vol. 77 (8), 2005, pp. 837–57

368. S. Shishodia *et al.*, 'Curcumin: Getting Back to the Roots', *Annals of the New York Academy of Sciences*, vol. 1056, 2005, pp. 206–17

369. G. B. Kudolo *et al.*, 'Short-term Oral ingestion of Ginkgo Biloba Extract (EGb 761) Reduces Malondialdehyde Levels in Washed Platelets of Type 2 Diabetic Subjects', *Diabetes Research and Clinical Practice*, vol. 68 (1), 2005, pp. 29–38

370. W. Zhou *et al.*, 'Clinical Use and Molecular Mechanisms of Action of Extract of Ginkgo Biloba Leaves in Cardiovascular Diseases', *Cardiovascular Drug Reviews*, vol. 22 (4), 2004, pp. 309–19. Review

371. X. Jiang *et al.*, 'Effect of Ginkgo and Ginger on the Pharmacokinetics and Pharmaco-dynamics of Warfarin in Healthy Subjects', *British Journal of Clinical Pharmacology*, vol. 59 (4), 2005, pp. 425–32

372. J. Biederman and S. V. Faraone, 'Attention-deficit Hyperactivity Disorder', *The Lancet*, vol. 366 (9481), 2005, pp. 237–48

373. T. Ford *et al.*, 'The British Child and Adolescent Mental Health Survey 1999: The Prevalence of DSM-IV disorders', *Journal of the American Academy of Child and Adolescent Psychiatry*, vol. 42 (10), 2003, pp. 1203–11

374. E. Costello *et al.*, '10-year Research Update Review: The Epidemiology of Child and Adolescent Psychiatric Disorders: II. Developmental Epidemiology', *Journal of the American Academy of Child and Adolescent Psychiatry*, vol. 45 (1), 2005, pp. 8–25

375. NICE Quick Reference Guide, 'Methylphenidate, Atomoxetine and Dexamfetamine for Attention Deficit Hyperactivity Disorder (ADHD) in Children and Adolescents', March 2006. Available at: http://www.nice.org.uk/download.aspx?o=TA098guidance

376. Drug Class Review on Pharmacologic Treatments for ADHD Final Report September 2005. Available from http://www.ohsu.edu/drugeffectiveness. See also: Health scepticism, accessed 19 September 2005, www.healthyskepticism.org/home.php? Also Medco Health Solutions, Associated Press, 15 September 2005

377. NIH Consensus Statement, 'Diagnosis and Treatment of Attention Deficit Hyperactivity Disorder (ADHD)', National Institutes of Health, Bethesda, 1998

378. C. A. Soutullo *et al.*, 'Bipolar Disorder in Children and Adolescents: International Perspective on Epidemiology and Phenomenology', *Bipolar Disorders*, vol. 7 (6), 2005, pp. 497–506

379. J. Wozniak and J. Biederman, 'A Pharmacological Approach to the Quagmire of Co-morbidity in Juvenile Mania', *Journal of the American Academy of Child and Adolescent Psychiatry*, vol. 35 (6), 1996, pp. 826–8

380. D. Papalos and J. Papalos, *The Bipolar Child*, Broadway Books, 2000

381. N. D. Volkow *et al.*, 'Therapeutic Doses of Oral Methylphenidate Significantly Increase Extracellular Dopamine in the Human Brain', *Journal of Neuroscience*, vol. 21 (RC121), 2001, pp. 1–5

382. J. Baizer, 'Methylphenidate Induces C-fos Expression in Juvenile Rats', poster presented at the Annual Meeting of the Society for Neuroscience, 11 November 2001

383. S. Nissen, 'ADHD Drugs and Cardiovascular risk', *New England Journal of Medicine*, vol. 354 (14), 2006, pp. 1445–8

384. J. Lumpkin, 'FDA Warns ADHD Drug May Be Associated with Thoughts of Suicide in Some Young People', Associated Press, 29 September 2005. This article is also available at www.adhdnews.com/forum/forum_posts.asp?TID=11785&PN=1&FID=5&PR=3

385. 'Polypharmacy in Children on the Rise in the US', as reported on the news site *Medical News Today*, 2 August 2005, available from: www.medicalnewstoday.com/medicalnews.php?newsid=28500

386. R. J. Prinz *et al.*, 'Dietary Correlates of Hyperactive Behaviour in Children', *Journal of Consulting and Clinical Psychology*, vol. 48, 1980, pp. 760–9

387. S. J. Schoenthaler *et al.*, 'The Effect of Randomised Vitamin-mineral Supplementation on Violent and Non-violent Antisocial Behaviour Among Incarcerated Juveniles', *Journal of Nutritional and Environmental Medicine*, vol. 7 (4), 1997, pp. 343–52

388. L. Langseth and J. Dowd, 'Glucose Tolerance and Hyperkinesis', *Food and Cosmetics Toxicology*, vol. 16, 1978, p. 129

389. I. Colquhon and S. Bunday, 'A Lack of Essential Fats as a Possible Cause of Hyperactivity in Children', *Medical Hypotheses*, vol. 7, 1981, pp. 673–9

390. L. J. Stevens *et al.*, 'Essential Fatty Acid Metabolism in Boys with Attention-deficit Hyperactivity Disorder', *American Journal of Clinical Nutrition*, vol. 65, 1995, pp. 761–8

391. A. Richardson and B. Puri, 'A Randomized Double-blind, Placebo-controlled Study of the Effects of Supplementation with Highly Unsaturated Fatty Acids on ADHD-related Symptoms in Children with Specific Learning Difficulties', *Progress in Neuropsychopharmacology and Biological Psychiatry*, vol. 26 (2), 2002, pp. 233–9

392. A. Richardson and P. Montgomery, 'The Oxford–Durham Study: A Randomized, Controlled Trial of Dietary Supplementation with Fatty acids in Children with Developmental Coordination Disorder', *Pediatrics*, vol. 115 (5), 2005, pp. 1360–6

393. D. Benton, 'Micro-nutrient Supplementation and the Intelligence of Children', *Neuroscience and Biobehavioral Reviews*, vol. 25 (4), 2001, pp. 297–309

394. W. Snowden, *Personality and Individual Differences*, vol. 22 (1), 1997, pp. 131–4

395. B. Starobrat-Hermelin and T. Kozielec, 'The Effects of Magnesium Physiological Supplementation on Hyperactivity in Children with Attention Deficit Hyperactivity Disorder (ADHD). Positive Response to Magnesium Oral Loading Test', *Magnesium Research*, vol. 10 (2), 1997, pp. 149–56

396. J. Penland *et al.*, 'Zinc Affects Cognition and Psychosocial Function of Middle-school Children', Experimental Biology meeting, San Diego, 4 April 2005

397. S. J. Schoenthaler *et al.*, 'The Effect of Randomised Vitamin-mineral Supplementation on Violent and Non-violent Antisocial Behaviour Among Incarcerated Juveniles', *Journal of Nutrition and Environmental Medicine*, vol. 7 (4), 1997, pp. 343–52

398. J. Bellanti *et al.*, 'Are Attention Deficit Hyperactivity Disorder and Chronic Fatigue Syndrome Allergy Related?' *Allergy and Asthma Proceedings*, vol. 26 (1), 2005, pp. 19–28

399. B. O'Reilly, Hyperactive Children's Support Group Conference, London, June 2001

400. M. D. Boris and F. S. Mandel, 'Foods and Additives are Common Causes of the Attention Deficit Hyperactive Disorder in Children', *Annals of Allergy*, vol. 72, 1994, pp. 462–8

401. N. I. Ward, 'Assessment of Clinical Factors in Relation to Child Hyperactivity', *Journal of Nutritional and Environmental Medicine*, vol. 7, 1997, pp. 333–42

402. N. I. Ward, 'Hyperactivity and a Previous History of Antibiotic Usage', *Nutrition Practitioner*, vol. 3 (3), 2001, p. 12

403. R. J. Theil, 'Nutrition Based Interventions for ADD and ADHD', *Townsend Letter for Doctors & Patients*, April 2000, pp. 93–5

404. C. M. Carter *et al.*, 'Effects of a Few Food Diet in Attention Deficit Disorder', *Archives of Disease in Childhood*, vol. 69, 1993, pp. 564–8

405. K. Blum and J. Holder, American College of Addictionology and Compulsive Disorders, *The Reward Deficiency Syndrome*, Amercol Ltd, Mattituck, USA, 2002

406. N. D. Volkow *et al.*, 'Therapeutic Doses of Oral Methylphenidate Significantly Increase Extracellular Dopamine in the Human Brain', *Journal of Neuroscience*, vol. 21, 2001, p. 121

407. See www.autismwebsite.com/ari/treatment/form34q.htm

408. K. L. Harding *et al.*, 'Outcome-based Comparison of Ritalin Versus Food-supplement Treated Children with AD/HD', *Alternative Medicine Review*, vol. 8 (3), 2003, pp. 319–30

Part 4

1. *Newsweek*, 5 July 1999, pp. 46–50

2. S. J. Eussen *et al.*, 'Oral cyanocobalamin supplementation in older people with vitamin B12 deficiency: a dose-finding trial', *Archives of Internal Medicine*, vol. 165 (10), 2005, pp. 1167–72

3. Food Standards Agency Newsletter, 'Bioavailability of folic acid and natural folates: studies using the functional marker plasma homocysteine', September 2004

4. See www.healthofthenation.com/focus2.htm

5. G. M. Shaw *et al.*, 'Maternal periconceptional use of multivitamins and reduced risk for conotruncal heart defects and limb deficiencies among offspring', *American Journal of Medical Genetics*, vol. 59 (4), 1995, pp. 536–45

6. See www.healthyoptions.co.nz/australia.pdf

7. World Cancer Research Fund, *Food Nutrition and the Prevention of Cancer*, 1997, p.138

8. B. Buijsse *et al.*, 'Plasma carotene and alpha-tocopherol in relation to 10-year all-cause and cause-specific mortality in European elderly: the Survey in Europe on Nutrition and the Elderly, a Concerted Action (SENECA)', *American Journal of Clinical Nutrition*, vol. 82 (4), 2005, pp. 879–86

9. R. B. Shekelle *et al.*, 'Dietary vitamin A and risk of cancer in the Western Electric study', *The Lancet*, vol. 2 (8257), 1981, pp. 1185–90

10. G. Omenn *et al.*, 'The Beta-Carotene and Retinol Efficacy Trial (CARET)', *New England Journal of Medicine*, vol. 334, 1996, pp. 1150–5

11. D. Albanes *et al.*, 'Alpha-tocopherol and beta-carotene supplements and lung cancer', *Journal of the National Cancer Institute*, vol. 88, 1996, pp. 1560–70 and 'The effect of vitamin E and beta-carotene on the incidence of lung cancer', *New England Journal of Medicine*, vol. 330 (15), 1994, pp. 1029–35

12. M. Caraballoso *et al.*, 'Drugs for preventing lung cancer in healthy people', The Cochrane Database of Systematic Reviews 2005, issue 4, article no.: CD002141

13. SuViMax study at news.bbc.co.uk/go/em/fr/-/1/hi/health/3122033.stm

14. J. Baron *et al.*, 'Neoplastic and antineoplastic effects of beta-carotene on volorectal adenoma', *Journal of the National Cancer Institute*, vol. 95 (10), 2003, pp. 717–22

15. S. Mannisto *et al.*, 'Dietary carotenoids and risk of lung cancer in a pooled analysis of seven cohort studies', *Cancer Epidemiology Biomarkers and Prevention*, vol. 13 (1), 2004, pp. 40–8

16. G. Bjekalovic *et al.*, 'Antioxidant supplements for prevention of gastrointestinal cancers: a systematic review and meta-analysis', *The Lancet*, vol. 364, 2004, pp. 1225–8

17. J. Baron, *et al.*, 'Neoplastic and antineoplastic effects of beta-carotene on volorectal adenoma', *Journal of the National Cancer Institute*, vol. 95 (10), 2003, pp. 717–22

18. P. Correa *et al.*, 'Chemoprevention of gastric dysplasia: randomised trial of antioxidant supplements and anti-helicobacter pylori therapy', *Journal of the National Cancer Institute*, vol. 92 (23), 2000, pp. 1881–8

19. Letter from Dr P. Correa, September 2004

20. M. J. Stampfer, *et al.*, 'Vitamin E consumption and the risk of coronary disease in women', *New England Journal of Medicine*, vol. 328 (20), 1993, pp. 1444–9

21. E. B. Rimm *et al.*, 'Vitamin E consumption and the risk of coronary heart disease in men', *New England Journal of Medicine*, vol. 328 (20), 1993, pp. 1450–6

22. S. Yusuf *et al.*, 'Vitamin E Supplementation and Cardiovascular Events in High-Risk Patients', *New England Journal of Medicine*, vol. 342, 2000, pp. 154–60

23. E. Miller *et al.*, 'Meta-analysis: High Dose Vitamin E Supplementation May Increase All-Cause Mortality', *Annals of Internal Medicine*, vol. 142(1), 2005, pp. 37–46. This study found that among people taking high-dose vitamin E (above 400iu), 34 more people in 10,000 died, while among those taking low-dose vitamin E (below 400iu), 33 fewer people died. This might sound like a lot of people, but in the control group, 1,000 out of 10,000 died. And these were people who were already sick. So, among those with cardiovascular disease, one in ten are expected to die within eight years, one in 300 will die before that if taking high-dose vitamin E, and one in 300 will live longer if taking a lower dose of vitamin E.

24. Department of Health, 'Dietary Reference Values for Food, Energy and Nutrients for the UK', RHSS 41, 1991

25. S. J. Padayatty *et al.*, 'Vitamin C Pharmacokinetics: Implications for Oral and Intravenous Use', *Annals of Internal Medicine*, vol. 140 (7), 2004, pp. 533–7

26. B. Auer *et al.*, 'The Effect of Ascorbic Acid ingestion on the Biochemical and Physico-chemical Risk Factors Associated with Calcium Oxalate Kidney Stone formation', *Clinical Chemistry and Laboratory Medicine*, vol. 36 (3), 1998, pp. 143–8

27. Food Standards Agency press release, 'New FSA advice on Safety of High Dose Vitamins and Minerals', 8 May 2003

28. See www.food.gov.uk/news/newsarchive/2004/dec/chromiumupdate

29. M. Rayner and P. Scarborough, 'The Burden of Food Related Ill Health in the UK', *Journal of Epidemiology and Community Health*, vol. 59, 2005, pp. 1054–7

30. P. H. Whincup, 'School Dinners and Markers of Cardiovascular Health and Type 2 Diabetes in 13–16 year olds: Cross Sectional Study', *British Medical Journal*, vol. 331, 2005, pp. 1060–1

31. S. E. Nissen *et al.*, 'Effect of Muraglitazar on Death and Major Adverse Cardiovascular Events in Patients with Type 2 Diabetes Mellitus', *Journal of the American Medical Association*, vol. 294 (20), 2005, pp. 2581–6

32. Report by the Expert Group on Vitamins and Minerals of the Food Standards Agency, 2003
33. See F. Lindberg, *The Greek Doctor's Diet*, Rodale, 2006
34. A. Trichopoulou *et al.*, 'Modified Mediterranean diet and Survival: EPIC – elderly Prospective Cohort Study', *British Medical Journal*, vol. 330, 2005, p. 991
35. N. Gordon, 'Effectiveness of Therapeutic Lifestyle Changes in Patients With Hypertension, Hyperlipidemia, and/or Hyperglycemia', *American Journal of Cardiology*, vol. 94, 2004, pp. 1558–61
36. G. Aldana, 'Effects of an Intensive Diet and Physical Activity Modification Program on the Health Risks of Adults', *Journal of the American Dietetic Association*, vol. 105 (3), 2005, pp. 371–81
37. D. Aaronovitch, 'The stomach for it' *Guardian* Weekend Magazine, 23 July 2005
38. P. Holford, K. Torrens and D. Colson, 'The Effects of a Low Glycaemic Load Diet on Weight Loss and Key Health Risk Indicators', *Journal of Orthomolecular Medicine*, vol. 21 (2), 2006, pp. 71–8
39. S. Hollinghurst *et al.*, 'Opportunity Cost of Antidepressant Prescribing in England: Analysis of Routine Data', *British Medical Journal*, vol. 330, 2005, pp. 999–1000
40. B. Gesch *et al.*, 'Influence of Supplementary Vitamins, Minerals and Essential Fatty Acids on the Antisocial Behaviour of Young Adult Prisoners. Randomised, Placebo-controlled Trial', *British Journal of Psychiatry*, vol. 181, 2002, pp. 22–8
41. W. Atkinson *et al.*, 'Food Elimination based on IgG Antibodies in Irritable Bowel Syndrome: a Randomised Controlled Trial', *Gut*, vol. 53 (10), 2004, pp. 1459–64
42. A. Majeed and P. Aylin, 'Dr Foster's Case Notes: The Aging Population of the United Kingdom and Cardiovascular Disease', *British Medical Journal*, vol. 331, 2005, p. 1362
43. S. Fairweather-Tait, 'Human Nutrition and Food Research: Opportunities and Challenges in the Post-genomic Era', *Philosophical Transactions of the Royal Society B: Biological Sciences,* vol. 358, 2003, pp. 1709–27
44. B. Unal *et al.*, 'Modelling the Decline in Coronary Heart Disease Deaths in England and Wales, 1981–2000: Comparing Contributions from Primary Prevention and Secondary Prevention', *British Medical Journal*, vol. 331, 2005, p. 614
45. B. Unal *et al.*, 'Modelling the Decline in Coronary Heart Disease Deaths in England and Wales, 1981–2000: Comparing Contributions from Primary Prevention and Secondary Prevention', *British Medical Journal*, vol. 331, 2005, p. 614
46. Available at www.hm-treasury.gov.uk/
47. H. Moore *et al.*, 'Improving Management of Obesity in Primary Care: Cluster Randomised Trial', *British Medical Journal*, vol. 327, 2003, p. 1085
48. Editorial, 'Full Engagement in Health Needs to Begin in Primary Care', *British Medical Journal*, vol. 329, 2004, pp. 1197–8
49. M. J. Reeves, 'Healthy Lifestyle Characteristics among Adults in the United States, 2000', *Archive of Internal Medicine*, vol. 165 (8), 2005, pp. 854–7. See also comment in *British Medical Journal*, vol. 330, 2005, p. 1044
50. R. Coombes, 'News extra: Public Distrusts Government Health Campaigns, Experts say', *British Medical Journal*, vol. 331, 2005, p. 70
51. Z. Kmietowicz, 'Too Many Heart Patients Discharged without Follow-up Care', *British Medical Journal*, vol. 330, 2005, p. 1346
52. R. Smith, 'Medical Journals Are an Extension of the Marketing Arm of Pharmaceutical Companies', *Public Library of Science: Medicine*, vol. 2 (5), 2005, p. e138
53. The House of Commons health committee, *The Influence of the Pharmaceutical Industry,*

March 2005, paragraph 328. See www.publications.parliament.uk/pa/cm200405/cmselect/cmhealth/42/42.pdf

54. Health Supplements Information Service survey reported in the OTC Bulletin, 16 December 2005

55. M. J. Heisler, 'When do Patients and their Physicians Agree on Diabetes Treatment Goals and Strategies, and What Difference does it Make?', *Journal of General Internal Medicine*, vol. 18 (11), 2003, pp. 893–902

56. S. Ebrahim and G. Davey-Smith, 'Multiple Risk Factor Interventions for Primary Prevention of Coronary Heart Disease', The Cochrane Database of Systematic Reviews 1999, vol. 2, article no.: CD001561

57. B. Unal *et al.*, 'Modelling the Decline in Coronary Heart Disease Deaths in England and Wales, 1981–2000: Comparing Contributions from Primary Prevention and Secondary Prevention', *British Medical Journal*, vol. 331, 2005, p. 614

58. D. Foggo, 'ADHD Advice Secretly Paid For by Drug Companies', *Daily Telegraph*, 9 October 2005

59. Editorial: 'The Flight from Science', *British Medical Journal*, vol. 289, 1980, pp. 1–2. This paper is hard to find unless you go to a medical library; a discussion of this issue is in A. Vickers, 'Complementary medicine' (Clinical review: Recent advances, under 'Attitudes' heading), *British Medical Journal*, vol. 321, 2000, pp. 683–6

60. S. Boseley, 'Keep Complementary Medicine out of NHS, say Leading Doctors', *Guardian*, 23 May 2006

Index

Note page numbers in **bold** refer to diagrams.

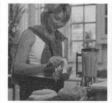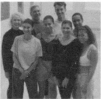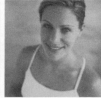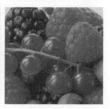
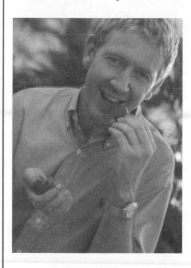